PRACTICAL PEDIATRICS

FIRST EDITION

Dr Surendra Nath Joshi MD FRCPCH (UK)
Chief Editor
Senior Consultant, Child Health and Metabolic Diseases
Sultan Qaboos University Hospital
Muscat, Oman

Dr Yasser Wali MD FRCPCH (UK)
Associate Editor
Associate Professor Pediatric Hematology & Oncology
Head of Child Health Department
Sultan Qaboos University Hospital
Muscat, Oman

authorHOUSE®

AuthorHouse™ UK Ltd.
500 Avebury Boulevard
Central Milton Keynes, MK9 2BE
www.authorhouse.co.uk
Phone: 08001974150

First published by AuthorHouse 1/15/2008

ISBN: 978-1-4343-1742-1 (sc)

Printed in the United States of America
Bloomington, Indiana

This book is printed on acid-free paper.

Medical knowledge is constantly changing. As new information becomes available, changes in treatment, procedures, equipment and the use of drugs become necessary. The volume editors, contributors and publishers have, as far as it is possible, taken care to ensure that the information given in this text is accurate and up to date. However readers are strongly advised to confirm that information, especially with regard to drug dose/usage, complies with latest legislation and standards of practice.

Preface:

While giving lectures to the undergraduate students, we observed that throughout the sessions many of them were busy in jotting down what was being said rather than focusing on understanding the concept. They had to be repeatedly assured that a copy of the lecture notes would be given at the end of the session. This prompted us to compile all the lecture notes and publish them in a book format. Subsequently the quest got bigger and broader and we decided to publish a practically useful book covering most of the common clinical scenarios encountered in Pediatric practice.

In this book we have tried to keep our focus on essential "core topics" in paediatrics and neonatology so as to meet the educational needs of *undergraduate students, interns and resident house officers*. We feel that junior doctors need to grasp basic facts, have a clear understanding of commonly encountered clinical conditions and develop a practical approach in ordering lab tests and treatment plans.

Each chapter is written by a specialist and represents a clear and practical approach to a real-life situation. All the unnecessary details of a didactic lecture have been omitted. We have tried to maintain a common format for each chapter. Firstly, the subject is defined and its incidence is mentioned to give an idea of how common the condition is. Secondly, the causes are classified in an order of priority rather than as a comprehensive theoretical list; a practical approach to differential diagnosis is discussed that is based on history, physical examination and primary investigations, followed by the mention of specific lab tests needed for confirmation of specific diagnosis. Thirdly, the management is outlined in a simple and practical form as it is practiced at our institution; wherever possible, we have used tables and algorithms and also tried to incorporate the standard ward protocols to make the management approach uniform and evidence based. Finally, the prognosis and common complications are outlined to understand the need for long-term follow-up. Family counselling issues are also listed to help students learn about this important aspect of patient management. Due care has been taken to avoid typing and spelling errors as well as the use of any copyrighted material. Any lapse in this regard is solely the responsibility of the individual author rather than the editors. We would appreciate it if our readers could kindly bring such instances to our attention by e-mail: **joshisnj@yahoo.com** for correction in subsequent editions.

To keep the format of this book practical, all rarities and superfluous details are omitted. We believe that the practice of medicine is a lifelong learning process and a committed student will surely refer to standard textbooks of paediatrics to enhance his knowledge.

As medical exams are an important part of student evaluation, we have included a chapter of guidance for students on how to prepare for MEQ and OSCE examinations.

We express our sincere thanks and appreciation to all contributing authors for maintaining the expected high standards in their write-ups. We acknowledge the efforts of Rashi Joshi and Ritu Joshi for their untiring assistance in compiling the manuscript. We also convey our gratefulness to our past medical students who have helped us in developing the practical teaching approach.

Muscat **Dr Surendra Nath Joshi**
Oman **Dr Yasser Wali**

CONTRIBUTORS

Dr Hamed Abdoon, MRCPCH (UK)
Senior Registrar in Pediatric Gastroenterology
Sultan Qaboos University and Hospital, Muscat, Oman.

Dr Reem Abdwani, FRCPC
Consultant, Pediatric Rheumatology,
Sultan Qaboos University and Hospital, Muscat, Oman.

Dr Mahmoud Fathalla Ahmed, DCH
Registrar in Pediatrics
Sultan Qaboos University and Hospital, Muscat, Oman.

Dr Shakeel Ahmed, MRCPCH (UK)
Ex Senior Registrar in Pediatrics,
Sultan Qaboos University and Hospital, Muscat, Oman.

Dr Amna Al Futaisi, MD, FRCPC
Consultant Pediatric Neurologist,
Sultan Qaboos University and Hospital, Muscat, Oman.

Dr Mohammed Al-Hosni, FRCPCH (UK)
Consultant, Pediatric Infectious Diseases and HOD, Pediatrics
Royal Hospital, Muscat, Oman.

Dr Saleh bin Mohammed Al-Khusaibi, FRCPCH (UK)
Dean Sohar campus, Oman Medical College, Oman.

Dr Hussein Al-Kindy, MD, FRCPC
Consultant, Pediatric Respiratory diseases,
Sultan Qaboos University and Hospital, Muscat, Oman.

Dr Zakia Al-Lamki, FRCPCH (UK)
Associate Professor, Pediatric Hematology and Oncology,
College of Medicine, Sultan Qaboos University, Muscat, Oman

Dr Muna Al-Saadoon, PhD Community Pediatrics
Assistant Professor, Child Health,
College of Medicine, Sultan Qaboos University, Muscat, Oman

Salah Salim Al-Shukaili, B.Sc.
Head of nutrition and dietetic services,
Sultan Qaboos University and Hospital, Muscat, Oman.

Dr Salem Al-Tamemi, MD, FRCPC
Consultant, Pediatric Clinical Immunology & Allergy,
Sultan Qaboos University and Hospital, Muscat, Oman.

Dr Saif Al-Yaarubi, MD, FRCPC
Consultant, Pediatric Endocrinology,
Sultan Qaboos University and Hospital, Muscat, Oman.

Dr Wafa Ahmed Bashir, MSc. Medical Genetics
Registrar in Pediatrics,
Sultan Qaboos University and Hospital, Muscat, Oman.

Dr Maria Flordeliz A. Bataclan, MD
Registrar in Neonatology
Sultan Qaboos University and Hospital, Muscat, Oman.

Dr Kamlesh Bhargava MD MRCGP (INT)
Consultant, Dept. of Family Medicine and Public Health
Sultan Qaboos University and Hospital, Muscat, Oman.

Dr Deepa Bhargava MS (ENT)
Senior Registrar, ENT Surgery
Sultan Qaboos University and Hospital, Muscat, Oman.

Dr Alexander Chacko, FRCPCH (UK)
Consultant, Pediatrics,
Sultan Qaboos University and Hospital, Muscat, Oman.

Dr Abdul Aziz Elamin, FRCPCH (UK)
Ex Associate Professor, Pediatric Endocrinology,
College of Medicine, Sultan Qaboos University, Muscat, Oman

Dr Mayada Samir El-Eraki, MD
Registrar in Pediatrics
Sultan Qaboos University and Hospital, Muscat, Oman

Dr Ibtisam B. Elnour, FRCPCH (UK)
Consultant, Pediatric Nephrology,
Sultan Qaboos University and Hospital, Muscat, Oman.

Dr Muhammad Fazalullah, DCH (Glasgow)
Registrar, Neonatology
Sultan Qaboos University and Hospital, Muscat, Oman.

Dr Hashim Javad, MRCPCH (UK)
Senior Registrar in Pediatrics
Sultan Qaboos University and Hospital, Muscat, Oman.

Dr Jaishree Joshi, MRCOG (UK)
Ex Medical Officer in Gynecology and Obstetrics
Sultan Qaboos University and Hospital, Muscat, Oman.

Dr Surendra Nath Joshi, FRCPCH (UK)
Senior Consultant, Metabolic diseases and Child Health
Sultan Qaboos University and Hospital, Muscat, Oman.

Dr Roshan Koul, FRCPCH (UK)
Senior Consultant and Pediatric Neurologist,
Sultan Qaboos University and Hospital, Muscat, Oman.

Dr Ghulam Qadir Pathan, MRCP (Ireland)
Registrar in Pediatric Hematology,
Sultan Qaboos University and Hospital, Muscat, Oman.

Dr Carmencita Galvez Remo, MD, DNM
Senior Registrar and In-Charge Pediatric ICU,
Sultan Qaboos University and Hospital, Muscat, Oman.

Dr Zenaida S. Reyes, MD
Senior Registrar, Neonatology and Pediatric ICU,
Sultan Qaboos University and Hospital, Muscat, Oman.

Dr Asad Ur-rahman, FCPS
Ex Registrar in Neonatology,
Sultan Qaboos University and Hospital, Muscat, Oman.

Aqeela Taqi, MSc (Clin. Pharmacy)
Sr. Pharmacist
Sultan Qaboos University and Hospital, Muscat, Oman

Dr Thomas Varghese, MRCP (UK)
Senior Registrar in Pediatrics,
Royal Hospital, Muscat, Oman

Dr P Venugopalan, FRCPCH (UK)
Ex Consultant Pediatric Cardiologist, SQ University & Hospital
Consultant, Pediatrics, University Hospital of Hartlepool, UK.

Dr Yasser Ahmed Wali, FRCPCH (UK)
Associate Professor, Pediatric Hematology and Oncology,
Head, Pediatric dept, Sultan Qaboos University and Hospital, Muscat, Oman.

Dr S.M. Wasifuddin, MD
Ex. Senior Registrar in Pediatrics
Sultan Qaboos University and Hospital, Muscat, Oman.

Elizabeth A. Worthing, MSc. (Clinical Pharmacy)
Ex. Sr. Pharmacist and training coordinator
Sultan Qaboos University and Hospital, Muscat, Oman

Dr Mathew Zaccharia, MD
Senior Registrar in Pediatrics
Sultan Qaboos University and Hospital, Muscat, Oman

Contents

1

General Pediatrics

1.1 Scope of Pediatrics

Pediatric Medicine is a clinical science that is concerned with the health of Infant, Children and Youth, making sure that they achieve their full Growth and Developmental potentials as adults.

Health means complete physical, mental and emotional well being, NOT just absence of disease.

How Pediatrics is different than adult medicine?
- Pediatric is a rapidly growing phase thus the needs are constantly changing
- Children are constantly maturing thus acquiring new developmental milestones
- Children are vulnerable to infections and accidents
- Children's response to disease and Stress is different then adults
- Children are dependent on adults for their daily needs
- Nutritional requirements are high and are ever changing
- Children are very sensitive to psycho-social impacts
- Children have a great regeneration power leading to quick recovery

Divisions of Pediatrics

Early Neonatal period	0 to 7 days
Late Neonatal period	8 to 28 days
Infancy	up to 1 year
Toddler period	2-5 years
Childhood	2 to 12 Year
Adolescence	12 year to adult

Some common causes for admissions in Pediatric ward
- Respiratory Diseases:
  - URTI: Pharyngo-Tonsillitis, Otitis Media
  - LRTI: Pneumonia, Bronchopneumonia
  - Bronchial Asthma
- Gastroenteritis with dehydration
- Blood disorders: Sickle cell disease, Thalassemia, G6PD, Bleeding Disorders, Childhood Malignancies
- Epilepsies, Febrile Convulsions, Meningitis, Cerebral palsy
- Congenital Heart Diseases and Heart failure
- Urinary tract infections
- Bacteremia, Septicemia, Soft tissue Infections
- Common Childhood infections
- Trauma, Poisonings and accidents
- Congenital anomalies
- Failure to thrive and Nutritional disorders

1.2   Pediatrics History and Physical Examination

Introduction

Clinical history is an important part of clinical assessment. Pediatrics patients usually cannot give the account of their own illness therefore one has to rely on observations made by mother or a close caretaker. A great deal of patience and skill is required to obtain an accurate history.

The history is generally less reliable if given by a person other then the primary caregiver of the child. The reason(s) for someone other than the mother or father giving the history should be noted. Language problem may also pose difficulty in obtaining accurate accounts of illness; use of interpreter may produce some disparities due to inaccurate translation.

In most developing countries where there is widespread ignorance because of lack of formal education, some parents are often ignorant of certain important information, such as the correct age of their children. They may also lack the ability to recall the duration of an illness. In such circumstances, the use of local historical events may help to establish the age of the child, or the duration of the symptoms, particularly if symptoms have been present for a long time. For example, in order to establish the age of child, a legitimate leading question may be asked, relating the birth of the child to a Moslem festival (Id al-Adha, Id al-fitr, etc).

It is important to take a complete account of child's illness without interrupting unless the person is deviating from the point. Clarification may be sought if some point is not clear, but leading questions should not be asked, as they tend to give the answer suggested within the question. During the history taking one should also closely observe the child's activity and general condition as this may give lot of important information about the child's development and the seriousness of illness.

In a chronic case, one should focus on: 1) the onset of disease, 2) the progress or course of the illness and 3) the current status of the patient.

Much of the information about the patient can be gathered accurately by thorough review of the 'pink card', previous discharge summaries, the patient's previous case notes and the referral letter.

While interviewing parents, one should observe certain "bed side manners", which include a courteous attitude, a helpful manner and professional behaviour and conduct so as to develop a proper parent-doctor relationship of trust and confidence.

The scheme and sequence given here is only a general guide in obtaining the fullest possible information about an individual child. More detailed information on a number of the sections of the schedule may be necessary for a particular child, depending on the presenting symptoms and the system involved.

At the end of history taking, the student should evaluate the reliability of the history and then write down sequentially, the development of the symptoms as well as his/her own impressions about the problem.

A. Demographic data

Name:
Age: (weeks, months or years)
Sex: (F/M)
Place of Origin:
Nationality:
Informant: Mother, father, or someone else, specify.
Previous hospitalization: (1st 2nd, etc)
Reason for Referral:

B. Present Complaint(s)

The complaints must be written in the *informant's own words*. A suggestion of medical terms to the informant should be avoided. If, for instance, the informant complains that the child's breathing is fast, students often state that the informant's complaint is dyspnoea. The symptoms should be written in chronological order as they evolved with dates and duration. Often the mother omits related symptoms that may occur in other systems; *systemic enquiry* should therefore, be made as set out below.

C. General and Systemic Review

Under this section, the student should ask <u>relevant</u> questions on possible related symptoms which the mother may not have volunteered. Positive as well as <u>relevant negative responses</u> to questions pertaining to different systems should be recorded.

1. **Alimentary System** Ask about *appetite, vomiting* (frequency and colour), *bowel habits,* (frequency, character of stools, any mucus or blood; is it offensive?) *abdominal pain* (location, nature; is it colicky? Does it radiate and to where? Is it relieved by anything? Has there been any associated abdominal distension or not?).

2. **Cardiovascular System** Symptoms of heart disease in infancy and early childhood are usually non-specific: *cough, breathlessness, excessive sweating, cyanosis, feeding problems* (easy fatigue which manifests by the child taking unusually long time over feeds) *vomiting, weight loss and failure to thrive,* etc. In older children, the symptoms are similar to those in adults; therefore, ask about *exertional dyspnoea, fatigue, palpitation, chest pains, cough and haemoptysis, squatting, fainting attacks,* etc.

3. **Central Nervous System**. Is there any *headache* and where is it located; character of the headache; any associated symptoms such as vomiting and fever? Can the child *hear and see* well? Are there any *convulsions*? (Type, duration, associated loss of consciousness, any incontinence of urine during attack, etc)

4. **Respiratory System**. Ask about *cough* (dry or loose, productive, colour of sputum, presence of blood), *chest pains* (stabbing or aching, is it worse on coughing and where is it located?) *breathlessness* – at rest or on exertion? any wheezing? Is the breathing noisy and is there any grunt?

5. **Genito–urinary System**: *Urine colour, frequency and volume, fever, bed-wetting, hematuria, dysuria, loin pains,* etc. In young children, symptoms are usually non-

specific and may consist of fever, vomiting, restlessness, febrile convulsions, etc. Is the *urinary stream* good or does the child dribble urine?

D.   Past History:

History of the past is of special relevance in Pediatrics. Details and elaboration of the information in this section may not be of much value in some patients. For example, in a previously well 5-year-old child, details and elaboration would be irrelevant on prenatal, perinatal and nutritional history.

1.   **Pregnancy and Birth History**: History about ***Prenatal, perinatal and postnatal events*** are highly necessary in a child with neurological or developmental disorder; this could be easily checked from the *"Pink Card"* or the neonatal discharge summary. Questions to be asked concern the mother's health during the pregnancy, any history of fever, specific infections or diseases (rubella, syphilis, renal or heart diseases, diabetes, hypertension, leaking membranes, drug ingestion, exposure to radiations, duration of labor, complications of labor, prolonged rupture of membranes etc. Inquire into problems of early and late neonatal periods e.g. did the child cry immediately after birth? What were the APGAR scores? Did the baby require any resuscitation? In the postnatal period did the baby develop any complications and for how long was the baby hospitalized? Did the baby required intensive care, ventilation or artificial feeding? Note the child's birth weight, length and head circumference.

2.   **Past Illness** The child's previous health should be noted; ask about *previous hospitalization* or *surgery*. Any relation of the past condition with present should be established. The discharge summaries or clinical notes from the past illness should be evaluated and summarized with relevant information. Also note and record any *drug allergies and blood transfusions*, etc.

E. Nutritional History

Most nutritional problems are generally seen between birth and 5 years age. Any recent and preceding illness, such as measles, diarrhea, that might have precipitated a nutritional disorder (e.g. marasmus) should be noted. Note how the child is fed – breast or bottle? Duration of breast feeding? What supplemental feeds and when started? If bottle-fed, when was it started and why? What type of milk formula is used, how the formula milk is prepared? How many bottles does the mother keep for use and how are these bottles sterilized? In an older child note what type of food is offered and does the child has access to 'junk food and fizzy drinks'?

F. Immunization History

This could also be obtained from the *'pink card'*. Note what inoculations child has received and when. Was there any reaction to any of these inoculations? If the child has received no immunization, ask for the reasons (which may include ignorance). Use this opportunity to educate parents.

G. Developmental History

Depending on the age of the child, ask and observe about milestones and record them with respect to the age at which they were achieved. This area is further elaborated in the relevant chapter of this book.

H. Family History:

The construction of a simple family tree should be carried out. Such a tree should include age, sex, and birth order of the patient and siblings. Note the cause of any unnatural death in the family. Record any parental consanguinity or multiple marriages. Make a specific note of familial conditions likely to affect the child e.g. diabetes, hypertension, asthma etc.

Monogamous   **Polygamous**

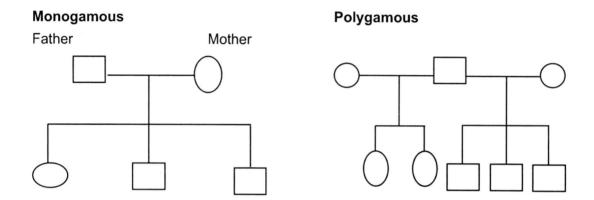

I. Social and Environmental History:

Record the interaction between the diseases and the social, cultural and environmental factors in the child's life. Ask about the parent's occupation and level of their education, financial status and how much housekeeping money they use per month. Are the parents divorced, what is the size and condition of their home and how many occupants are there? Are there any conditions, which may provoke jealousies or fears in the child, such as a new baby, absence of parents from home? Note the type and size of house, electricity, water supply, sewage system, overcrowding, any animals in the house, and social habits like smoking, alcohol and narcotics use by the family members.

In a child with chronic illness also assess how the child's disease affects other family members and vice versa and how the family copes with the illness and regular attendance to the hospital. Note how far away the child lives from the medical facility and the mode of transport available. Does the father live away from the family for his work?

Physical Examination

Examination of infants and young children in particular, is an art that requires patience, tact and understanding. The student learns this art not from reading textbooks, but by careful observation of how experienced physicians carry out their examination and by his/her frequent practice.

An infant or a young child can be examined in any comfortable position mostly in the mother's lap. The sequence of the examination should be varied according to the clinical impression as suggested by the history. In older and cooperative children, examination should be undertaken as in adults. Uncomfortable or distasteful procedures, such as BP measurement, examination of the ears or throat, should be performed last.

During the examination, it is a good ethical practice to explain the process and nature of examination to the child reassuring him/her so as to gain the best co-operation. The child may be given the stethoscope or patellar hammer to play with for reassurance. One must talk to the child with a firm but friendly voice and maintain the privacy of older children by using appropriate covering of private areas.

A. General Examination

Much can be learnt on general observation of the child while taking the history.

Observe the child's appearance, signs of sickness, interest in the surroundings, state of nutrition, growth of the child in relation to age, level of activity, facies and dysmorphic features, type of breathing and any associated cough, strider, whooping, and any deviation from normal behaviour.

Note the following signs (**JARCCOLD**) on general examination:

Jaundice, **A**nemia, **R**ashes, **C**yanosis, **C**lubbing, **O**edema, **L**ymphadenopathy, **D**ehydration signs

Vital signs and compare them with normal for the age:
1. Temperature
2. Pulse
3. Respiration
4. Blood pressure (BP). This can be difficult to measure in small children. Use an appropriate cuff size that should cover approximately 2/3 of the upper arm. Use of the new electronic devices is encouraged if available.

Normal vital signs

	RR	HR	B.P
Newborn	40 (35-45)	120 (120-260)	80/50
Infants	30 (25-35)	110 (80-140)	80/50
Young child	25 (20-30)	100 (80-120)	85/50
Older children	20 (15-25)	90 (70-110)	90/60

Anthropometrics measurements and plot them on a graph
1. Weight
2. Height (length, in infants)
3. Head circumference
   (See appendix for description and normal values)

B. Systemic Examination

The systemic examination consists of *Inspection, Palpation, Percussion and Auscultation* of various systems. The examination should start with the affected system as suggested by the history. Following order of examination is recommended.

Examination of Head and Neck
Note the shape of the head, which may be hydrocephalic, microcephalic, etc. Examine the fontanels and suture in a small child, noting whether it is patent or closed, depressed

as occurs in dehydration, or bulging as in raised intracranial pressure. Note any abnormal facies, as well as any abnormalities in the nose and ears. In the mouth, examine the mucosa, noting whether it is moist or dry, normal coloured, anemic or cyanosed. Look for ulcers, bleeding spots, etc. Assess the teeth for the number, size, shape, caries, discoloration, e.g., the yellow discoloration of primary dentition in Kernicterus, or tetracycline ingestion. Examination of the neck should include the front and the back, looking for any swelling (thyroid) and its characteristics. There may be webbing of the neck. Examine the throat and the ears. In small children, the examination may include percussion of head for 'cracked pot signs', palpation for 'craniotabes' and auscultation for 'bruit'. Trans-illumination is required if hydrocephalus is suspected.

Chest and Lungs

Count the respiratory rate, note the type of respiration, which may be fast and deep, as occurs in acidosis, or fast and shallow as in pneumonias. Note any deformity in the chest wall, including the sternum (e.g. pectus deformity), ribs (rickety rosary and Harrison's sulcus of rickets), and the spine (scoliosis, gibbous of spinal tuberculosis). The precordium may be prominent or bulging due to right ventricular hypertrophy. Examine the trachea and chest movements; percuss for resonance and auscultate for breath sounds and any adventitious sounds.

Chest signs and their interpretation

	Consolidation	Hyperinflation	Collapse	Effusion	Pneumothorax
Mediastinal shift	None	None	Towards the same side	Away to opposite side	Away to the opposite side
Vocal Fremitus	Increased	Diminished	Diminished	Markedly Diminished	Diminished
Percussion	Dull	Hyper resonance	Dull	Stony dull	Tympanitic
Breath sounds	Bronchial	Diminished with prolonged expiration	Absent or bronchial	Diminished	Diminished or amphoric
Adventitious sounds	Fine crepitations (in early stage and during resolution)	Expiratory wheezes	None	Rub in early stages	None

Cardiovascular System

Assess the pulses, noting the rate, volume and rhythm (small volume, full, bounding, or large and collapsing, regular or irregular). In describing any irregularity, state precisely the type of irregularity that is present. In childhood, irregularities most likely encountered include sinus arrhythmia, an innocent phenomenon due to variation by respiration phases. Note any ectopic beats and atrial fibrillation. The student should note any delay between pulses in upper and lower extremities, as in coarctation of the aorta. Assessment of the jugular venous pressure (JVP) is not practicable in infants, because of their short neck and lack of cooperation.

On inspection of the precordium, note whether it is quiet or overactive with pulsations, as seen in right ventricular hypertrophy. Determine the apex beat (AB), defined as the "Outermost, lowermost point at which the cardiac impulse is most distinctly felt or seen". An estimate of the size of the heart should be undertaken using the position of the AB (a displaced

AB indicates left ventricular hypertrophy in the absence of a mediastinal shift) as well as the presence of a thrust or heave, either of which indicates right ventricular hypertrophy. Percussion is of no value in the evaluation of the heart size. Auscultate for heart sounds in the conventional areas (apex, tricuspid, pulmonary and aortic). Heart sounds should be described as either normal or abnormal and abnormalities specified as loud or accentuated, reduced or absent. Besides the normal first and second heart sounds, there may be a third sound that is common and best heard at the apex in normal children. A triple or gallop rhythm may also be present and is usually associated with heart failure.

Auscultation for heart murmurs should similarly be undertaken in the conventional areas as well as in the neck, back of the chest, and the axillae for radiation. Note the area of maximum intensity and grade of the murmur, this ranges from 1-6; only grade 4 and above are associated with thrill (palpable murmur). Note any variation in either the intensity or disappearance of the murmur with change of position. In timing, murmur may be systolic (early or late) or diastolic (early, mid diastolic, or presystolic). A continuous murmur is one that occurs both in systole and diastole. It is characteristically associated with a wide pulse pressure as occurs in persistent ductus arteriosus (PDA). Auscultation may reveal other adventitious sounds, such as pericardial friction rub.

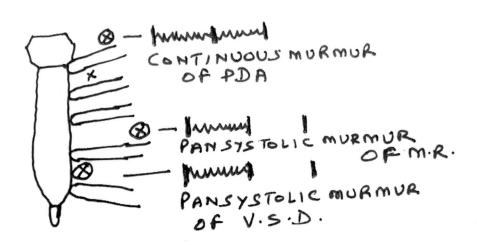

AUSCULTATORY FINDINGS

Abdominal Examination

By inspection, the student should note whether there is distension that may be associated with a shiny, tense abdominal skin. Abdominal breathing is normal in children and loss of this sign, indicates a serious intra-abdominal problem such as peritonitis. Note whether the abdomen is uniformly distended and test for ascites. Look for distended veins, umbilicus and peristalsis. Palpate first superficially for tenderness and guarding followed by deep palpation for liver, spleen and any other intra-abdominal mass. Examine the femoral, inguinal region for hernia and hydrocele. Examine external genitalia for ambiguity; examine testes and their normal descent. Rectal examination is performed only if indicated and using the little finger. Abdominal findings can be usefully represented diagrammatically as follows:

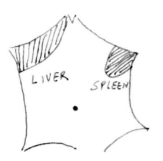

ABDOMINAL EXAMINATION

Differential diagnosis between renal and splenic swellings

	Splenic swelling	Renal swelling
1) Direction of enlargement	Oblique	Downwards
2) Hand insinuation between swelling and costal margin	cannot be done	Hand can be insinuated
3) Ballottement	-Ve	+Ve
4) Notch	+Ve	-Ve
5) Traube's area	Dull	Resonant
6) Movement with respiration	Freely movable	Limited movement
7) Percussion	Dull	Dull with a band of colonic resonance

Methods of examination for ascites
1. **Shifting dullness**

   The patient lies supine. Percuss and note dullness in the flanks. Turn the patient to the opposite side; allow time for the fluid to gravitate down and percuss again. If the flank becomes resonant ⇒ sign is +ve for ascites.
2. **Knee chest position**

   This method is used for minimal amount of ascites. The dullness is elicited in the periumbilical area.
3. **Fluid thrill** for tense ascites.

   The patient lies supine. Place one hand flat over the lumbar region of one side; get an assistant to put the side of his hand firmly in the midline of the abdomen and then tap the opposite lumbar region. A fluid thrill or wave is felt as a definite impulse by the hand held flat in the lumbar region. The purpose of the assistant's hand is to dampen any impulse that may be transmitted through the fat of the abdominal wall.

Central Nervous System (CNS): *Please refer to the neurology chapter*
On inspection, note the state of consciousness of the child, especially the degree of alertness, interest in the surroundings, activity, unresponsiveness, drowsiness and semi-consciousness, or unconsciousness. The posture and any abnormal movements should be noted. Look for obvious palsies, such as facial palsy or Erb's Palsy. Test the cranial nerves, muscle tone and power and reflexes. An attempt should be made to localize the abnormality; whether it is a central or peripheral aspect of the CNS.

Musculo-skeletal system
Although this system is separately itemized, some of its aspects can be examined under CNS. Observe the child while he is walking and note the gait, which may be characteristic of specific conditions, such as a hemiplegic gait. Look for muscle wasting and its distribution e.g. asymmetrical muscle wasting in paralytic poliomyelitis.

Urine analysis
If facilities are available, always do urinalysis using the dipstick method and present its findings at the end of the physical examination before the final summary.

Case Summary
Summary is the most important part of the doctor's ability to analyse and interpret various points in the history and physical examination with their relevance to the patient's illness. The summary should take account of all problems discovered in the history not just the presenting complaint. In a long and complicated case it may be useful to present them as *'Problem List'*.

Summarize all relevant features of the case, identify the problems and make a clinical diagnosis or list of possible differential diagnoses.

Suggest the **essential investigations**, keeping in mind that unnecessary X-rays and lab tests are disadvantageous to everybody including the patient, lab staff and the hospital budget.

Finally outline a **clear plan of management** dealing with all essential problems not just the primary disease.

1.3   Developmental Assessment and early warning signs

Definitions:
> **Growth =** Growing in terms of size
>
> **Development =** Maturation of functions.
>
> **Neurodevelopment**
>
> Is an orderly & sequential process from fetal to adult life. Anatomically fetus at 5 months has full adult's numbers of 12 billion neurons but future skills depend on neuronal interconnections & myelination process.

Principles of Development
- Development is continuous process from intrauterine fetal life
- Development is related to maturity of CNS (myelination)
- Sequence of development is same but rate of development varies
- Development always occurs Cephalo-caudally
- Primitive reflexes have to be lost before voluntary functions are acquired
- Gross activity matures to fine coordinated activity
- **Sensitive period** – Is the time when if given a chance, the learning comes automatically. If this period is missed for some reason then the milestone is either difficult or can not be achieved e.g.
  - ❑ Prolonged tube feeding leading to loss of sucking and feeding
  - ❑ Unrecognized deafness or cataract leading to loss of speech and amblyopia respectively.
  - ❑ Uncorrected cleft palate leading to feeding and speech problems
  - ❑ Emotional deprivation leading to delayed development

Developmental Delay: Slow progress leading to delay in one or more areas significantly below average it is Non progressive disease also known as Static encephalopathy. It could be either
> **Global** involving all areas of development
>
> **Specific:** Involving specific area like cognitive (mental retardation) or motor (cerebral palsy)

Developmental Regression: Loss of acquired milestones: This is more serious as it signifies an underlying progressive neuro-degenerative or metabolic disease

Factors Affecting Development:
> **1) Genetic Factors:** Genetic potentials inherited from parents
>
> **2) Prenatal Factors**

Fetal	- Metabolic Diseases. – PKU, Hypothyroidism
	- Chromosomal Anomaly –Down syndrome
	- Multiple Pregnancies, Abnormal presentation
	- Pre or post maturity & Low birth weight babies
Maternal	- X-Ray Irradiation
	- Drugs & Toxins – Antiepileptic, Warfarin, anticancer,
	- Smoking, alcohol, stress
	- Infections – TORCH
	- Diseases of pregnancy – Diabetes, Hypertension, APH, Toxemia of pregnancy, Placental insufficiency,
	- Uterine anomalies

3) **Natal Factors:** Any factor leading to Perinatal anoxia
   -Difficult delivery, prolonged labor
   -Meconium aspiration
   -Cord around the neck
4) **Postnatal Factors**
   -Birth injuries
   -Neonatal convulsions
   -Neonatal illness – RDS, meningitis, sepsis, IVH
   -Hypoglycemia, Hyper-bilirubinemia
   -Chronic illness, drugs
5) **Environmental Factors**
   -Socioeconomic - Learning opportunity v/s Deprivation, Unwanted child
   -Poverty, Age & nutrition of parents,
   - Cultural practices, nutrition, care, love & security

Instructions on performing the developmental testing

History taking:
- Take a good history of **Pre, Peri and Postnatal period** (Gestation, Perinatal complications, Type of delivery, **APGAR score**, Admission to NICU, Ventilation, Complications etc)
- **Family history** of any Genetic, Metabolic disease death or Neuro regression
- **Social and environmental factors** (neglect, poor opportunity to practice a skill, chronic illness and Prolonged or repeated hospitalization)
- While you are taking the history from the mother, leave the child free to observe his activities. Offer various test objects individually to play, this way you will save time as well as learn more about his developmental abilities.
- **Prematurity allowance** should be given up-to two years age.
- Note any familial pattern of delay especially in walking, speech, toilet training etc.
- Note that a child with bottom shuffling is usually delayed in walking.
- Mother's observations are very important about vision, squint, hearing etc.

Examination:
- **Prematurity allowance:** If the child was born premature then deduct the number of months he was born early from the actual age. This is important until child reaches 2 years of age
- First perform a routine **Neurological exam**, take a note of **Head size** (Micro or macrocephaly, Hydrocephalus)
- Note any **dysmorphic features** and signs of **Neuro-cutaneous markers** (Café au let or white macules)
- Hearing and vision should always be separately
- Postpone the test if the child is sick, hungry, sleepy or unwilling.

Developmental Testing:
- Use a quiet room with minimal distractions, use one test item at a time, and keep others hidden.
- Child should not be sleepy, Hungry, in need of diaper change or sick, if so then repeat the test at a later date
- Even if child doesn't succeed in a task, give credit to interest and ability to try

- **Developmental testing is done by 3 methods:**
  - **Checking mile stones from mother** e.g. social smile, climbing stairs, toilet training
  - **Direct Observation of mile stones** e.g. grasping, sitting, standing, walking, speech
  - **Performing a test** item e.g. use of cubes, scissors, pencil, picture, color identification
- **Test Items used:**
  - Nine one inch size cubes
  - Bell, Rattle, Cup & spoon for hearing check
  - Torch, small red ball on thread to check vision
  - Small sweets to check pincer grasp and fine vision
  - Paper & pencil, Beads and thread, Scissors: to test fine movements
  - Simple picture and color book / cards
  - Large Ball to throw and catch
- If not known, roughly estimate child's age and start with items from corresponding row in the developmental table, if failed, go to previous row until a pass is achieved. Do the same in all five columns. Report the Developmental age for "Each Area" if different.
- If an item is failed, give another chance with more encouragement, check with mother if child usually can do it and note the interest and willingness to perform.

Interpretation of the Test:
- Report if delay is **Global or Isolated** in **One or More areas**
- **Report if there is a delay or regression**
- **Report the developmental age in each area**
- **Developmental quotient (DQ)** for each area can be calculated by:

$$\frac{\text{Developmental Age}}{\text{Actual Age}} \times 100$$

Degree of Mental Retardation	DQ	Expected Mental Age as an Adult
Dull normal	80-90	-
Borderline	70-79	-
Mild (educable)	55-69	9-11 Years
Moderate (Trainable)	40-54	5-8 Years
Severe	25-39	3-5 Years
Profound	below 25	below 3 Years

- The gross motor milestones are related to Neuro-muscular functions,
- Fine motor milestones to co-ordination and vision
- Speech and social milestones relate more to intelligence
  Therefore in cerebral palsy motor milestones are predominantly affected while in mental retardation speech and social milestones are affected.
- **Differentiate between Developmental delay and Regression,** later is more significant in terms of presence of some underlying progressive neurological disease that may be treatable e.g. Hypothyroidism, Metabolic disease, Uncontrolled seizures, Wilson disease, Tumors, Hearing or visual defect etc.

Developmental Milestones

AGE	GROSS MOTOR	FINE MOTOR	SOCIAL	HEARING & SPEECH	VISION
BIRTH	**Prone** - Pelvis high Knees under abdomen **Ventral Suspension-** Elbows flexed & hips partially extended	Tight grasp Reflex **NN Reflexes: Birth - to** Stepping – 2 m Gallant – 2 m Palmer – 4 m Moro – 4 m ATNR – 4 m Plantar – 9 m			Pupil Reflex + Eye closes to bright light
6 W	**Prone** – Lifts head **V S** - Head in line with body **Pull to sit** – Head lag+		**Social smile**	Quiets to sound Startle to sound	Fixate & Follows ball to ¼ circle
3m	**Prone** -Weight on forearms **Pull to sit**- slight head lag	Holds object placed in hand	Recognizes parents	Cooing, Laughs	Follows ball to ½ circle
4 m	**Head control**	**Hand regard**			Responds to Visual threat
5m	**Prone** - Weight on wrist	Feet to mouth **Reaches & grasps**	Puts objects in mouth (Mouthing-up to 15 Months)		
6m	Turns **Prone to Supine** **Sits with arm support** Standing-Supports full weight on legs	**Transfer objects Chews/sucks on biscuit**	Enjoys Mirror	**Babbling** (Ba, Da, Ma) **Distraction Test +**	**No squint** Fixate on small objects
7m	Turns **Supine to Prone**		**Stranger anxiety**		
8m	**Sits alone**		Respond to name Understand "No"		
9m	**Crawl**	**Poking with index finger**	Peak – A –Boo **Clapping,** Finds hidden toy	Joining syllables (Dada, Mama (Nonspecific)	Pokes at small Object (sweets)
10m	**Pull to stand**	**Early Pincer grasp**	**Waves Bye, Helps in dressing**	Dada, Mama, specific	Picks up small sweets
11m	**Walk around furniture or with 2 hands held**	**Mature Pincer grasp Release on demand**		**One word with meaning**	
12m	Stands alone Walk with one hand held	Bangs 2 cubes Casting (Throwing objects, normal up to 18m)	Respond to simple questions (where?) Enjoys picture book Shy to strangers	2-3 words with meaning	
13m	**Walks alone**				
15m	Creep upstairs	**No Mouthing/ drooling** Tower of **2 cubes,** **Uses cup**	**Domestic mimicry (copying mother in house work)**	**Jargon speech** (unclear speech)	

18m	Throws ball without falling Bends & picks toy from floor	**3 cubes tower** Uses spoon Turns 3-4 pages Holds pencil, Scribbles	Points to 2 body parts Identify 1 picture card **Follows simple command**		
2 y	Runs, throws & kicks Walks backwards Up & down stairs – 2 feet	**6 cubes (tower/ train)** Unscrew Lids Turns single page Vertical line Horizontal at 2y 6 mo.	Points to 4 body parts Identify 4 Picture cards Doesn't leave mother Plays alone & possessive **Undress** **Dry by day**	**Joins 2 words** Uses I, Me, You 50 words	
3y	Jumps, Tip toe walk Upstairs – alternate feet, downstairs with 2 feet Can stand on 1 foot Pedals tricycle	**Handedness** **9 cubes tower** **Imitates Bridge** Thread beads Copies- **O**	Point to 8 Pictures 1-2 color Play with others & shares **Dresses** **Fasten buttons** **Dry by night**	**Sentences** Name & sex, Questions **Count to 10** Understand On, In & under	STYCAR toy matching test
4 y	Up & Downstairs alternate feet, Can Hop	Cubes- Bridge & 3 steps Use Scissor, Copies **+**	Names 3 colors Quarrels, Brushes Washes	Conversate well Tells Poems Tells Age	
5y	Can skip rope	Cubes- 4 steps Copies Cross & Triangle		Tells Story, Knows address & Birth date	Snellen' s chart

Important early developmental warning signs

1. General

- Head size too large or small
- Presence of congenital anomalies, dysmorphic features or genetic syndrome
- Persistent neonatal reflexes after 6 months of age.
- Tight fisting or adducted (Cortical) thumb after the second month of age.

2. Gross Motor

5 m	Can not roll over
8 m	Can not sit without support
10 m	Can not stand with support
18 m	Can not walk alone
2 yr	Can not climb stairs
3 yr	Can not stand on one foot momentarily
5 yr	Can not walk a straight line or balance on one foot

3. Fine Motor

5 m	Cant hold objects
7 m	Cant transfer objects
12 m	No pincer grasp
2 yr	Cant scribble
3 yr	Cant draw straight line
4 yr	Cant copy a circle
5 yr	Cant copy a cross

4. Language

6 m	No babbling
9 m	No syllables "da" or "Ba"
18 m	No words with meaning
2 yr	Cant join 2 words
3 yr	No clear speech, uses gestures instead.
4 yr	Does not ask simple questions or tell a simple story.
5 yr	Cant construct proper sentences

5. Psychosocial

3 m	No social smile, poor alertness
6-8 m	Does not respond to playful situations
1 yr	Persistent cry and stiffness on handling
2 yr	Poor social activity and eye contact
3-5 yr	Persistent rocking motion

6. Cognitive

3 m	Poor attention or visual contact
9 m	Doesn't like social contact
12 m	Doesn't search for hidden object
3 yr	Doesn't know own full name
4 yr	Cant pick shorter or longer of two lines
4-½ yr	Cant count
5 yr	Cant recognize colors or any letters

1.4   Vision and Hearing assessment

A.   Vision testing:

Risk factors for blindness or poor vision:
- **Diseases:**
  - Congenital anomalies
  - Glaucoma
  - Cataract – TORCH, Galactosemia, Mucopolysaccharidoses
  - Retinopathy of Prematurity
  - Trauma, Non accidental injuries
  - Birth asphyxia

- **Parental concern**

- **Presence of searching nystagmus**

- **Delayed fine motor coordination**

Test Methods

A: **Birth Onward:**
   Clinical: -Pupillary response
   -Response to bright light
   -Face regard
   -Following a red ball

   Testing: -VEP by flash electric stimuli

B: **6 Months Onward**
   - **STYCAR graded ball test (Sheridan)**
   -1/8 to 2 ½ inches white balls rolled on black cloth at 3 meters
   -Near Vision – by placing colored sweets of various sizes

C: **2 Year – 3 Years**
   STYCAR Miniature Toys Matching: Two sets of toys are used (Chair, car, doll, spoon, fork etc.) one set is with child and another with examiner sitting 10 feet apart. Examiner picks one toy without speaking the name and child is supposed to pick same toy from his set

D: **Over 3 years**
   STYCAR letter (VOXHT) matching: by using two sets and sitting 10 feet away.

E: **Over 6 years:**
   Snellen's chart can be used.

B.   Hearing Tests:

Risk factors for deafness:
- Speech delay
- TORCH infections
- Ototoxic drugs
- Hyperbilirubinemia
- Family history of deafness
- Birth asphyxia
- Meningitis, head injury.
- Syndromes and congenital malformations
- Recurrent otitis media, glue ear or perforated drums

•**Parent's concern- Mother is usually right about child's vision or hearing**

Testing Methods:
A: Birth to Any Age
-Clinical: response to noise, turning to voice
-BAER: needs sedation

B: 8 Months to 2 years (Distraction Test)
- Baby sits on mother's lap
- Distracter sits in front with a toy to attracts child's attention
- Examiner produces sounds at ear level 45 cm away while distracter removes the toy.
- Distracter notes reaction (turning towards the sound) and response
Sound Used in the test:
-Voice – high tone (Pssss), low tone (ooo')
-High pitch rattle or Spoon rotated inside a tea cup
-Sound produced by crumpling a paper.
Test is done on each side – pass if respond to 2 out of 3 times, on each side.

C: From 3-3 ½ year (McCormick Toy Test)
- 7 pairs of toys with similar sounding names are used (e.g. tree/key; cup/ duck)
- Child identifies and shows the toy named by examiner at sound level of < 40db.

D: Over 5 years (Pure Tone Audiometry)
Head phone sound used from 0.5 to 8 KHZ on each ear at various db threshold
Child responds by raising the hand when sound is heard
Quietest Volume at different frequencies is recorded.

1.5 Infant nutrition and Weaning

In order to improve infant morbidity and mortality, WHO has recommended that till 6 months of age exclusive breast feeding must be given for all infants.

Advantages of breastfeeding
- Colon pH is lower in breast fed babies that inhibits colonization of gram negative organisms.
- The lower stool pH of breast fed infants promotes growth of gut flora thus inhibiting pathogenic bacterial growth.
- Anti staphylococcal factors are present in breast milk.
- The presence of lactoperoxidase thiocyanates in breast milk helps kill streptococci.
- Non specific anti viral substances provide protection against viral illnesses.
- Presence of lysozyme, leucocytes and macrophages in breast milk help active phagocytosis of bacteria.
- Lactoferrin in breast milk binds with iron thus depriving bacteria inhibiting their multiplication.
- Secretory IgA, IgG and IgM antibodies protect against gram negative pathogens in small bowel.
- Breast milk causes less solute load on the neonatal renal system.
- Breastfeeding provides better bonding between mother and child.
- Artificial feeds can cause obesity in later life.

Reasons for decline in breast-feeding
- Changing life style and urbanization
- Working women with minimum maternity leave.
- Promotion of artificial feeding.

Complementary diet / Weaning
Process of introduction of any non milk food into the infant's diet, irrespective of whether breast fed or bottle fed. Weaning should start after 6 months.

Principles of weaning
- The whole process of weaning should not take more than 3-4 months.
- By one year the child should be able to cope with normal family diet.
- Breast feeding should continue throughout the weaning process.
- Weaning is to supplement extra amino acids, minerals, vitamins and iron to the infant's diet.
- Refusal and rejection of feeds are normal responses of the infant, demanding patience.
- By 9 months, teeth appear and the desire to bite should be fulfilled by giving biscuits and rusks.
- Cereals should be the first food to be introduced in liquid form and then mixed with milk into semisolid diet. Rice is better to begin with, than wheat based cereal, because of risk for gluten enteropathy in sensitive individuals.

The order/Sequence of type of weaning food introduction:
- Cereals (e.g. Rice)
- Vegetables (Pureed)
- Mashed fruits (Banana, apple)
- Chicken, fish or Meat (Pureed)
- Eggs (Yellow part first)
- Fruit juice

Replace the milk feed once the solid meal is fully accepted

Introduce only one thing at a time and continue in increasing quantity over the week in order to look for food allergy or intolerance. Try to give variety of food groups of different flavor, consistency and texture.

By one year the infant should bet adjusted to about five meals per day.

Hazards of weaning

Weaning diarrhea: generally caused by lack of hygiene, infected water, unclean vessels, improper or high osmolar food or rarely due to food allergy due to gluten sensitivity

Malnutrition: deficiency of proteins and calories can lead to kwashiorkor, marasmus and vitamin deficiencies.

Hypernatremia: too much sodium content in the weaning diet can lead to this.

Composition of 100 ml of milk:

Milk	Proteins (g)	Fat (g)	Carbohydrates (g)	Kilocalories
Breast milk	1.3	4	7	74
Cow's milk	3.3	3.5	4.5	70
Infant formula	1.8	3.5	7	70

Milk requirements for babies on full feeds from birth:

Age in days	ml/kg/day
1	60
2 – 3	90
4 – 6	120
7 days to 6 months	130 to 190 (Average 150)

Number of milk feeds required:

Age	Number of feeds
Birth to 1 week	6-10
1 wk to 1 mo	6-8
2-6 mo	5-6
6-12 mo	3-4

Nutritional Requirements in children:

Age	Fluids ml/ Kg	Calories/Kg	Proteins Gram/Kg
0-3 mo	150	110	2.1
3-6 mo	130	95	1.6
6-12 mo	120	95	1.5
1-3 y	95	95	1.1
4-6 y	85	90	1.1
7-12 y	70	70	1.0

1.6   Child with Failure to Thrive (FTT)

Definition:
Growth failure, or failure to thrive (FTT), is a descriptive term and not a specific diagnosis. Although there is no clear consensus about the definition, many authors define FTT as Growth (height or weight) less than third percentile for age and sex on more than one occasion.

FTT can also be termed if height or weight measurements fall crossing two major percentile lines.

All authorities agree that only by comparing height and weight on growth chart over time can FTT be assessed accurately.

Frequency:
- Ten percent of children seen in the primary care settings show signs of growth failure
- In underdeveloped countries, malnutrition manifesting as FTT is more common.

Classification:
> **Organic FTT** – Is caused by some other underlying medical condition
> **Non-Organic FTT** – Children with no known medical condition
> **Mixed FTT**– Child has features of both organic and non-organic failure to thrive

History: Most important part of the evaluation of FTT may be by obtaining a detailed history.

Neonatal History:
- Maternal smoking or alcohol consumption during pregnancy
- Use of antenatal medications
- Any illness during pregnancy
- Prematurity / IUGR / Significant neonatal illness

Feeding History:
> Assess details of breast or formula feeding, timing and introduction of solids,
> Feeding pattern, who feeds the infant, position and placement.
> Detailed account of feeding with calculation of Protein, calories and other nutrients

Developmental History:
> To assess for associated developmental delay

Psychosocial History:
> Should include family composition, employment status, financial status
> Availability of food and child rearing practice
> Stress isolation, child-rearing beliefs, and history of maternal depression
> Possible child abuse or neglect.

Family History:
> Should include height, weight of parents and any significant familial illnesses

Detailed systemic enquiry:
To uncover any underlying systemic disease as per the table given below

Major Organic Causes of FTT:

System	Causes
Prenatal causes	Prematurity with complications, maternal malnutrition, Toxic exposure in utero, Alcohol, smoking, medications, infections, Intra Uterine Growth Retardation (IUGR), multiple pregnancies Chromosomal anomalies
Gastrointestinal	Gastro esophageal reflux, Celiac disease, Pyloric stenosis, Cleft palate/cleft lip, Lactose intolerance, Hirschprung's disease,Milk protein intolerance, Hepatitis, Cirrhosis, Pancreatic Insufficiency, Biliary disease, inflammatory bowel disease, Malabsorption
Renal	Recurrent or silent Urinary tract infections, renal tubular acidosis, diabetes insipidus, chronic renal insufficiency
Cardiopulmonary	CHD and CHF, Asthma, BPD, CF, Obstructive upper airway disease
Endocrine	Hypothyroidism, Diabetes, Adrenal insufficiency, Pituitary disorders Hyper-parathyroidism, Growth hormone deficiency
Neurology	Mental retardation, Cerebral palsy, Degenerative brain Disorders, any neurological disease leading to chronic disability
Infections	Parasitic or bacterial infections of the gastrointestinal tract, Tuberculosis, Human immunodeficiency virus disease
Metabolic	Inborn error of metabolism
Genetics	Chromosomal abnormalities, congenital syndromes
Miscellaneous	Lead poisoning, Malignancy, Collagen vascular disease, Recurrently infected adenoids and tonsils

Non-organic causes of FTT:
- Poor feeding or feeding-skills disorder
- Dysfunctional family interactions
- Difficult parent-child interactions
- Lack of support (e.g. no friends, no extended family)
- Lack of preparation for parenting
- Family dysfunction (e.g. divorce, spouse abuse, chaotic family style)
- Difficult child
- Child neglect, Emotional deprivation syndrome

Pathophysiology of FTT:

Inadequate Intake:
- Lack of appetite (e.g. iron deficiency anemia, CNS pathology, chronic infection)
- Inability to suck or swallow: CNS or muscular diseases
- Vomiting (e.g. CNS, metabolic, obstruction, renal diseases)
- Gastro esophageal reflux and esophagitis

Poor absorption:
- GI disorder (e.g. celiac disease, chronic diarrhea), Malabsorption
- Liver diseases
- Pancreatic diseases
- Inborn error of metabolism
- Chronic infection: (e.g. HIV, tuberculosis, parasites)

Increased Nutritional demand:
- Hyperthyroidism
- Chronic disease (e.g. Heart failure, BPD)
- Chronic inflammatory conditions
- Renal failure
- Malignancy

Combined Organic and Non-organic FTT:

FTT in a patient can result from the combination of both organic and non-organic reasons. Half of the cases with organic etiology had psychosocial factor contributing to the FTT, Children suffering from chronic illnesses also suffer from family stresses. Presence of a chronic illness can result in resistance or noncompliance in many aspects of a child's life.

Approach to Failure to Thrive Based on Age:

Age of onset	Major diagnostic considerations
Birth to 3-month	psychosocial failure to thrive, perinatal infections, gastro esophageal reflux, inborn errors of metabolism, cystic fibrosis
3-6 months	psychosocial failure to thrive, HIV disease, GE reflux, IEM, Milk protein intolerance, Cystic fibrosis, renal tubular Acidosis
7-12 months	psychosocial failure to thrive, Delayed weaning, GE Reflux, intestinal parasites, renal tubular acidosis
12 months +	Psychosocial failure to thrive, GE Reflux

Physical Examination:

The first thing that the pediatricians should do in all health assessments is to plot the growth chart. Every effort should be made to obtain as many previous growth parameters as possible to detect trends in growth rather than to rely on measurements on one particular visit.

If weight, height, and head circumference are all less than what is expected for age, this may result from in utero insults, genetic or chromosomal factors.

If weight and height are delayed with a normal head circumference, Endocrinopathies or constitutional delay should be suspected. This pattern also can occur in long-standing FTT. Ultimately head circumference is also delayed. When only weight is delayed, this usually reflects recent energy (caloric) deprivation.

Marasmus characterized by severe wasting or cachexia without edema and is caused by extreme food shortage (caloric deprivation), while **Kwashiorkor** is an extreme failure to thrive with edema and dermatosis due to eating poor quality food, which is severely deficient in proteins.

The physical examination of children with FTT may show the following:
- Edema
- Wasting (Loss of subcutaneous fat followed by muscle mass)
- Hepatomegaly
- Rash, skin and hair changes
- Altered mental status
- Signs of vitamin deficiency

Diagnostic Testing:

History and physical examination usually give a clue to the diagnosis; Laboratory assessment has a limited value in determining the etiology except that occasionally, laboratory results are unexpectedly abnormal in cases like blood dyscrasias, chronic urinary tract infections, chronic acidosis, and renal failure. Following tests may be ordered as initial work up in all cases:
- Complete blood count, ESR
- Urinalysis, Urine culture
- Renal profile
- Liver function tests

More specific tests may be indicated (depending on findings from the history and physical examination), including the following:
- HIV testing
- Sweat chloride test
- Thyroid function tests
- Stool studies for parasites and Malabsorption
- Immunoglobulins
- Montoux test for tuberculosis
- Radiologic determination of Bone Age: if the bone age is normal, it is unlikely that the infant has a systemic chronic disease or a hormonal abnormality as the cause of poor weight gain.

Treatment:

Interdisciplinary team approach combining pediatrician, Nutritionist, and Social expertise is required. If neglect is suspected, child protective services should be involved
Sub specialists should be involved for the treatment of organic illness when identified.

Dietary Management:

The cornerstone of therapy is aggressive dietary management.
The normal, healthy infants require an average of 100 kcal/kg of body weight per day; nutritional requirements in children with FTT usually go up-to 150 kcal/kg and Protein intake increased to 2-3 G/Kg day. Balanced, palatable and easily digestible diet should be designed

For older infants and young children with psychosocial FTT, mealtimes should be
Approximately 20 – 30 min, solid foods should be offered before liquids, environmental

distractions should be minimized, and the children should eat with other people and force-feeding should always be avoided.

For children with organic FTT, the underlying medical condition should be treated.

Medical care:
Most children with FTT can be treated as outpatients; home visits and close
Clinical follow-ups often help determine the reason for the FTT. Hospitalization is necessary for
diagnostic and therapeutic reasons. Diagnostic benefits of admission may include observation of feeding, parent-child interaction, dietary habits and ability to perform other specific tests

Prognosis:
Ultimate physical growth may be decreased in children with FTT.

FTT in the first year of life, regardless of cause is particularly ominous because maximal postnatal brain growth occurs during this time.

Cognitive development may be affected in children younger than 5 years that may not be completely reversible. Children with FTT attain lower intelligence, speech and language development, less developed reading skills, lower social maturity, and a higher incidence of behavioral disturbances.
Non-organic FTT results in more cognitive deficits then organic. Approximately one third of children with Non-Organic psychosocial FTT will have developmental, behavioral and emotional problems.

The prognosis for children with organic FTT is more variable depending on the underlying cause

Infants with faulty feeding and delayed weaning require aggressive caloric supplementation and correction of feeding practices that will lead to a good outcome.

In developing countries, malnutrition is a significant cause of mortality and morbidity either directly or secondary to complications (e.g. infections).

1.7 Childhood obesity

Definition:
Obesity is not equivalent to overweight, *overweight* may be due to fat or other tissue (like muscles and bones) in excess in relation to height. **Obesity denotes excess body fat (Adiposity).**

Obesity is a global nutritional concern. An increased prevalence of obesity is now found in many developing countries where the major nutritional disorder previously was malnutrition but now obesity coexists due to poor food choices and decreased activity.

The Body Mass Index (BMI) is the commonly accepted index for classifying adiposity:

> **Body mass index (BMI) = Weight (in kg)/Height (in m)²**

High BMI correlates well with excess body fat at all ages and in both genders.

For adults, BMI > 25 is defined as overweight
BMI > 30 is defined as obesity.

For children, BMI changes with age and sex as given in BMI percentile curves:
- **BMI** above the 85th percentile but less than 95th percentile is labeled: "at risk of overweight."
- **BMI** above the 95th percentile is labeled as "obesity" by most health care providers

Causes of Childhood Obesity:

1. Idiopathic obesity: This is the most common and often is multifactorial (the result of complex interactions of multiple genes and environmental factors) influencing food intake (↑ **energy input**) and energy expenditure (↓**energy output**): There are important **contributing factors** to idiopathic obesity:
- ♦ Lack of information on proper nutrition for parents
- ♦ Attractive commercials about "junk food" in the media (TV, etc.)
- ♦ Trying to compensate the physical absence of the parents through junk food
- ♦ Lack of exercise program
- ♦ Lack of promotion of health nutrients in the schools.
- ♦ Indiscriminate increase of fast food restaurants.
- ♦ TV or computer interactive games.

2. Endogenous Obesity:

♦ **Endocrine causes**: e.g. Hypothyroidism, Cushing's syndrome, Primary hyper insulinism and hypothalamic syndrome due to hypothalamic tumor, infection, trauma or vascular lesion.

♦ **Genetic** or syndromic causes e.g. Prader Willi and Laurence Moon Biedl syndromes

Characteristics of Idiopathic and Endogenous Obesity:

Idiopathic obesity	Endogenous obesity
• > 90 percent of cases • Tall stature (usually>50th percentile) • Family history common • Mental function normal • Normal or advanced bone age • Physical examination otherwise normal	• <10 percent of cases • Short stature(usually <5th percentile • Family history uncommon • Often mentally impaired • Delayed bone age • Associated stigmata on physical examination

Childhood Obesity has a Tendency to Continue into adulthood:

Chubby infant will not necessarily grow to be an obese adult. However, an overweight child is more likely to be obese adult, especially if it is acquired at late childhood. It is proven that more severe the obesity, higher is the risk of it's persistence.

Complications of Obesity in Childhood and Adolescence:

Childhood obesity is not a benign condition. Obese children and adolescents are at risk of many health problems. Immediate concerns include social and psychological stress, metabolic and physical disorders, and future complications in adulthood.

Main complications of obesity are:
- Psychosocial problems as insecurity, social discrimination and rejection, low self –esteem
- Easy fatigability
- Hypertension
- Dyslipidemia
- Hyperinsulinemia and type 2 diabetes.
- Orthopedic problems (tibial torsion, bowed legs, slipped capital femoral epiphysis)
- Skin problems (stretch marks, heat rash, intetrigo, monilial dermatitis, acne, etc)
- Adulthood obesity
- Premature atherosclerosis

Counseling parents on prevention of childhood obesity:

> ### IT IS MUCH EASIER TO PREVENT OBESITY THAN TO TREAT IT

Treating childhood obesity relies on positive family support and lifestyle changes for the whole family. Children learn to be active or inactive from their parents. In addition, physical activity (or more commonly, physical inactivity) habits that are established in childhood tend to persist into adulthood. Following are some tips that may help families to prevent obesity in their children.
- Encourage breast feeding
- Respect the children's appetite - do not force feed.
- Avoid pre-prepared and sugared foods when possible
- Limit the amount of high – calorie foods kept at home
- Provide a healthy diet with <30 percent calories from fat, ample fiber in the child's diet

- Skimmed milk may safely replace whole milk at 2 years of age
- Do not provide food as a reward, Do not offer sweets in exchange for a finished meal.
- Limit amount of television viewing to 2 hours /day
- Encourage active play and regular family activities like walks, ball games etc.

Treatment of Childhood Obesity:

The most important goal is to prevent the development of obesity related morbidities in adulthood. *The lines of treatment include:*

1. **Reduction of energy intake and to improve dietary quality:** Balanced hypo-caloric diet with high complex carbohydrate, low fat, adequate protein and low in energy density.
2. **Increase physical activity to** increase energy expenditure through increased general activity and play rather than vigorous exercise.
3. **Behavioral therapy** :
   - The most essential long term line of treatment in childhood
   - It includes self-monitoring nutritional education, eating behavior, etc.
4. **Drugs**: Drugs do not cure obesity and should be discouraged in pediatrics.

1.8   Rickets in Pediatrics

Definition:
Failure of mineralization of growing bones or osteoid tissue is called rickets.
Osteomalacia is Under-mineralization with normal bone volume
Osteoporosis on the other end is Normal mineralization with reduced bone volume

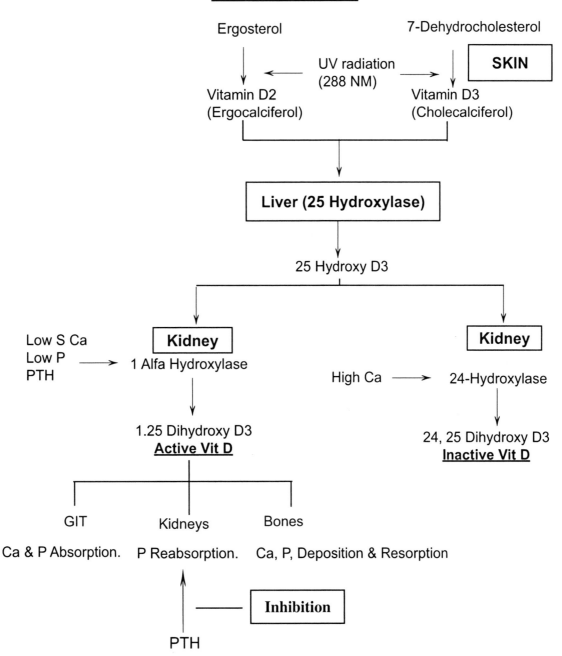

Vitamin D Metabolism

Etiology:

A: **Simple Rickets**

1. **Nutritional**
-Breast fed infants of Vit D deficient mothers
-Use of unfortified cow's milk
-Increased requirements- Rickets of prematurity (breastfed babies)
-Poor exposure to sunlight – dark skin (black children)

2. **Malabsorption – Fats malabsorption – steatorrhea**
-Celiac Dis
-Pancreatitis
-Cystic Fibrous
-Liver Dis – cirrhosis, biliary atresia, NN Hepatitis

3. **Anticonvulsant Therapy – Phenobarbitone & Phenytoin**
-Stimulation of microsomal oxidase - ↑ Vit D Catabolism
-GI Calcium Absorption Inhibition

B: **Vitamin D – Dependant Rickets**
-Type I – Defective one hydroxylation
-Type II – End organ resistance

C: **Vitamin D – Resistant Rickets**
X-Linked dominant hypophosphatemic rickets. (↓ P. Reabsorption)

A. Simple Rickets

Pathology –
Growing bone ends- Osteoblast tissue → matrix → Poor mineralization

Clinical Manifestations –
Mostly onset is at the end of first or during 2nd year. Signs can be divided from head to toes

Head	-craniotabes -large & delayed closure of ant. Fontanel -delayed teething, caries
Thorax	-rachitic rosary -pigeon breast -Harrison sulcus -kyphoscoliosis
Extremities	-lax ligaments- Hypotonia -bowing of legs -enlarged wrist & ankle (double malleoli) -short stature
Muscles	hypotonia – delayed walking, pot belly

Diagnosis:

History of Vit D Deficiency (See aetiology factors)

Biochemistry: -↓↓ Phosphorus
- Calcium is usually normal due to PTH stimulation.
- ↑↑ Alkaline Phosphatase (due to ↑ osteoblastic activity)
- Aminoaciduria
- Iron Deficiency may be coexisting

Radiology: - **Wrist x-ray** shows following signs:
Widening
Cupping
Fraying
Osteopenia
Green stick fractures

Treatment:

One Alfa: (1α D3) = 2 μgm/ml = 0.1 μgm/drop
Dose 0.05 μgm/kg/day

Vit D3 : 4000 IU (100 μgm) daily
600,000 IU (15000 μgm) one stat dose if compliance is poor

Remember to look for vitamin D dependent or Vitamin D resistant types of rickets if patient fails to respond to adequate vitamin D treatment. Avoid giving repeated mega doses of Vitamin D, as this will cause nephrocalcinosis.

Signs of Recovery/Healing:
- Healing begins in few days and is Complete in 6 weeks.
-X-Ray– initially shows a line of preparatory calcification at the terminal end of bone
followed by progressive mineralization of osteoid tissue
- Alkaline Phosphatase & PTH levels drop to normal

Prevention –

•Sun exposure
•Vit D 400 IU (10 μgm) added to the milk – Fortified milk

B. Vitamin D Dependent Rickets

Type I Vitamin D dependent Rickets

Autosomal Recessive deficiency of renal 1- hydroxylase ⟶ ↓ 1, 25 Vit D3

Differences from simple rickets

•Early onset – 3 to 6 months
•History of adequate intake of Vit D & sun exposure

- Needs very high doses of Vit D for healing (though small doses of 1 Alfa is adequate)
- Low serum calcium - ↑ PTH, Patient may present with Hypocalcemic Tetany or Convulsions
- Severe tooth enamel hypoplasia & caries
- Normal 25 hydroxy Vit D but Very low 125 Dihydroxy D3

Treatment:
- 0.5 to 4 μgm/day of 1.25 Vit D3
- Maintenance dose 0.25 – 2 μgm/day

Type II Vitamin D dependent Rickets

- End organ resistance to 1.25 Vit D3 (abnormal receptor)
- Clinically same as in Type I except Generalized **ALOPECIA** occur in 50 % of cases.
- Normal or V. high 1.25 Vit D3 levels.

Treatment:
- V. difficult esp. when ALOPECIA is present.
- 5-60 μgm/day of 1.25 Vit D
- Parenteral calcium infusions.

C. Vitamin D Resistant Rickets – familial hypophosphatemia

Proximal tubular phosphaturia leading to hypophosphatemia is the major factor
Also there seems to be some element of ↓ed 1 hydroxylation defect associated

Etiology: X linked Dominant – severe in males, Females – short stature, AR, Sporadic

Clinical Features
Early onset Rickets – By the end of first yr.
Severe Deformities,
Short Stature, Severe dental caries
No tetany/seizures
Normal PTH levels: Normal Calcium levels
No aminoaciduria
No response to usual dose of Vit D
Phosphaturia in presence of hypophosphatemia

$$\% \text{ TRP} = 1 - \boxed{\frac{\text{U.Ph} \times \text{S Cr}}{\text{S. P} \times \text{U.Cr}}} \times 100$$

TRP= Fractional Phosphate reabsorption, U=Urine, Ph=Phosphate, S=Serum, Cr=Creatinine
↓ % TRP   normal = > 80%, Patients = < 70%

Treatment:

> Oral Phosphate therapy is very important
> Rickets may not heal with calcium and vitamin D alone.

Oral phosphate is given as 1 to 4 gm/day in 5 DD, 4 hourly, Most important side effect is Diarrhea – improves with time.

Small dose of active vit. D is also needed, 1.25 Vit D3 given as 0.025 – 0.05 μgm/kg/d

Phosphate Therapy alone causes hyperparathyroidism.
Excessive Vit D Therapy ↑es Ca absorption leading to hypercalciuria & nephrocalcinosis.

Corrective osteotomy may be needed after healing is complete

Prevention
- Family Screen
- Screening of children of affected individual in infancy to prevent short stature & deformities

SUMMARY OF BIOCHEMICAL FEATURES OF VARIOUS TYPES OF RICKETS:

Type	CA	P	AP	PTH	25 Vit D	125 Vit D	Amino Aciduria
CALCIPENIC—							
1. Nutritional R	↓/N	↓/N	↑	↑	(↓)	N	+
2. Vit D Dep Type I	↓	↓/N	↑↑	↑	N	(↓↓)	+
3. Vit D Dep Type II	↓	↓/N	↑↑	↑	N	(↑↑)	+
PHOSPHOPENIC— **4. Vit D Res**	N	↓↓	↑	(N)	N	↓	No.

↑ Increased, ↓ Decreased, N = Normal, AP = Alkaline Phosphatase

1.9 Childhood immunization

Introduction

WHO launched the expanded program of immunization **(EPI)** in 1974; as a result, three million lives are being saved each year. ***In Oman EPI was launched in 1981***. Immunization is the most cost effective means of preventing infectious diseases. Immunization has eradicated deadly disease like Small pox.

In 1970s, <10% of worlds children were immunized, this increased to 80% by 1980.

In Oman only 10 % of children were immunized in 1981, by 2001 near 100% coverage has been achieved.

Definition:

Immunization is the process of inducing immunity artificially either by vaccination **(active)** or by administration of antibody **(passive)**

Active Immunization:

By giving a live or Inactivated Vaccine, It is called active because of active role played by body's own immune system to provide immunity in response to a vaccine.

Examples of Live Vaccines: (Mainly viral)
1. OPV (Oral Polio Vaccine)
2. BCG (For Tuberculosis)
3, Measles
4. MMR (Measles mumps and Rubella)

Examples of Inactivated Vaccines: (mostly bacterial)
1. Hepatitis B (Hep-B)
2. DPT (Diphtheria, Pertussis and Tetanus)
3. Hib (Haemophilus influenza)
4. Tetanus toxoid (TT)
5. Penta vaccine (DPT, Hep B & Hib)
6. IPV (Inactivated Parenteral Polio Vaccine)

Passive Immunization:
By using preformed immunoglobulins (Specific Ig or Pooled Ig):
1. Varicella Zoster immunoglobulin. (Chicken pox)
2. Hepatitis B Immunoglobulin (Hepatitis B)
3. Tetanus Ig (TIG)

Vaccination recommended for a country is based on:
a. Epidemiology of the disease
b. Age specific morbidity and mortality
C. Vaccine immunogenicity
d. Cost effectiveness

IMMUNIZATION PROGRAM IN OMAN (1/8/2006)

First year of life

Age	Vaccine
At birth	BCG OPV HBV
6 Weeks	OPV 40 plus PENTA-1 or HBV, DTP, Hib
3 Months	OPV-1 PENTA-2 or HBV, DTP, Hib
5 Months	OPV-2 PENTA-3 or HBV, DTP, Hib
7 months	OPV-3 Vitamin A 100,000 IU
12 months	MMR-1 Vitamin A100, 000 IU

Note: The current immunization program in Oman uses PENTA vaccine (A mix of DTP, Hib and HBV vaccines) in place of individual DTP, Hib and HBV vaccines as given previously).

Second year of life

18 months	MMR-2 DTP Booster OPV Booster

School Immunization schedule

Primary School, Level 1 (6-7 Years)

Vaccine	Schedule
OPV Booster	One dose
DT Booster (1 dose) DT (2 doses)	One dose to all children OR Give TWO DOSES at an interval of 4 to 6 weeks if NOT vaccinated previously, or if no documentary evidence available i.e. immunization card.

Primary School, Level 6 (12-13 Years)

Vaccine	Schedule
Td Booster (One dose) Or Td (2 doses)	For GIRLS & BOYS who have been fully immunized before with DTP and DT Give a Booster dose (One dose) If not fully immunized as above or NO records available give 2 doses of Td at an interval of 4-6 weeks.

Secondary School Level 2 (17 – 18 Years)

Vaccine	Schedule
TT Booster (One dose) OR	If the Student is fully immunized in class 6 Primary school give one dose
TT (2 doses)	If NOT fully immunized as above or if no records available give 2 doses of TT at an interval of 4-6 weeks
OPV Booster (one dose)	To be given to all students at this level

Tetanus Toxoid for Adults

Vaccination status	Action
If Immunized as per schedule &documentary evidence available	Give one Booster of TT every 10 years
If not immunized as per schedule above OR Immunization status unknown	-Give 2 doses of TT at an interval of 4-6 weeks apart -Give 3rd dose of TT with a minimum interval of 6 months after 6 months after the 2nd dose. -Give the 4th dose with a minimum interval of one year after the 3rd dose followed by a 5th dose after one year Subsequently give one booster dose every ten years.

Route, site, and dose of various vaccines:

Vaccine	Route	Site	Dose
BCG	ID	Left deltoid-Insertion	0.05 ml
OPV	Oral	Mouth	2 drops
DTP	IM	Lt. Anterolateral thigh	0.5 ml
Hib	IM	Left/ Rt. anterolateral thigh	0.5 ml
Hep-B	IM	Left/ Rt. anterolateral thigh	0.5 ml
Measles	IM	Rt. anterolateral thigh	0.5 ml
MMR	IM	Rt. anterolateral thigh	0.5 ml
DT	IM	Lt. Deltoid	0.5 ml
Td/ TT	IM	Lt. Deltoid	0.5 ml
TT	IM	Lt. Deltoid	0.5 ml

BCG = Bacille Calmette Guerin, DTP = Diphtheria, Tetanus and Pertusis, DT = Normal dose diphtheria and tetanus, Hib = Haemophilus Influenzae B, HBV =Hepatitis B vaccine, IPV =Inactivated polio vaccine, OPV = Oral polio vaccine, Td = Vaccine with low dose diphtheria, TT = Tetanus toxoid,

Contraindications to Vaccination

Vaccines	Specific Contraindications
BCG	Clinically Symptomatic HIV infection or known immunodeficiency
DTP	History of uncontrolled seizures (Not febrile convulsions) (Especially if these occurred after a previous dose of DPT) or any progressive and evolving neurological disease, severe local or general reaction to pertussis vaccine. In all such cases use either DT or DTaP (With acellular pertussis vaccine)
OPV	Immune-compromised patient – e.g. HIV, SCID
Hib	None

Measles/MMR	None
TT	None
DT	None
Hepatitis	None

Immunization policies for specific situations
Recommendation for the Immunization of HIV-infected Children

| Vaccine | HIV INFECTION | |
	Asymptomatic	Symptomatic
BCG	No	No
DTP	Yes	Yes
IPV	Yes	Yes
Measles	Yes	Yes
Hepatitis B	Yes	Yes
Yellow fever	Yes	No

Note: In severely symptomatic HIV, do not administer measles vaccination

Cold chain for vaccine storage:
A network of Freezer rooms, refrigerators, and cold boxes that is organized & maintained by teams of people throughout the world to ensure that vaccine is kept in the right temperature at all times to retain its potency from the moment it leaves the manufacturer until the moment it is administered.

Adverse events following immunization (AEFI): All reactions should be reported

1. **Local adverse reactions.**
   a. Injection site abscess
   b. Lymphadenitis
   c. Severe local reaction

2. **Central nervous system adverse events.**
   1. Acute paralysis: Within 4 -30 days of OPV or within 4-75 days after contact with vaccine recipient or neurological deficit remaining 60 days after onset.
   2. Guillian-Barre Syndrome (GBS): Within 30 days after immunization
   3. Encephalopathy: Within 72 hrs after vaccination.
   4. Encephalitis: Within 1-4 weeks following vaccination.
   5. Meningitis.
   6. Seizures: for > 15 minutes and not accompanied by neurological deficit, (Febrile or Afebrile)

3. **Other Adverse Events**
   1. Anaphylactic reaction- within 2 hrs.
   2. Arthralgia - Persisting for 10 days.
   3. BCG- adenitis: Within 1-2 months   following vaccination.
   4. Persistent un-consolable high-pitched screaming lasting at least 3 hrs.
   5. Toxic- Shock Syndrome- Acute diarrhea and shock causing death in 24-48 hrs.

6. Any other severe adverse events occurring within 4 weeks after immunization and not specified in the above description **should also be reported**.

New vaccines

Can be searched on WHO website:

http://www.who.int/vaccine_**research/documents/new_vacc.../index/. htm**

Some new vaccines of interest:

1. Pneumo coccal Vaccine (Prevenar): Used before Splenectomy in Sickle cell disease
2. Rota virus vaccine: Oral live attenuated vaccine, not yet used routinely
3. RSV Vaccine: Delivered to the respiratory mucosa is under trial.
4. HIV Vaccine: Still there is no effective and safe vaccine.
5. Herpes Virus type 2 Vaccine: Still under trial
6. Malaria Vaccine: Still there is no established vaccine.
7. Anthrax Vaccine: Under trial because of fear of biological weapons.
8. Activax: Combined multivalent vaccine for traveler's diarrhea against Entero toxigenic E. Coli, Shigella & Campylobacter.

1.10   Child Abuse and Neglect

Child abuse is a spectrum of abusive actions (acts of commission), and/or neglect in child care (act of omission) that is detrimental to child's physical, emotional or psycho-social health resulting in morbidity or even death.

Any maltreatment of children or adolescents by their parents, guardians, or other caretakers is considered as child abuse. It is becoming a major health problem all over the world, with an estimation showing that 40,000,000 children aged 0 to 14 years suffer from abuse and neglects (WHO report on child abuse 1999). It is estimated that as many as one in 5,000 to one in 10,000 children under the age of five dies each year from the effect of physical violence (WHO report on child abuse 1997).

Classification:
- Child maltreatment: Neglect
- Physical abuse **(Non accidental injury)**
- Sexual abuse and
- Emotional abuse

Recognition of abuse is important especially in young children due to the risk of fatality. The duty of physician is to detect report and prevent child abuse.

The prevalence of abuse is unknown and under-reported due to many factors (variation in the definition, cultural effect, not reported by children or parents, failure of doctors and other professionals to diagnose it)

In Western countries laws require physicians to report suspected cases of child abuse or neglect to a local child protection agency. Laws also protect physicians from liability should their suspicions be unsubstantiated.

Definition
The definition of child abuse is variable from one culture to another but in general the following definitions can be used.

Neglect is failure to provide for child's basic needs. This may be:
- ❑ **Physical** (e.g., lack of appropriate supervision or physical care).
- ❑ **Educational** (e.g., failure to educate a child or attend to special education needs).
- ❑ **Emotional** (e.g., inattention to a child's emotional needs or exposure to domestic violence).

These situations do not always mean that a child is neglected. Sometimes cultural values, the standards of care in the community, and poverty may be contributing factors, indicating that the family is in need of information or assistance. When a family fails to use information and resources, and the child's needs continue to be unmet, then further child welfare professional intervention may be required.

Physical abuse (also known as non-accidental injury, NAI) is physical injury (ranging from minor bruises to severe fractures or intracranial trauma and deaths) as a result of punching, beating, kicking, biting, shaking, throwing, stabbing, chocking, hitting (with a hand, stick, strap, or other object), burning, or otherwise harming, such injury is considered abuse regardless of whether the caretaker intended to hurt the child or not.

Sexual abuse (Also refer to chapter15.2) This includes activities by a parent or caretaker such as fondling a child's genitals, penetration incest (within the family), rape, sodomy, indecent exposure, and commercial exploitation through prostitution or the production of pornographic materials. It is most often over looked.

Emotional abuse is any pattern of behavior that impairs a child's emotional development or sense of self-worth. This may include constant criticism, threats, or rejection, as well as withholding love, support, or guidance.

Munchausen's Syndrome by Proxy (fictitous illness): in this syndrome the care provider, invariably the mother simulates or fakes or induces a disease in a child in order to gain attention

Risk factors of child abuse
Although all the causes of child abuse and neglect are not known, a significant body of research has identified several risk factors and protective factors associated with child abuse (figure 1). Studies also have shown that when there are multiple risk factors present, the risk is greater.

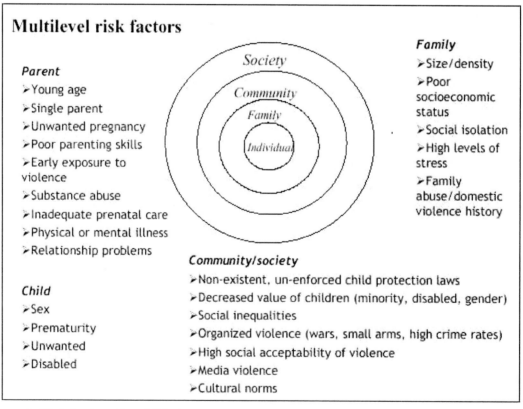

Figure 1. Risk factors for child abuse

Clinical characteristics of Non accidental injury:
- Delayed presentation.
- Unexplained injury/Explanation is offered but is implausible.

❏ Inconsistency. Change of story with time or by different people.
❏ Unusual parental reaction to injury (Under or over reaction).
❏ Repeated injury.
❏ Site/shape/type of injuries (buttocks lower back).
1. Bruising on head and face and lumbar region (often finger marks).
2. Small circular bruises (finger marks).
3. Bruising around wrists and ankles (swinging)
4. Bruising inside and behind pinna (blow with hand).
5. Ring of bruises (bite mark).
6. Two black eyes.
7. Torn frenulum of the tongue (blow or force feeding).
8. Small circular burns (cigarette burns).
9. Burns or scalds to feet and/or buttocks (with well defined line or splashes).
10. Fractured ribs (shaking).
11. Epiphyses torn off (swinging).
12. Subdural hematoma (shaking).
13. Retinal hemorrhages (shaking).
14. Multiple injuries and injuries of different ages.

Abnormal child behavior as a warning sign:
❏ Nervousness around adults.
❏ Aggression toward adults or other children.
❏ Inability to stay awake or to concentrate for extended periods.
❏ Sudden, dramatic changes in personality or activities.
❏ Acting out sexually or showing interest in sex that is not appropriate for his or her age.
❏ Frequent or unexplained bruises or injuries.
❏ Low self-esteem.
❏ Poor hygiene.

Pitfalls in diagnosis:
❏ Mongolian spots over the buttocks seen usually in colored races can be misinterpreted as bruises.
❏ Bruises from a bleeding disorder.
❏ Fracture from a bony disorder (Osteogenesis imperfecta).

Management
Ideally a full detailed history should be written in the file. All visible lesions should be photographed as evidence in court.

Investigations:
1. Skeletal survey (especially if the child is younger than 2 years).
2. Coagulation studies (to rule out bleeding diathesis).
3. Cranial CT scan (MRI might also be needed) in the case of badly injured infant even when the CNS examination is normal.
4. In the case of sexual abuse, swabs for sexually transmitted diseases, sperms should be sent. Child also should be screened for HIV and hepatitis B. pregnancy test for adolescent girls.
5. In the case of non organic failure to thrive prior to any extensive laboratory evaluation

the child should be admitted and given unlimited feeding of a diet appropriate for age for a minimum of 1 week. Gaining weight will confirm the diagnosis and no further investigations are needed.

6. When Munchausen's Syndrome by Proxy (factious illness) is suspected observation of the child and mother in the hospital with careful review of documents from other health services might be the only investigation needed.

Other investigations might be needed depending on the nature of injury.

In countries with child protection regulations a **case conference** will normally be called soon after admission to collect information and plan further management, which may be either of the following:

*   Appoint a key social worker to monitor the case and placing the child's name on the **register of "at risk" children**.
*   In a grievous injury, make recommendations to the police about prosecution
*   To place the child remove the child from the family to other caretakers

In more minor cases of injury where there is significant doubt about the diagnosis, careful recording of the history, findings and discussions with the parents is essential. The register of children at risk should be consulted. The general practitioner, and health visitor or school nurse should be consulted. A referral to social services might be thought appropriate.

In Oman until now there is no protocol to deal with such cases and the usual approach of depends on the severity of the abuse and care provider and institute resources. However, the care of the physical injuries, attending the psychological effect of the abuse, counseling parents about consequences of abuse and other options of disciplinary methods should be emphasized to help such children.

Consequences
Abused children possibly undergo substantial social, emotional, and environmental changes and disruptions during their development. There is evidence that abused and neglected children have significantly lower IQ scores.

Physically abused children also tend to suffer from serious psychological problems and are at greater risk of being involved in crime, self-inflicted or interpersonal violent actions. They also develop major depression, post-traumatic stress disorder, antisocial behavior, drug abuse-dependence, suicidal ideation, and suicidal tendencies.

Fatalities
Despite the efforts of the child protection system, child maltreatment fatalities remain a serious problem. Although untimely deaths of children due to illness and accidents have been closely monitored, deaths that result from physical assault or severe neglect can be more difficult to track. Research indicates very young children (ages 3 and younger) are the most frequent victims of child fatalities

Child abuse prevention:
Primary prevention involves identifying families at risk before any injury occurs. There may be a "cry for help" from the mother, such as frequent visits to the doctor for minor problems or complaints of excessive crying or difficult feeding. The mother may say that she thinks she will injure the child; this should always be taken seriously and steps taken to relieve

the crisis by admitting the child to hospital if necessary. Once recognized as a family at risk, additional support from health visitor or social worker may prevent the crisis leading to actual injury

Secondary prevention means identifying children who have been injured and taking steps to prevent further injury. Subsequent injury is likely to be more severe. Plans will normally be made at a case conference and may mean removing the child from home at least temporarily, but many children perhaps 35-45% can be reunited with their parents when situation improves. Child abuse can be prevented through the efforts to build on family strengths. This could be achieved through activities such as Parent education, Home visits, Parent support groups or Public education campaigns.

1.11   Common ambulatory Pediatric Problems

Enuresis

Definition:
Repeated voluntary or involuntary passage of urine into clothes or bed after a developmental age when bladder control should have been established (5 years).

Prevalence of enuresis

Age (years)	Male	Female
5	7%	3%
10	3%	2%
18	1%	Very rare

Classification:
1. **Primary (Developmental)** Child has never been dry (90% of all cases)
2. **Secondary (Regressive)** Child who has been dry for at least 6 months to 1 year begins to wet again. It occurs secondary to stress in the child's life and is typically transient and has a better prognosis compared to primary enuresis.

Another classification is:
1. **Nocturnal enuresis**: voiding urine while a sleep. (Strong genetic predisposition)
2. **Diurnal enuresis**: voiding urine while awake.
3. **Nocturnal/diurnal**: mix of the two types.

Patho-physiological factors:

Nocturnal enuresis
- Delayed cortical maturation of the mechanisms that allow voluntary control of the micturition.
- Sleep disorder: deep sleepers
- Reduced antidiuretic hormone production at night, resulting in an increased urine output.
- Genetic predisposition (positive family history of enuresis in siblings/parents)
- Psychological factors (as the case in secondary enuresis)
- Organic factors: UTI, obstructive Uropathy.
- Sleep apnea (with snoring) secondary to enlarged adenoids.

Diurnal enuresis
The most common cause is unstable bladder (uninhibited bladder, bladder spasm) other causes include: Infrequent voiding, detrusor-sphincter dyssynergia, cystitis, bladder outlet obstruction (posterior urethral valves), ectopic ureter, traumatic, constipation, behavioral.

History
Explore the type of enuresis.
- Severity (number of wet nights, amount of urine passed).
- The effect of environmental and psychosocial factors on the symptoms.
- Parental reaction to the events/child response.

Screening for contributing factors
- Fluid intake/urine output: diabetes insipidus, diabetes mellitus, chronic renal disease, may have a high obligatory urinary output and compulsive polydipsia.
- Snoring at night
- Urinary symptoms: Urgency, dysuria, dribbling (UTI)
- History of encopresis/constipation.

Examination
- Complete general examination (high BP and failure to thrive due to renal diseases)
- Examination of the genitalia (Epispadias, phimosis, abnormality in urethral opening).
- Abdominal examination (distended bladder)
- Neurological and spinal abnormalities (Spina bifida)

Investigations: To rule out organic causes
1. Urinary dipstick for (proteins, glucose, specific gravity, signs of UTI) to rule out diabetes insipidus, diabetes mellitus and UTI.
2. Urine microscopy/culture (looking for signs of UTI, glucosuria)
3. Urea and electrolyte (renal dysfunction)
4. Abdominal US for bladder/kidney abnormalities
5. X-ray lumbar spine for spina bifida

If there are abnormalities in the above investigations then invasive investigations to reach a diagnosis might be needed (e.g. voiding cystourethrogram, cystoscopy).

Treatment
To treat the cause If there is an organic problem. If there is no organic problem:
1. Reassure the parents that it is a self-limiting problem in most of the times
2. Parents should avoid punishment (verbal/physical)
3. Restriction of fluid intake in the evening and prior to sleep
4. Voiding before bed time
5. Waking the child a few hours after they go to sleep to void
6. Star chart (praising dry nights/rewards)
7. Conditioning therapy (use of bed wetting alarm)
8. Desmopressin (symptomatic treatment not curative)

The participation of the child in the treatment plan is very important (explain the problem and the management plan to the child not only the parents). The parents should be counseled fully regarding the problem and progression of it with special emphasis on the involuntary nature of the symptoms. Such steps usually remove any sense of guilt and allow the child to develop an optimistic perspective. It also allows the parents to provide maximum emotional support to the child and will reduce the struggle between them.

If the enuresis is severe enough to the degree of affecting the child's social, emotional, or cognitive development, therapy beyond reassurance and supportive counseling is indicated. However, both parents and child should be alerted to the potential for relapse and, thus, the need for a "second dose" of treatment.

Breath Holding Spells

Usually occurs in children 6 months to 5 years old (most of the cyanotic spells occurs between 12-18 months). They are due to autonomic nervous system dysregulation (involuntary and reflexive). They usually cause no harm. Child may use them in an attempt to control the parents to fulfill his demands.

They are triggered by injury (often trivial), anger, frustration and fear. Usually the attacks start by vigorous crying (expiratory phase) until the breath is held that may end up with loss of consciousness or termination of the attack due to muscle relaxation. However, some children might develop tonic/clonic convulsive movements thus causing confusion with epileptic attack. Epilepsy can be excluded by history and EEG (cyanosis occur during or after the attacks in epilepsy not before as in breath holding spells).

It is unlikely for a child to have more than one attack/day and it is not associated with increased predisposition to epilepsy.

Figure 1 Clinical sequence of spell.

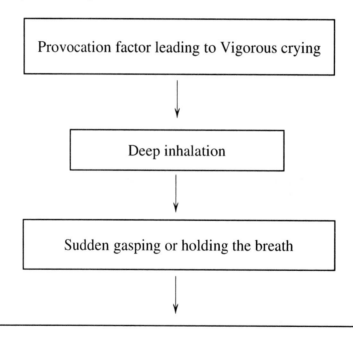

Pallid syncope (precipitated by fear or minor injury) differs from the cyanotic spell by the initial brief or silent cry. Children with these spells also have higher risk of syncopal attacks as adults (vasovagal response) such as fainting at the sight of blood or when injured.

Management
- There is no effective medical therapy
- Iron deficiency anemia has been associated with the spells and treating it can reduce the spells in these children.
- Counseling the parents and supporting them to cope with the problem/behavior modification is very important. Parent should not give in to unreasonable demands or attention seeking behavior. Child should be left alone if behaving unreasonably
- Neurological and psychological assessment of the child might be needed to rule out organic problems and assurance to the parents.

Nappy rash

Is a general term describing inflammatory skin conditions affecting the diaper area.

Classification:

1. Rashes directly or indirectly caused by diapers. This includes dermatoses, such as **Irritant contact dermatitis, Candidal diaper dermatitis**

2. Rashes that appear elsewhere but can be exaggerated in the groin area due to the irritating effects of wearing a diaper. This category includes **Atopic dermatitis, Seborrheic dermatitis and Psoriasis.**

3. Rashes that appear in the diaper area irrespective of diaper use. This category includes rashes associated with **Bullous impetigo, Langerhans cell histiocytosis, acrodermatitis enteropathica (zinc deficiency), cong. syphilis, scabies, and HIV.**

Pathophysiology:

Contact / irritant or ammoniacal nappy rash likely result from a combination of factors that begin with prolonged exposure to moisture and the contents of the diaper i.e. urine and feces, the enteric bacteria in stool produce urease enzyme that degrade urea in urine to produce ammonia which increases alkalinity which in turn activate lipase and proteases to damage the skin by irritant effect. The infrequent diaper changes, improper cleansing and drying of the diaper area, failure to apply topical preparations to protect the skin and Diarrhea aggravate this phenomenon.

It is not unusual for every child to have at least 1 episode of diaper rash by the time he or she is toilet-trained. The incidence is lower among breastfed infants perhaps due to the less acidic nature of their urine and stool. Diaper rashes can start in the neonatal period as soon as the child begins to wear diapers and peaks in those aged 7-12 months, then decreases with age. It stops being a problem once the child is toilet trained, usually around 2 years of age.

Candida is a common cause of secondary infection. Other possible sources of secondary infection include species of *Staphylococcus, Streptococcus,* and enteric anaerobes (*Bacteroides* and *Peptostreptococcus* species).

Diagnosis

Diagnosis of diaper rash is based largely on the physical examination. A careful history, however, could elicit clues that aid in narrowing the differential diagnosis. Important points to obtain on history include: Onset, duration, and change in the nature of the rash, Presence of rashes outside the diaper area, Associated scratching or crying, Contact with infants with a similar rash, recent illness, diarrhea, or antibiotic use. Assessment of diapering practices (e.g. change frequency, type of diapers used, creams or ointments applied, methods used to clean the diaper area).

Mild forms consist of shiny erythema with or without scale, Margins are not always evident. Moderate cases have areas of papules, vesicles, and small superficial erosions. It can progress to well-demarcated ulcerated nodules that measure a centimeter or more in diameter. It is found on the prominent parts of the buttocks, medial thighs, mons pubis, and scrotum. Skin folds are spared or involved last.

Intertrigo occurs when wet skin, which is more fragile and has a higher coefficient of friction, becomes damaged from maceration and chafing. This occurs in skin creases where skin surfaces are in apposition. It is characterized by slight to severe erythema in the inguinal, intergluteal area or inguinal folds. Pustules or erosions are not present.

Candidal diaper dermatitis

Once the skin is compromised, secondary infection by *Candida Albicans* is common. Between 40-75% of diaper rashes that last for more than 3 days are colonized with *Candida Albicans*. It is Painful with distinctive clusters of erythematous papules and pustules, which later coalesce into a beefy red confluent rash with sharp borders. **Satellite lesions** are frequently found beyond these borders. Skin folds are commonly involved due to proliferation of Candida in warm and moist spaces. The oropharynx should be inspected for the associated white plaques of thrush.

Other Differential diagnosis:

1. Atopic dermatitis
Pruritic lesions, Associated with current or previous flares of rash on the face and extensor limb surfaces

2. Seborrheic dermatitis
Usually occurs in infants aged 2 weeks to 3 months, Consists of an Asymptomatic, well-demarcated erythematous patches or plaques with an occasional *greasy yellow scaly eruption* over the face, retro auricular regions, axilla, and presternal areas. In the groin area, the skin creases show more severe involvement. Crusty deposits of scales over the scalp is called **Cradle Cap**

3. Acrodermatitis enteropathica
Erythematous, well-demarcated, scaly plaques and erosions associated with diarrhea, hair loss, and erosive perioral dermatitis. Patient may have a predisposition for malabsorption (i.e., cystic fibrosis) or malnutrition.

Treatment:
Irritant contact dermatitis and intertrigo often can be treated non-medically through frequent changes in diapers. Skin in the diaper area should be kept as dry as possible. Exposing the skin under the diaper to open air and avoiding tight-fitting diapers and excessive scrubbing is quite helpful in healing.

The use of barrier creams, such as zinc oxide paste or petroleum jelly, is recommended to minimize urine and fecal contact with the skin. Other useful creams include vitamin A & D ointment and Burrow solution. For the typical irritant dermatitis or intertrigo, a Non fluorinated, low-potency corticosteroid ointment or cream (i.e., 1% hydrocortisone) can be prescribed for no longer than 2 weeks. The ointment or cream should be applied to the affected area 4 times daily with diaper changes. Parent should be advised to avoid fixed combination medications containing potent steroids as they can cause skin atrophy, striae, adrenal suppression, and Cushing syndrome on prolonged and indiscriminate use, care should be taken to warn mother about these dangers as some times mothers may purchase them without prescription.

If Candidal infection is suspected, topical ointments or creams, such as nystatin, clotrimazole, miconazole, or ketoconazole can be applied to the rash with every diaper change. If oral thrush or perianal candidiasis is present or if repeated bouts of Candidal dermatitis have occurred, oral nystatin should also be prescribed.

For mild bacterial infections, a topical antibiotic ointment (i.e., bacitracin) should be prescribed. More severe infections caused by gram-positive organisms and anaerobes can be treated with a broad-spectrum oral antibiotic.

Prognosis:
- Most cases completely resolve and subsequently prevented by counseling mothers toward diaper hygiene.
- The time to resolution is typically a few days for uncomplicated irritant dermatitis; Candidal infections may last a few days after treatment is begun.
- At least one half of the cases of atopic dermatitis resolve by the third year of life.

Scabies

Scabies is caused by mite parasites called *Sarcoptes scabiei* that burrow under the skin causing intense itching 6-8 weeks after they have initially affected the skin. It is highly contagious infestation.

Life cycle:
The mite remains viable for 2-5 days on inanimate objects; therefore, transmission through fomites, such as infected bedding or clothing, is possible, but less likely. The female mite burrows into the epidermis of the host using her jaws and front legs, where she lays up to 3 eggs per day for the duration of her 30- to 60-day lifetime. Affected host harbors approximately 11 adult female mites during a typical infestation. The eggs hatch in 3-4 days. The larvae leave the burrow to mature on the skin. Fewer than 10% of the eggs laid result in mature mites.

Clinical presentation:
Tiny red raised papules are often found on the palms and soles in infants and children. Other common locations are armpits, face, and waist. Secondary lesions resulting from the excessive scratching includes excoriations and post-inflammatory Hyperpigmentation and

pyoderma. The itching (usually worse at night) is part of a delayed type IV hypersensitivity reaction of the human body to the waste products deposited by the mite under the skin. Usually itching spares the head and neck but can be localized anywhere else on the body. However, in infants and young children, the lesions are localized to the face, neck, trunk, palms, and soles. Sometimes scabies can cause scaling looking like eczema. It is often treated with steroids, which then can alter its appearance and is then more difficult to diagnose.

Diagnosis:
Confirmed by curettage of a burrow followed by KOH microscopy of the arthropod, its scat or eggs. This technique is often unyielding leaving clinical judgment is the best diagnostic test. Inquiry as to the source of infection can be an important clinical correlate. Such personal contacts should be evaluated and treated for scabies to avoid re-infection.
Elevated immunoglobulin E and eosinophilia may be demonstrated in some patients with scabies. Defective immune function, especially in individuals with HIV disease, may be associated with hyperkeratotic scabies.

Treatment: Treat with a chemical scabicide and symptomatic relief for pruritus by antihistamines.
Antibiotics may be needed for treatment of secondary infections. For crusted scabies, crust and scale removal is necessary for scabicide penetration. All family members and close contacts must receive treatment simultaneously. Instruct patients to wash bed linens, clothing, and towels in warm water following the completion of scabicidal treatment.

Kwell lotion given twice daily for 3 days, repeated weekly for 3 weeks, **Eurax** cream or lotion (Geigy) twice a day, and the old-fashioned remedy of 10% sulfur ointment applied at night for four nights in a row and washing it off in the morning are effective. The best treatment is **benzyl benzoate**, used as 25% emulsion applied from the neck down (Particular attention should be paid to body folds) after a hot bath while the skin is still damp, and then left on, is effective if repeated for three nights after which the bedding clothing is removed and cleaned in hot water. Treatment should be repeated a week later.

Permethrin, a crysanthenum derivative applied neck down, left overnight and repeated in a week is sufficient when combined with hot water laundry of linen. Permethrin have no neurotoxicity.

Neonates or pregnant women should only be treated if the benefit exceeds the risk and if the diagnosis is confirmed by skin scraping.

Common Helminthic Infestations

1. Ascariasis (Ascaris lumbricoides)

It is the most prevalent human helminthiasis in the world.
Life cycle of ascaris lumbricoides (From CDC Web site):

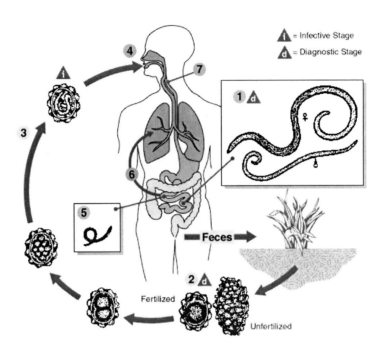

Adult worms live in the lumen of the small intestine. A female may produce up to 240,000 eggs per day, which are excreted with the feces. Fertile eggs embryonate and become infective after 18 days to several weeks, depending on the environmental conditions (optimum: moist, warm and shaded soil etc). After infective eggs are swallowed, the larvae hatch, invade the intestinal mucosa, and are carried via the portal, then systemic circulation to the lungs. The larvae mature further in the lungs (10-14 days), penetrate the alveolar walls, ascend the bronchial tree to the throat, and are swallowed. Upon reaching the small intestine, they develop into adult worms. Between 2 and 3 months are required from ingestion of the infective eggs to oviposition by the adult female. Adult worms can live for 1 to 2 years. (DPDx, the CDC Parasitology Website)

Clinical manifestations: Depends on the intensity of infection and the organs involved. Most individuals have no symptoms or signs.

> **Pulmonary disease:** transient respiratory symptoms such as cough and dyspnea, pulmonary infiltrates, and blood eosinophilia. Larvae may be observed in the sputum.
> **Intestinal manifestations:** vague abdominal pain, acute bowel obstruction (vomiting, abdominal distention, cramps).
> **Biliary and pancreatic disease:** cholecystitis or pancreatitis

Diagnosis: Fecal examination to detect excreted eggs.

Treatment: Albendazole (400 mg oral dose once), mebandazole (100 mg BD for 3 days).

Piperazine citrate (150 mg/Kg PO initially, followed by six doses of 65 mg/Kg at 12-hr intervals PO) is the treatment of choice for intestinal or biliary obstruction and is administered as syrup through a nasogastric tube. There is no effective treatment for the pulmonary phase of the infection.

Prevention: Anthelminthic chemotherapy programs can be implemented to prevent the disease. Improving sanitary conditions and sewage facilities, discontinuing the practice of using human feces as fertilizer, and health education.

2. Enterobiasis (Enterobius vermicularis) or Pin Worms

Pinworms typically inhabit the caecum, appendix, and adjacent areas of the ileum and ascending colon.
Life cycle of Enterobius vermicularis (From CDC web site):

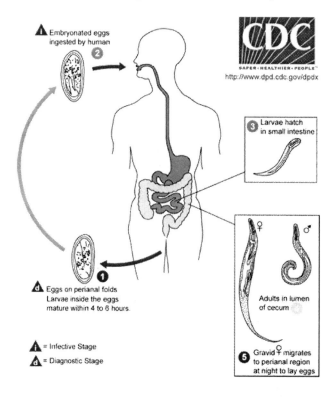

Eggs are deposited on perianal folds. Self-infestation occurs by transferring infective eggs to the mouth with ones own hands after scratching the perianal area. Person-to-person transmission can also occur through contaminated clothes or bed linens. Small number of eggs may become airborne and inhaled. Following ingestion of infective eggs, the larvae hatch in the small intestine and the adult worms establish themselves in the colon. The time interval from ingestion of infective eggs to oviposition by the adult females is about one month. The life span of the adult worms is about two months. Gravid females migrate nocturnally outside the anus and oviposit while crawling on the skin of the perianal area. The larvae contained inside the eggs develop (become infective) in 4 to 6 hours under optimal conditions. Retro infection or migration of newly hatched larvae from the anal skin back into the rectum may sometimes occur.

Clinical manifestations: This infection rarely causes serious medical problems. The most common complaints include itching and restless sleep secondary to nocturnal perianal or perineal pruritus. Rarely perianal granulomas containing live or dead worms or eggs develop that may require surgical excision. Aberrant migration occasionally may lead to appendicitis, chronic salpingitis, peritonitis, hepatitis, and GI ulcerations.

Diagnosis: history of nocturnal perianal pruritus strongly suggests the infection. Definitive diagnosis requires identification of parasite eggs or worms on microscopic examination of adhesive cellophane tape pressed against the perianal region early in the morning. Routine stool samples rarely demonstrate Enterobius ova.

Treatment: anthelminthic drugs should be administered to patient and family members. Use *Mebandazole* 100 mg stat, repeat same dose after 2 weeks

Prevention: repeated treatment every 3-4 months may be required in circumstances with repeated exposure, such as with institutionalized children. Although personal cleanliness with trimming of nails and protective clothing to avoid anal itching at night. There is no evidence that it has a role in the control or prevention of Enterobiasis.

3. Schistosomiasis

Life cycle of Schistosoma (From CDC Web site):

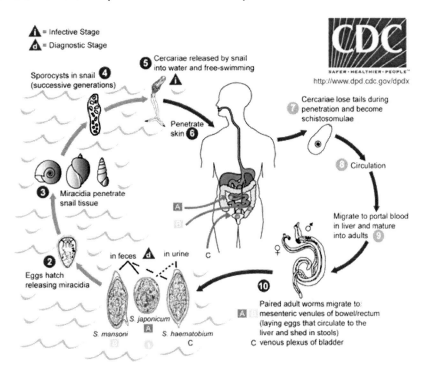

Eggs are eliminated with feces or urine. Under optimal conditions the eggs hatch and release miracidia, which swim and penetrate specific snail intermediate hosts. The life cycle in the snail include 2 generations of sporocysts and the production of cercariae. Upon release from the snail, the infective cercariae swim, penetrate the skin of the human host, and shed their forked tail, becoming schistosomulae. The schistosomulae migrate through several tissues and stages to their residence in the veins. Adult worms in humans reside in the mesenteric venules in various locations (as described above). The females deposit eggs in the small venules of the portal and perivesical systems. The eggs are moved progressively toward the lumen of the intestine (S. mansoni and S. japonicum) and of the bladder and ureters (S. haematobium), and are excreted out with feces or urine respectively.

Adult worms migrate to specific anatomic site that is characteristic of each schistosome species:

1. **Perivesical and periureteral venous plexus in S. haematobium**
2. **Inferior mesenteric veins in S. mansoni, and**
3. **Superior mesenteric veins in S. japonicum.**

The early manifestations of the disease are immunologically mediated (papular pruritic rash, Katayama fever and granuloma formation)

Pathology of *S. mansoni* and *S. japonicum* schistosomiasis includes: Katayama fever, hepatic perisinusoidal granulomas, Symmers' pipe stem periportal fibrosis, portal hypertension, and occasional embolic egg granulomas in brain or spinal cord. Pathology of *S. haematobium* includes: hematuria, scarring, calcification, squamous cell carcinoma, and occasional embolic egg granulomas in brain or spinal cord. Human contact with infested river water is thus necessary for infection by schistosomes. Various animals, such as dogs, cats, rodents, pigs, horse and goats, serve as reservoirs for *S. japonicum*, and dogs for *S. mekongi*.

Clinical manifestations:

Schistosomal dermatitis/swimmer's itch: popular pruritic rash which is more pronounced in previously exposed individuals and is characterized by edema and massive cellular infiltrates in the dermis and epidermis.

Katayama fever: serum sickness-like syndrome manifested by the acute onset of fever, chills, sweating, lymphadenopathy, Hepato-splenomegaly, and eosinophilia.

Chronic Schistosomiasis haematobia: Causes urinary symptoms like frequency, dysuria and hematuria, urine examination shows erythrocytes, parasite eggs, and occasional leukocytes. The terminal stage of the disease is associated with chronic renal failure, secondary infections, and cancer of the bladder.

Intestinal disease: colicky abdominal pain, bloody diarrhea, Hepato-splenomegaly, portal hypertension, Ascites, and Hematemesis. Liver disease is due to granuloma formation and subsequent fibrosis; Hepatic function may be preserved for a long time.

Lung disease: pulmonary hypertension and core pulmonale.

Brain disease: localized brain lesions and transverse myelitis.

Diagnosis: eggs are found in the excreta of infected individuals.

Treatment: praziquantel (40 mg/Kg/24 hr).

Prevention: reducing the parasite load in the population by using chemotherapeutic agents. Improving sanitation and focal application of molluscacides.

Squint (strabismus)

Squint is a misalignment of the two eyes so that they are not looking in the same direction. It is one of the most common eye problems encountered in children affecting approximately 4% of all children younger than 6 years.

It is important to remember that the eyes of a newborn are rarely aligned at birth. Most establish alignment at 3-4 weeks of age. Therefore squint in any child who is more than six weeks old must be taken seriously and be evaluated by an ophthalmologist.

Types of Squint:

Paralytic squint: Means one of the six extra ocular muscles is weak or paralyzed and the affected eye may turn in/out/up/down depending on the muscle involved i.e. the eye movement is restricted in the direction of the action of the weak muscle. This can be congenital or caused by direct trauma to the muscle e.g. injury during forceps delivery or any other injury. It may also be caused by certain nerve palsies, which in turn may be caused by peripheral neuritis or diseases of the CNS, e.g. meningitis, encephalitis etc. Treatment of paralytic squint depends on the cause and many time paralytic squints may not be completely cured. In such cases spectacles with prisms are prescribed.

Non-Paralytic Squint: A loss of coordination between the muscles of the two eyes leads to misalignment. This misalignment may be the same in all direction of gaze, or in some conditions the misalignment may be more in one direction of gaze. The exact cause of non-paralytic squint is not really known.

Latent Squint: In this condition eye remains straight in normal gaze but gets squinted on strain and tiredness. Squint is seen on covering one eye - the covered eye becomes squinted. Actually the imbalance in this case is not so much to cause obvious squint. Eye muscles try to maintain binocular vision. This causes strain and headache. Mostly it is due to refractive error and correction may give relief from headache

Extra ocular eye muscles:

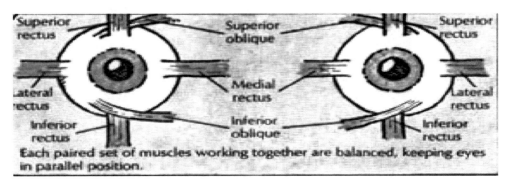

Each paired set of muscles working together are balanced, keeping eyes in parallel position.

Sometimes a refractive error hypermetropia (long sight) may lead to inward deviation of the eye. Poor vision in an eye because of some other eye disease like cataract, etc. may also cause the eye to deviate. Therefore it is important in all the cases of squint, especially in children, to have a thorough eye checkup to rule out any other cause of loss of vision. When the eyes are not aligned properly two different images will reach the brain leading to confusion and may have either of the following effects:
- Suppress one image (if prolonged, the squinting eye becomes amblyopic).
- Development of an abnormal head posture.

Remember that children after six month's of age would never grow out of squint. Any delay in treatment may decrease the chances of getting a good alignment and vision and squint can also have a negative effect on a child's self-confidence.

Clinical examination

- **Corneal light reflex test** (Normally light reflux should fall on identical point on two cornea, if not, the squint is likely) is the most rapid and easily performed diagnostic tests for strabismus.
- **Cover tests** for strabismus require a child's attention and cooperation, good eye movement capability, and reasonably good vision in each eye.
- In a child with strabismus assessment of **visual acuity** is mandatory.
- **CNS examination** in case of paralytic Squint.

Cover-uncover test:

Child looks at an object in the distance, preferably 6 m away, the examiner covers one eye and watches for movement of the uncovered eye. If no movement occurs, then there is no apparent misalignment of that eye. The test should be repeated for the other eye

Alternate cover test:

Examiner rapidly covers and uncovers each eye, shifting back and forth from one eye to another. If the child has any ocular deviation, the eye rapidly moves as the cover is shifted to the other eye.

Both of the tests should be performed at both distance and near fixation, with and without glasses.

Management:

The aims of treatment of squint in order of importance are:
- To preserve or restore vision
- Straighten the eyes
- Restore binocular vision

First: correct refractive error. (Glasses)

Second: eyes are checked for presence of amblyopia. It is important to treat it before the surgery for squint. Generally speaking, the younger the age at which amblyopia is treated; better is the chance of vision recovery

Third: squint is treated by surgery of either one or both eyes. The surgery involves weakening or strengthening of the relevant muscles to restore balance and coordination.

Dental caries

Dental caries is one of the most common of all disorders, second only to common cold. It usually occurs in children and young adults. It is the most important cause of tooth loss in younger people. The development of dental caries depends on the relationship between the tooth surface, dietary carbohydrates and oral bacteria (mutans type streptococci, lactobacilli). Organic acids produced by bacterial fermentation of dietary carbohydrates reduce the pH of dental plaque adjacent to the tooth to a point at which demineralization and decay occurs.

Dental caries is common among children due to following factors:

        Nursing bottle of a sweetened drink

        Sticky candies or frequent carbohydrate consumption

        Not brushing teeth prior to night sleep

It is important to examine the oral cavity of all children and to look for dental caries for counseling (child and parents) about dental care, referral to dentist at an early stage to prevent complications and avoid further caries in adulthood.

Where to look for dental caries:
- In the pits and fissures
- Contact surfaces between the teeth

Symptoms
Toothache -- particularly after sweet, hot, or cold foods and drinks
Visible pits or holes in the teeth

Signs and tests
Most cavities are discovered in the early stages during routine checkups. The surface of the tooth may be soft when probed with a sharp instrument. Pain may not be present until the advanced stages of tooth decay. Dental x-rays may show some cavities before they are visible to the eye.

Complications
1. Destruction of the tooth/ discomfort or pain /tooth sensitivity
2. Pulpitis
3. Dental abscess
4. Peri-apical abscess
5. Facial space infection
6. Disruption of normal development of the successor permanent tooth
7. Sepsis

Prevention of dental caries
- Optimizing the fluoride content of communal water supplies
- Oral hygiene: This consists of regular professional cleaning of teeth (every 6 months), brushing at least twice a day, and flossing at least daily. Chewy, sticky foods (such as dried fruit or candy) are best if eaten as part of a meal rather than as a snack. If possible, brush the teeth or rinse the mouth with water after eating food. Minimize snacking, which creates a constant supply of acid in the mouth. Avoid constant sipping of sugary drinks or frequent sucking on candy and mints. Avoid milk bottle during sleep. Brush before sleep and don't eat anything after brushing. Use good fluoride toothpaste. Learn to brush as soon as teeth erupt
- Decreasing the frequency of sugar ingestion (nursing bottle of a sweetened beverage and bedtime bottle should also be discouraged)
- Plastic dental sealants (thin plastic-like coating applied to the chewing surfaces of the molars) are effective in preventing the pit and fissure caries.
- Identification of high-risk patients with early referral to dentists

Treatment
Destroyed tooth structure does not regenerate. However, the progression of cavities can be stopped. The goal is to preserve the tooth and prevent complications. In filling teeth, the decayed material is removed (by drilling) and replaced with a restorative material such as silver alloy, gold, porcelain, or composite resin.

- Silver amalgam or plastic restorations and crowns
- Partial removal of the pulp (pulpotomy)
- Complete removal of the pulp (pulpectomy)
- Tooth extraction (with or without space maintainer)
- Oral antibiotics depending on the severity of infection (penicillin, clindamycin, erythromycin)
- Oral analgesics

Developmental Dysplasia of the Hip (DDH)
(Congenital dislocation of the hip joint)

Ortolani, an Italian pediatrician in the early 1900s, evaluated, diagnosed and first began treating hip dysplasia. At birth the hips are rarely dislocated but dislocation tends to occur after delivery this is why now a day it is called "DDH." And not CDH

Classification: 2 major groups:
1. Typical DDH: occurs in infant with normal neurological system (common form)
2. Teratologic: usually there is an underlying neuromuscular disease (Myelodysplasia or arthrogryposis multiplex congenital) and the dislocation occur in utero.

The definition of DDH is not universally agreed upon. It is simply an abnormal growth of the hip joint affecting various structures such as the acetabulum, proximal femur, labrum, capsule, and other soft tissues. It may occur at any time, from conception to skeletal maturity. More specific terms are often used to better describe the condition:
- Subluxation is incomplete contact between femoral head and acetabulum.
- Dislocation is complete loss of contact between articular surface of the femoral head and acetabulum.
- Instability is the tendency to subluxate or dislocate with passive manipulation.
- Teratologic dislocation is antenatal dislocation of the hip.

The overall frequency is 1 per 1000 individuals, although it is believed that the instance of hip instability during newborn examinations is as high as 1 case per 60 newborns, more than 60% become stable by one week of age and 88% became stable by age 2 months, leaving only 12% (of the 1 in 60 newborns, or 0.2%) with residual hip instability.

Etiology:
The etiology of typical DDH is multifactorial: generalized ligamentous laxity, maternal estrogens and other hormones associated with pelvic relaxation, intrauterine positioning female sex, first-born child, and breech positioning are all associated with an increased prevalence of DDH.
An underlying genetic disposition also appears to exist in that a 10-fold increase in the frequency of hip dysplasia occurs in children whose parents had DDH.

Oligohydramnios: This is believed to be due to the common intrauterine position of the left hip against the mother's sacrum, forcing it into an adducted position. Children in cultures in which the mother swaddles the baby, forcing the hips to be adducted, also have similar effect

Hip dysplasia can be associated with underlying neuromuscular disorders, such as cerebral palsy, myelomeningocele, arthrogryposis, and Larsen syndrome, although these are not usually considered DDH.

Clinical features:
Early clinical manifestations of DDH is identified during routine examination of the newborn. The classic examination finding is revealed with the **Ortolani maneuver** (a test to reduce a dislocated hip); a palpable "clunk" is felt when the hip is reduced back into the acetabulum from adducted position. It is most likely to be positive below 1-2 month of age. After 2 months a manual reduction usually not possible because of the development of soft tissue contractors.

To perform this maneuver correctly, the patient must be relaxed. Only one hip is examined at a time. The examiner's thumb placed over the patient's inner thigh, and the index finger is placed over the greater trochanter. The hip is abducted, with gentle pressure over the greater trochanter. A clunk sound, similar to turning a light switch on or off, is felt when the dislocated hip is reduced into acetabulum by abduction. This should be performed gently, such that the fingertips do not blanch.

Barlow' sign is a provocation test to first dislocate an unstable hip by putting backward pressure in the adducted position thus encouraging the hip to dislocate out of acetabulum with a "Clunk" if it was dislocatable.

Late clinical signs: After age 3-6 months the hip, if dislocated, is often dislocated in a fixed position. The **Galeazzi sign** is a classic sign for unilateral hip dislocation. This is performed with the patient lying supine and the hips and knees flexed. Examination should demonstrate that one leg appears shorter than the other. Additional physical examination findings for late dislocation include asymmetry of the gluteal thigh or labral skin folds, decreased abduction on the affected side, standing or walking with external rotation, and leg length inequality, limping, waddling, increased lumbar lordosis, toe walking etc. Bilateral dislocation of the hip, especially at a later age, can be quite difficult to diagnose. This often manifests as a waddling gait with hyper-lordosis. Careful examination is needed, and a high level of suspicion is important. Once the diagnosis is made, the patient should be examined to be sure he or she has no underlying medical or neuromuscular disorder.

Radiographic evaluation: in neonates and infants hip stability as well as acetabular development may be assessed accurately by **dynamic ultrasonography**. In older infant **X-Ray of the pelvis** can be used to determine the relationship of femoral head to the acetabulum. **CT and MRI** scans may be beneficial in complicated cases.

Treatment depends on age of the patient:
- Birth: maintenance of the hip in the position of flexion and abduction for 1-2 months is usually sufficient (using bracing or **double or triple nappies**)
- 1-6 months: with instability upon examination are treated with a form of bracing (**Pavlik harness**). If this method is not successful (less than 20% of the cases) then the child should be treated as in the next age group.
- 6-18 months: Closed reduction, often with traction prior to the reduction.
- 18 months-8 years or with failure of the previous treatment needs: open reduction

Complications of treatment:
1. Avascular necrosis of the capital femoral epiphysis.
2. Re-dislocation
3. Residual subluxation

Prognosis:
Overall, the prognosis for children treated for hip dysplasia is very good, especially if the dysplasia is managed with closed treatment. If closed treatment is unsuccessful and open reduction is needed, the outcome is less favorable, although short-term outcome appears to be satisfactory. If secondary procedures are needed to obtain reduction, then the overall outcome is significantly worse.

1.12 Child with Chronic Arthritis

Chronic arthritis in children describes a group of disorders, mostly caused by collagen vascular or rheumatic disease.
Incidence 1 per 10,000 and prevalence 1 per 1000 children

Definition:
Chronic arthritis in children is defined as arthritis of more than six weeks duration occurring before 16 yrs of age.

Arthritis is defined by presence of joint swelling or effusion or presence of 2 or more of following three criteria:
- Increased heat or redness
- Joint pain with limitation of range of movement;
- Tenderness on direct palpation.

Juvenile rheumatoid arthritis is one of the most common rheumatic diseases in children. It's cause is unknown but presumed to be due to an abnormal host immunologic response to multiple environmental factors like viruses (parvovirus B19, Rubella, EB virus), bacteria, mycobacterium or autoimmune process

ACR (American College of Rheumatology) classification of Juvenile Rheumatoid Arthritis: Based on the disease presentation within the first 6 months of illness, the disease is divided into 3 main types:
- Pauciarticular / Oligoarticular JRA
- Polyarticular JRA
- Systemic JRA

Characteristic features:

Characteristics	Polyarthritis	Oligoarthritis	Systemic
Percent of cases	30	60	10
Number of joints	> 4	<4	Variable
Type of joints	Large and small (Hands)	Large	Large May present as PUO +/- rash
Sex ratio (F:M)	3:1	5:1	1:1
Age at onset	Throughout childhood;	Throughout childhood; Peak 1-2 yrs	Throughout childhood; No peak age
Chronic Uveitis	5%	5-15%	Rare
Rheumatoid Factor	10%	Rare	Rare
Antinuclear Antibody (ANA)	40-50%	70-80%	10%

Complications	Joint damage esp. in RF positive cases	Chronic eye involvement and joint damage	Amyloidosis Failure to thrive Serositis
Prognosis	Guarded – moderate	Excellent	Moderate – poor

Etiology of chronic arthritis in children:

1. Trauma

2. Infections / Reactive arthritis :
  Septic arthritis
  Tuberculosis
  Viral – varicella, coxsackie, EBV, Herpes simplex, rubella, Hep B
  Acute rheumatic fever
  Post streptococcal arthritis
  Arthritis secondary to enteric pathogens
  Transient synovitis of the hips
  Lyme disease

4. Immune arthritis:
  Connective tissue disease
  Serum sickness
  Henoch Schonlein Purpura
  Inflammatory Bowel Disease
  Sarcoidosis

3. Malignancy : Leukemia, Lymphoma, neuroblastoma
  Ostoesarcoma, Ewing's

5. Non-Inflammatory arthritis:
  Storage – Mucopolysaccharidoses, Gaucher and Farber disease
  Growing pain
  Benign hypermobility syndrome
  Legg calve perthe's disease
  Slipped capital femoral epiphysis
  Synovial hemangioma
  Hemophilia

Clinical evaluation:

History: Note following points in history
  Onset: insidious or abrupt?
  Proceeding viral illness? (Possibility of reactive arthritis)
  Trauma?

Chronological course of disease?
Pattern of joint involvement?
Joint swelling, redness or warmth?
Morning stiffness?
Limping? Degree of disability due to pain at home or school?
Fever?
Rashes?
Contact with TB?
GI symptoms? (Possibility of Inflammatory Bowel Disease)
Very severe joint pain? (Possibility of infection or malignancy)
Visual complaints?
Complete review of systems to exclude other differential diagnosis

Physical Examination:

Growth,
Vital signs, note the pattern of fever
General: Rashes (evanescent, psoriasis)
Nail changes
Generalized lymphadenopathy
Eyes: Redness, discharge, Synechia, cataract (sequalae of uveitis)
Cardiorespiratory: evidence of serositis
Abdominal: Hepatosplenomegaly
Posture, stance, gait
Identify all affected joints: Note
Tenderness
Swelling/ effusion, redness, warmth
Range limitation (active/passive)
Deformity
Muscles strength, bulk/atrophy, deep tendon reflexes

Investigations:

Investigations are used to support the diagnosis of JRA, help monitor disease activity and drug toxicity.

CBC
ESR, CRP
LFT
RFT
ANA: positive in 25% JRA who have increased risk of uveitis.
RF: only positive in 5-10% JRA
Synovial joint fluid aspirates – help distinguish infective arthritis

Imaging:

X-ray findings include: soft tissue swelling, periarticular osteopenia, joint space narrowing, erosions, periosteal new bone formation, subluxation and ankylosis.

MRI with gadolinium to enhance synovitis, early detection of cartilage loss, as well as other intra-articular pathology.

Management:

Necessitates a multidisciplinary approach designed to address progression of joint disease as well as child's functional, nutritional as well as emotional well-being. The goals are to relieve the pain, reduce the complications, increase the mobility, and encourage the normal living as much as possible.

Medical treatment:

First line: NSAID's: Naproxen, Ibuprofen, Indomethacin

Second line: Methoteraxate, lefluonomide, Sulfasalzine, Cyclosporin, Immunoglobulins, Gold

Biologic agents: Infliximab, Etanercept, Anakinra

Physical and Occupational therapy:

Objective is to:

Minimize pain: Heat/cold therapy

Maintain and restore function: splints, exercises

Prevent deformity and disability: Balanced physical activity

Orthopedic surgery:

Although procedures like soft tissue releases, tendon lengthening, synovectomies and reconstructive surgery with joint replacement do not alter the course of the disease but they could improve function and relieve pain.

1.13   Henoch-Schonlein Purpura (HSP)

HSP is an acute Ig A (Immunoglobulin-A) mediated vasculitis that affects primarily children (peak 3-10 years). It is twice more common in males. In one half to two thirds of children, an upper respiratory tract infection precedes the clinical onset by 1-3 weeks.

Clinical Manifestations:

The dominant clinical manifestations of HSP include:

Cutaneous rash

Arthritis

Abdominal visceral pain, Malena

Nephritis

Skin lesions are characteristic of disease and present in 100% cases. Typically, the rash is present on the posterior aspects of legs and buttocks accentuated at pressure areas. Classic lesions consist of urticarial wheals, erythematous maculopapules and larger, palpable ecchymosis-like lesions. The purpuric areas evolve from red to purple, become rust-colored with a brownish hue before fading.

Abdominal pain occurs in up to 65% of cases. Most common complaint is colicky abdominal pain, which may be severe and associated with vomiting. Stools may show gross or occult blood; hematemesis may also occur. Severe cases may proceed to Intussusception, hemorrhage and shock.

Joint symptoms occur in 70 percent of cases, affecting mainly large joints, are transient and leave no permanent deformity. Joint symptoms may precede the rash in 25 % cases

Renal disease is the most serious complication and occurs in up to 50% of older children and in 25% of younger children. 1% cases progress to end-stage renal disease. Risk factors for renal disease include persistence rash, presence of proteinuria and/or hematuria leading to nephrotic or nephritic syndrome.

Other rare systemic manifestations: may include hepatosplenomegaly, myocardial infarction, pulmonary hemorrhage and pleural effusion. Central nervous system involvement may manifest as behavioral changes, seizures, headache and focal deficit. Peripheral nerves may be involved leading to mononeuropathies. Genital involvement such as scrotal swelling and testicular torsion has also been reported.

Treatment and prognosis:

There is no specific treatment. Bed rest and supportive care, such as assuring adequate hydration are helpful. Nonsteroidal anti-inflammatory drugs can relieve joint and soft tissue discomfort. Corticosteroids have dramatic role in relief of patients with severe abdominal pain. However, corticosteroids are not recommended for treatment of rash, joint pain or renal disease alone. Immunosuppressive therapy and renal transplantation may be required for severe chronic nephritis with end stage renal failure.

HSP is generally a benign disease with an excellent prognosis. More than 80% of patients have a single isolated episode lasting a few weeks. Approximately 10-20% of patients have recurrences. Fewer than 5% of patients develop chronic HSP. End stage renal disease occurs in just 1% patients after several years, therefore, any patient with persistent hematuria, Proteinuria and hypertension must be followed for long term.

1.14 Kawasaki Disease

Kawasaki disease is the most common cause of childhood vasculitis. It is most prevalent in young children below five years of age. Its etiology remains unknown although infectious etiology has been postulated.

Up to 25% of untreated children can develop coronary artery aneurysms as a complication but this could be reduced to less than 5-10% in patients treated with intravenous gamma globulin provided it is started before 10th day of illness.

The risk of coronary aneurysm is high if:
Fever persist for more than 16 days
Recurrence of fever after an afebrile period of at least 48 hours,
Males, who are younger than 1 year age
If cardiomegaly is present.

Diagnostic Criteria: Diagnosis should be considered in any child with fever of >5 days duration with 4 out of following 5 signs: *(Muco-cutaneous-lymph node syndrome)*
- Skin Changes
Initial: Redness and edema of palms and soles
Later: desquamation and peeling of skin of hands and feet
- Polymorphous exanthematous skin rash esp. localized on the back
- Bilateral non-exudative conjunctivitis
- Redness of oropharynx, tongue or lips
- Nonpurulant cervical lymphadenopathy (>1.5 cm)

Other organ involvement include: arthritis, sterile pyuria, aseptic meningitis, diarrhea, pancreatitis, hydrops of gallbladder, otitis media, myopericarditis, congestive heart failure, peripheral ischemia.

Diagnosis is generally of exclusion, **Differential diagnosis** include:
Other viral infections such as adenovirus, measles, EBV
Bacterial infection such as Scarlet fever and Toxic shock syndrome.
Other rheumatic conditions: Systemic JRA, Polyarteritis nodosa and Serum
sickness.

Investigation:

CBC: expected finding include leucocytosis, normocytic anemia and thrombocytosis usually during the second or third week of illness. (Thrombocytopenia is associated with risk of severe coronary artery disease and myocardial infarction)

Raised acute phase reactants.

Raised Liver enzymes in 40% of affected patients.

Urinalysis: Mild-to-moderate sterile pyuria of urethral origin and proteinuria may occur.

Cardiac enzymes (CK mB) levels are elevated during a myocardial infarction. ECG and Echocardiogram should be preformed initially as baseline and then at 6 weeks to assess for presence of coronary aneurysms.

Treatment:

Aspirin: High dose (100 mg/kg/day) until fever subsides, then low dose (3-5 mg/kg/day) until thrombocytosis and acute phase reactant normalize.

Intravenous Immunoglobulin: 2 gm/kg single dose; if patient does not improve after 48 hrs; a second dose of IVIG can be given. If patient is still resistant to therapy a single pulse dose of methyl prednisone followed by short course of oral prednisone can be considered.

Regular follow up with cardiologist if coronary aneurysm exists

1.15   Common Childhood Poisonings

Accidental poisoning in children accounts for more than 2 million reported cases every year in the United States, 50% of them are less than 5 years of age.
90% occur at home and are caused by a single substance.
75 % substances are ingested and 60% are non-drugs.
75% of cases can be managed at home.

Principles of management:

History must be as accurate as possible - quantity, time of exposure and progression.

Initial management should be directed at airway, breathing and circulation (ABC). Shock, arrhythmia, respiratory failure and seizures are life threatening complications.

1. Prevention of absorption by
Emesis - Syrup of Ipecac:
Doses: 6-9 months: 5 ml, 9-12 months: 10 ml, 1-10 years: 15 ml, Over 10 years: 30 ml
Contraindications: less than 6 m of age, severe vomiting, significant hematemesis, neurologically impaired children. Corrosives and hydrocarbons ingestion,
Gastric lavage: Contra indications in corrosives and hydrocarbon ingestion, and if convulsions are present.
Activated charcoal
This adsorbs most organic poisons and is very effective in the treatment of ingestion of sustained release substances with entero-hepatic recirculation; however it is ineffective in alcohols, corrosives, caustics and metals. Dose: 1-2 grams /kg/dose.
Catharsis:
Used to speed transit time of the remaining toxin through the gastrointestinal tract. Magnesium sulfate (250 mg/kg/dose) and Sodium sulfate (250 mg/kg/dose) are used commonly. Contraindicated in paralytic ileus, intestinal obstruction and renal failure.

2. Enhance elimination by
Diuresis: By using a fast acting diuretic and increasing the pH of the urine with IV bicarbonate. Weak acids like salicylate and Phenobarbitone can be rapidly eliminated.
Dialysis:
Dialyzable poisons include methanol, ethylene glycol and salicylate.
Hemoperfusion:
Passing blood through activated charcoal, e.g. Salicylate & Theophylline

3. Evaluate drug levels in the laboratory.

4. Use antidotes if available: Commonly used antidotes are
- N Acetyl cysteine for Acetaminophen (Paracetamol)
- Atropine & Pralidoxime for Organophosphorus compounds
- Dimercaprol for Arsenic, Mercury

- Desferoxamine for Iron
- Dimercapto succinic acid, CaEDTA, d Penicillamine for Lead
- Flumazenil for Benzodiazepines
- Naloxone for Narcotics (morphine and opioids)
- Physostigmine for Ant cholinergic agents

5. Notification

Notify the ward pharmacist and fill in the Accidental poisoning form.
The Pharmacy Department would forward it to the National Poison Control Centre, Ministry of Health Tel: 24566510. National guidelines for management of accidental poisoning are available there.

6. Prevention

- Use child-resistant containers to store medicines/toxic substances.
- Keep all medicines and chemicals locked, out of reach of children.
- Keep products in original containers.
- Do not take medicines in front of children.
- Read labels on household products and medicines carefully.
- Discard/ Return to Pharmacy unused medicines and toxic products after use.
- Do not store kerosene or insecticides in Pepsi/Coke/Water bottles.
- Teach children not to eat anything given by strangers.

Some commonly encountered poisons

1. Paracetamol

Poisoning occurs when > 150mg/kg ingested. Fatality is unlikely with < 225 mg/kg.
Nausea, vomiting and abdominal pain in the first 24 hours
Liver enzymes begin to rise 48 and peak 72-96 hours after ingestion
Renal impairment may occur
Resolution after 4 days unless liver failure develops
Most serious effect is liver damage, which may not be apparent for the first 2 days.

Management

1. **Gastric lavage /induce vomiting with ipecac** if patient is conscious.
    Protect airway by intubation in an unconscious patient before lavage.
    Not suitable if ingestion >4 hours
2. **Measure the plasma Paracetamol level** at 4 hours after ingestion and 4 hourly.
3. **Other investigations:**
    RBS/LFT/PT/PTT/RFT daily for 3 days
3. **IV N-Acetyl-cysteine is used if** four hours plasma Paracetamol level exceeds 150 mcg/ ml.
Give 150mg in 200 mls D5 over 15 min, followed by 50mg/kg in 500 mls D5 over 4 hours, then 100mg/kg in 500 mls D5 over 16 hours. It is much less effective if given later than 15 hour after ingestion. Toxicity levels of plasma Paracetamol after 4 hours of ingestion can be obtained from Rumack-Mathew nomogram (see fig.). If patients on enzyme inducing

drugs, they should be given acetylcysteine if the levels are 50% or more of the Standard reference line. If IV preparation is not available, then use oral N-Acetylcysteine 140 mg/kg stat followed by 70 mg/kg every 4 hours for 17 doses.

4. Give oral methionine 50mg/kg 4 hourly for 4 doses if patient can tolerate orally as an alternative to IV N-acetylcysteine.
5. Keep patient warm and quiet.
6. If PT ratio exceeds 3.0, give **Vitamin K** 1-10mg IM. FFP or clotting factor concentrate may be necessary.
7. Treat complication of acute hepatorenal failure.

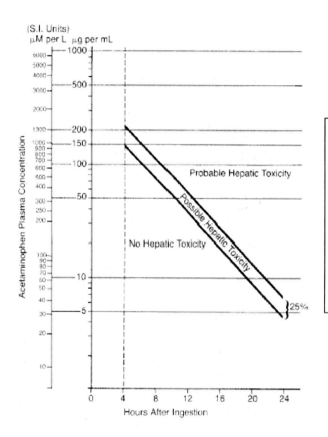

Rumack-Matthew nomogram for acetaminophen poisoning. Semi logarithmic plot of plasma acetaminophen levels versus time. *Cautions for the use of this chart:* (1) The time coordinates refer to time after *ingestion*. (2) Serum levels drawn before 4 hr may not represent peak levels. (3) The graph should be used only in relation to a single acute ingestion. (4) The lower *solid line 25%* below the standard nomogram is included to allow for possible errors in acetaminophen plasma assays and estimated time from ingestion of an overdose. (From Rumack BH, Hess AJ (eds): Poisindex. Denver, 1995. Adapted from Rumack BH, Matthew H: Acetaminophen poisoning and toxicity. Pediatrics 55:871, 1975.)

Prognosis:
Without treatment, 2/3 will develop severe liver and/or renal damage and 5 % will die. If treatment given within 15 hours post ingestion, prognosis is excellent.

2. Salicylate (Aspirin)

Ingestion of > 150 mg/kg will cause toxic symptoms. The fatal dose is estimated to be 200 – 500 mg/kg. Its main effects are as a metabolic poison causing metabolic acidosis and hyperglycemia

Clinical features
General: Hyperpyrexia, profuse sweating and dehydration
CNS: Delirium, seizures, cerebral edema, coma, Reye's syndrome

Respiratory: Hyperventilation
GIT: Epigastric pain, nausea, vomiting, upper GI bleeding, acute hepatitis
Renal: Acute renal failure
Metabolic: Hyper/hypoglycaemia, high anion gap metabolic acidosis, hypokaliemia
CVS: Noncardiogenic pulmonary edema

Investigation:
FBC, PCV, Renal profile, LFT/PT/PTT, RBS and ABG
Serum salicylate level at least 6 hours after ingestion

Management
1. Gastric lavage useful up to 12 hours post ingestion with 15 ml/kg of normal saline till the aspirate is clear and use activated charcoal 1-2g/kg/dose 4-8 hourly.
2. Correct dehydration, hypoglycaemia, hypokaliemia, hypothermia and metabolic acidosis.
3. Give vitamin K if there PT is high
4. Plot the salicylate level on the nomogram.
5. **Forced alkaline diuresis:** For moderate to severe cases (as per the nomogram) in 1st hour give 30 ml/kg pediatric saline + 1ml/kg 8.4% NaHCO3 and Frusemide 1 mg/kg/dose) every 8 hourly. Then, continue at 10 ml/kg/hr till the salicylate level is at the therapeutic range. Add 20 mmol KCl to each 500 mls 1/5 DS to the above regime (discontinue KCl if S. K+ > 5 mmol/L). Aim for pH of >7.5 and urine output of > 3 –6 ml/kg/h.
Repeat renal profile/RBS/ABG every 6 hrs.
Treatment of Hypoglycaemia (5 ml/kg of 10% dextrose IV)

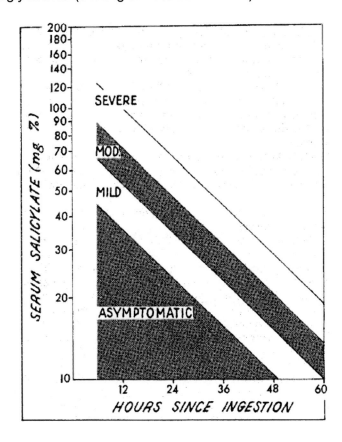

5. Hemodialysis is needed if:
   a. Severe cases, blood salicylate level > 100mg/dl
   b. Refractory acidosis
   c. Renal failure
   d. Noncardiogenic pulmonary edema
   e. Severe CNS symptoms e.g. seizures

Prognosis: Depends on presence of coma, severe metabolic acidosis and high blood Salicylate levels.

3. Iron

Dangerous dose of iron can be as small as 30mg/kg. The toxic effect of iron is due to unbound iron in the serum

Clinical features

1st Stage: (6-12 hrs) - GI Bleeding, vomiting, abdominal pain, diarrhea, hypotension, dehydration, acidosis and coma.

2nd Stage: (8-16 hrs) - Symptom-free period.

3rd Stage: (16-24 hrs) - Cardiovascular collapse, acute iron encephalopathy, Hepatic failure.

4th Stage: (2-5 wks) - Gastrointestinal scarring with pyloric obstruction.

Management:

1. Gastric lavage may be used to remove the pieces of tablets.
2. FBC, Se iron level, renal profile
3. Correct Hypovolemia and electrolyte disturbance.
4. **IV Deferoxamine** 15 mg/kg/hr (Max 6 G/24 hr) given as infusion in symptomatic or if serum iron > 500 mcg/dl. (Beware; Desferrioxamine may cause hypotension, rashes and anaphylaxis, minimized by slow infusion). Infusion should be continued until patient is a-symptomatic or till urine loses the orange/red color of desferrioxamine iron complex excretion.

Prognosis:

GI. hemorrhage, hypotension, metabolic acidosis, coma and shock indicate poor prognosis

4. Kerosene and Hydrocarbon ingestion

Most hydrocarbons cause two types of symptoms:
   1. Aspiration pneumonia during ingestion or later following vomiting. Chest X-Ray may not show pneumonia until 8-12 hours after aspiration. Persistent coughing is first symptom that may progress to respiratory failure in severe cases, therefore always admit and observe the patient for 24 hours. Fever and leucocytosis may appear even without infection and are therefore no guide to antibiotics use.
   2. CNS depression due to systemic absorption

Gastric lavage and emesis are strict contraindication because of increased risk of chemical pneumonitis.

Prophylactic Antibiotics and steroids are of no value but may be useful in lipoid pneumonia (esp. liquid paraffin).

5. Tricyclic Antidepressants

Clinical features:
Anti-cholinergic effects: fever, dry mouth, mydriasis, urinary retention, ileus
Central nervous system: agitation, confusion, convulsion, drowsiness, coma
Respiratory system: respiratory depression
Cardiovascular system: sinus tachycardia, hypotension, complex arrhythmias

Management:
1. There is no specific antidote.
2. Gastric lavage till clear and repeated doses of activated charcoal 1-2 g/kg/dose 4-8 hourly are used even up to 12 hours post ingestion because of re-excretion of drug in to the GI tract for prolong period.
3. Put patient on continuous ECG monitoring.
4. Treatment should be instituted for prolonged QRS and wide complex arrhythmias
5. Correct metabolic acidosis. Give bicarbonate (1-2 mmol/kg) to keep pH 7.45 – 7.55 to prevent development of arrhythmias
6. Convulsions should be treated with diazepam.
7. Use Propranolol to treat life-threatening arrhythmias.
8. Treat hypotension with Norepinephrine. (Dopamine is not effective).
9. Hemodialysis/PD is not effective as tricyclics are protein bound.
10. Only completely a-symptomatic cases are discharged after 6 hours observation.

6. Organophosphates

Clinical features:
Cholinergic effects: Miosis, sweating, lacrimation, muscle twitching, urination, excessive salivation, vomiting, diarrhea
Central nervous system: convulsions, coma and pinpoint pupils
Respiratory system: bronchospasm, pulmonary edema, respiratory arrest
Cardiovascular system: bradycardia, hypotension

Management:
1. Remove contaminated clothing and wash with soap and water.
2. Gastric lavage and activated charcoal.
3. Protect the airway by early intubation. Use only non-depolarizing neuromuscular agents
4. Give **IV atropine** 0.05 mg/kg every 15 minutes till fully atropinized. (Control of respiratory secretions). Keep patient well atropinized for the next 2-3 days.
Continuous infusion of atropine can be started at 0.05 mg/kg/hr and titrated.
5. Give **IV Pralidoxime** 25-50mg/kg over 30 min, repeated in 1-2 hrs and at 10-12 Hr intervals as needed for symptom control (max 12g/day) till nicotinic signs resolves.
6. Treat convulsions with diazepam.
7. IV Frusemide for pulmonary congestion after full atropinization

7. Chronic Lead Poisoning

Is important diagnosis to be considered in any child who has raised ICP or Encephalopathy.

Clinical Features

History of ingestion is usually negative.

• Colicky abdominal pain, constipation, lethargy, anemia, drowsiness, vomiting, headache, fits, coma due to encephalopathy.

• Behavioral changes.

Investigations:

1. Increase blood lead levels >45 microgram/dl.
2. Lead lines (lines of increased density) at growing ends of long bones.
3. Basophilic stippling of red cells.
4. Increased urinary coproporphyrin excretion.

Management

1. Identify source and prevent further ingestion.
2. Decrease cerebral edema - Dexamethasone 0.2-0.4 mg/kg ± Mannitol.
3. Chelating agents - **Dimercaprol** 4 mg/kg IM 4 hourly, gradually decreasing over next few days; Calcium EDTA 50mg/kg/day in divided 4 hourly doses IV/IM.
4. Oral penicillamine 40 mg/kg/day when the child recovered.

8. Caustic agents/ cleaners

These are strong acids, alkalis or oxidizing agents that cause tissue damage on contact.

Local burns, drooling, white plaques of necrosis, swelling, vomiting refusal to swallow.

Burns in esophagus and pylorus may cause stricture and late obstructions needing surgical correction or dilatation procedures.

Gastric lavage and emesis are contraindicated

Thorough flushing of lesion with water is required, Absence of oral lesion does not rule out esophageal injury. In symptomatic cases keep NPO and surgical opinion is asked for.

Use of Steroid to prevent strictures is controversial.

1.16 Snake bites and Scorpion stings

A. Snake bites

About 3,000 known species of snakes exist in the world. Snakes are air-breathing reptiles without eyelids, ear openings and functional limbs. Most species lay eggs. Sea snakes are exceptions. Snakes are sensitive to vibrations rather than sounds. Only 200 species are poisonous to humans. Poisonous species belong to one of three families.

1. Elapidae are deadly snakes, they include the Cobra and the Mamba. They have non-mobile fangs of 3-5 mm length.
2. Viperidae: Vipers and Pit viper (have heat sensitive pits between eyes and nose). Pit vipers are rattlesnakes and Copper heads.
3. Hydrophidae: Poisonous Sea snakes

Snake Venom Is species specific and contains a complex mixture of polypeptides, proteolytic enzymes and toxins. Toxins include anticoagulants, procoagulants, neurotoxins, cardiotoxins, cholinesterases and hyaluronidase. Venom usually shows affinity for a particular system.

300,000 poisonous snakebites occur worldwide per year. Only 10% bites result in death. Cobra bites are commoner in South East Asia while viper bites are commoner in other parts of the world.

Snakes in Oman

Vipers: venom is hematotoxic
Vipers have hinged front fangs. Venom leads to tissue necrosis, vascular leak, hemolysis and coagulopathy. Death is from hemorrhage, shock and renal failure. Three species are seen in the Gulf. All are very dangerous and are *nocturnal*. When alarmed they make a hissing sound.

Cobra: venom is Neurotoxic

Hydrophidae (sea snake): venom is myotoxic and neurotoxic. They act by blocking the neuronal transmission at neuromuscular junction. Death is by respiratory depression.

Effects of snake venom on coagulation.
Spontaneous oozing happens because of the direct endothelial damage by the venom component hemorrhagin. The victim's blood fails to coagulate due to consumptive coagulopathy. DIC by procoagulants. Procoagulant venom directly depletes fibrinogen. Prothrombin (Factor II), Labile Factor (Factor V), Antihemophilic factor (Factor VIII), Stuart Prower factor and Fibrin stabilizing factor are also depleted. Thrombocytopenia may be seen due to local consumption and aggregation.

Symptoms of snakebite envenomation:

Hemotoxic Symptoms	Neurotoxic Symptoms
Intense Pain	Minimal pain
Edema	Ptosis
Weakness	Weakness
Swelling	Paresthesia (often numb at the bite site)
Numbness or tingling	
Rapid pulse	Diplopia
Ecchymosis	Dysphasia
Muscle fasciculations	Sweating
Paresthesia (oral)	Salivation
Unusual metallic taste	Diaphoresis
Vomiting	Hyporeflexia
Confusion	Respiratory depression
Bleeding disorders	Paralysis

Pathophysiology of venomous snakebites
- Local swelling, necrosis
- Systemic effects
  - Non-specific early symptoms
  - Shock
  - Bleeding disorders
  - Neurotoxic, Myotoxic, Cardiotoxic and Nephrotoxic effects

Evaluation and Treatment of Envenomation

Degree of envenomation	Clinical Observation	Antivenin Treatment	Other treatment	Disposition
0. None	Fang marks may be seen. No local or systemic manifestation after 6-8 hours of observation.	None	Local wound cleaning. Tetanus prophylaxis if needed. Antibiotics prophylaxis value unknown	Discharge with follow up after 12 hours of observation
1. Mild	Minimal local swelling and discomfort. No systemic symptoms. Normal lab findings. No blister or ecchymosis or necrosis. No progression after 6 hours of observation.	None	Same as above	Same as above

II. Moderate	Progression of swelling beyond area of bite. Moderate to severe pain. Petechiae and ecchymosis of bite area. Minor systemic symptoms. Minor lab abnormalities.	5-15 vials Depending on the severity	Tetanus prophylaxis if needed. Broad-spectrum antibiotics. Vital signs and cardiac monitoring. IV fluids, pain medication. Follow up lab results	
Severe	Progressive swelling and pain. Blisters, Ecchymosis and Necrosis. Vomiting, Weakness, Fasciculations, Tachycardia, Hypotension, Epistaxis, Hematuria. Abnormal clotting studies Bleeding tendencies. Hemolysis and Renal failure.	15-25 vials	Same as above	Admit to ICU

Laboratory workup of Envenomation case

CBC PT APTT Fibrinogen FDP Blood type and Cross match S. Electrolytes S. Glucose Blood Urea and Creatinine	LFT Bilirubin Creatine kinase Urine exam Arterial blood gas, If respiratory symptoms

Pitfall and Errors in management
1. Not considering snake poisoning in the case of an edematous, ecchymotic extremity in a child who was playing in an area where snakes are seen.
2. Not looking for fang marks at the site of pain
3. Not considering that an envenomation grade can change with time and thus the clinical status of the patient may worsen over a period of time.
4. Not checking initial coagulation studies and repeating these later
5. Not considering the diagnosis of envenomation because the offending snake was not seen
6. Not administrating antivenin early in envenomation with the presence of progressive signs and symptoms.
7. Not considering the administration of broad-spectrum prophylactic antibiotics.
8. Not realizing the antivenom can successfully reverse coagulopathy even more than 24 hours after envenomation.

9. Leaving a constriction band or tourniquet on an extremity for a prolonged period of time can cause more damage

10. Not considering hypovolemia due to presence of massive tissue edema or bleeding in a child not adequately dehydrating.

Treatment

First Aid

The immediate first aid measures include *immobilizing* the bitten extremity and quickly transporting the victim to the nearest hospital. A wide flat *constriction band* may be applied proximal to the bite to block only superficial venous and lymphatic flow and should be left in place until antivenin therapy, if indicated, begins. One or two fingers should easily slide beneath this band since any impairment of arterial blood flow could increase tissue death.

An attempt should be made to *identify the type of snake* if possible. Once the patient is admitted to the hospital, the wound should be cleaned and tetanus toxoid should be considered for under immunized or non-immunized patients. Intravenous fluid should be given and blood should be collected from the unaffected extremity. Full work up of laboratory evaluation must be done as given in the table above. At least 25% of snakebites do not result in envenomation.

Patients with *asymptomatic viper bites* should be observed for 12-24 hours before discharge. If there is no proximal progression of local signs on the extremity and no coagulopathy after 12-24 hours of clinical observations, the patient can be sent home with the instruction to return to hospital immediately if symptoms worsen. Patients with bites from snakes with neurotoxic venom should be observed for 24 hours.

Equine derived antivenin to snake poison has been the mainstay of hospital treatment for last 35 years. **In Oman 3 types of antivenin are available.**
1. Saudi National Guard antivenin covers the vipers in Oman but not the Arabian cobra
2. Pasteur Institute (French) antivenin covers the vipers in Oman and the Arabian cobra.
3. Haffkine Institute (India) antivenin covers 80% of vipers in Oman, but is not recommended for use.
None of the above covers sea snake bites.

Ideally, antivenin to be administered as early as possible, but should be given anytime if we fear envenomation has occurred. A physician should be present for antivenin administration and adrenaline and antihistamines should be available at the bedside.

Performing skin test with horse serum is a matter of controversy because it delays therapy and can itself cause anaphylaxis and serum sickness. There are 30% false negative and false positive results. In the event of a significant anaphylaxis patient should be managed with adrenaline, antihistamines and steroids and should restart antivenin slowly undercover of the above medication. Sometime it may be necessary to do desensitization prior to antivenin treatment. All patients should receive antivenin because no other treatment can reverse the venom effect. If allergic to one antivenin try to use another type of antivenin.

The decision to use antivenin requires a careful analysis of the risks and benefits. In moderate envenomation (swelling beyond bite, impaired coagulation (viper), ptosis (cobra) give 50-

100 ml of antivenin diluted in 100 ml normal sale and to run as fast as possible according to age and weight of the patient. In severe envenomation give 100-150 ml antivenin diluted in 200 ml normal saline and give as fast as possible. Can give undiluted directly in severe cases.

It should be noted that the dose of antivenin does not depend on per kilo weight or age but on severity of envenomation

The coagulation profile should be checked after one hour and repeat the dose if not corrected. The antivenin should be repeated again every 4-6 hours till the abnormality is corrected.

Cobra: 50-100 ml antivenin diluted and given as above. Anti-cholinesterase (neostigmine) is also indicated.

Toxicity of Antivenin
Early Fever, rigors, hypotension (can be treated with paracetamol and anti-histamines)
Late (5 days to 3 weeks): Serum sickness- fever, itching, urticaria, arthralgia and lymphadenopathy. If coagulopathy is present, consult a hematologist, you may need cryoprecipitate, FFP, packed cells or platelets transfusion.

B. Scorpion Stings

There are more than 350 species of scorpion about 15 of which are dangerous. Dangerous ones in the Middle East include *Leiurus quinquestriatus* and *Androctonus* and *Buthus*.
Most scorpion stings produce severe local pain with swelling without systemic effects.
Envenomation induces arrhythmias, hypertension, hypotension, and rarely pulmonary edema. Most of the effects are due to outpouring of catecholamine into circulation.
Pancreatitis, myocarditis and convulsions are rarely seen.
Child may have leukocytosis, mild hyperglycemia, and hypocalcemia. Normal coagulation with a mild elevation of serum amylase is commonly observed.

Management
Local infiltration of 0.5% Xylocain to reduce pain can be used.
Tetanus toxoid is given.
Observe for a few hours and, if no signs of envenomation seen, discharge the patient.

If envenomation signs appear
Saudi National Guard or Pasteur polyvalent anti scorpion antivenin is administered.
Test dose is not required. 2-5 vials in 20 ml 0.45 normal saline to run over 30 minutes.
Repeat after two hours if no improvement.

1.17 Drowning & Near Drowning

Definitions:

Drowning: Means death within 24 hrs due to submersion in water.

Near-Drowning: Complete or temporary survival beyond 24hrs after a submersion

Epidemiology

In US it accounts for 2nd leading cause of injuries-related deaths in children aged 1-14yrs

1500-children die/yr

Males 4 times more affected then females

Age distribution: Bimodal, < 4yrs, 15-19yrs

Children < 5 years accounts for 87% of all drowning cases

Site of drowning
> < 1yr: Bathtubs
> 1-5 yrs: Swimming pools, Septic tanks
> Older children: open bodies of water (lakes, ponds, streams)

Types:

- Cold water / Warm water drowning
- Salt water / Fresh water drowning

Pathophysiology:

Water aspiration (wet drowning) / Laryngospasm (dry drowning)

↓oxygenation → hypoxemia

Multi-organ failure

Severity of hypoxemia is determined by:
> - Duration of submersion and presence of pulmonary Aspiration

Duration of submersion:

Critical time is 3-5 mints

Complete survival has been reported even after submersion for 10-40 mts.

Pulmonary Aspiration:

Occurs in 80-90% of wet drowning, usually 1-3ml/kg.

There is no significant difference observed in prognosis in cases of fresh & seawater drowning although the mechanism differs.

Aspiration of stomach contents occurs in 25%of cases, esp. after CPR

Sea water (hyper tonic)

Draws water into lungs from plasma

↓

Pulmonary edema

↓

Hypoxia

Fresh water (hypo tonic)

Draws water into plasma
↓
Disruption of lung surfactant
↓
Atelectasis
↓
Hypoxia

CVS effect:

Hypoxia: - increased capillary permeability
↓
Hypovolemia
↓
Arrhythmias
↓
Myocardial damage.

Fluid / Electrolyte imbalance:

Seen only in 15%of pts.
Hypernatremia in sea water drowning.
Hyponatremia in fresh water drowning.
Hyperkalemia due to hemolysis
Hypercalcemia.
Hypoglycemia/hyperglycemia

Other metabolic effects:

Hypothermia:
Bradycardia, decreased myocardial contractility, hypotension → shock
CNS →hypoventilation →apnea →Hypoxic encephalopathy
Thrombocytopenia, platelets dysfunction
DIC
Impair neutrophil function →infections
Diving reflex→ Bradycardia → Peripheral vasoconstriction

Clinical Evaluation:

History:

A symptomatic
Symptomatic: - cough
                 - dyspnea
                 - wheeze
                 - vomiting
                 - altered level of consciousness
Cardiopulmonary arrest and Death

Past Medical History:

Trauma, Seizure (4-10 times increase risk), Cardiac disease, Syncope and Alcohol or drug use

Lab studies:

ABG
CBC
Renal & Hepatic profile
Drug screen
ECG
CXR
Cervical spine X-Ray, CT if indicated

Management:

Immediate rescue:

ABC
Cervical spine stabilization
Remove patient from water as soon as possible
Rescue breathing
Chest compression
Heimlich maneuver not effective in removing aspirated water

In A/E:

Correction of hypoxemia /acidosis:
100% O2
IV fluids
Correction of hypothermia
Correction of Hypovolemia / Inotropic support

Indications for admissions:

Respiratory symptoms
Altered ABG, Hypoxia- Low SaPo2
Altered level of consciousness

Indications for Intubation/mechanical ventilation/ use of artificial Surfactant:

Poor respiratory effort
Altered sensorium
Severe hypoxemia
Severe acidosis

Corticosteroids have no role

Routine Antibiotics prophylaxis is not indicated unless child submerged in grossly contaminated water

Prognosis:

Brain damage: Mental retardation in 20% in hospitalized patient & is usually due to cardiopulmonary failure/ arrest.
Unfavorable prognostic factors:

Prolonged submersion. > 25mints
Prolonged resuscitation > 25mints
Apneic / comatose patient at presentation
Initial blood PH <7.1

1.18   Shock

Definition:
Shock is a life threatening condition characterized by extreme degree of tissue hypoperfusion leading to generalized cellular hypoxia and multiorgan failure. It accounts for the high morbidity and mortality rate.

In children hypovolemic shock is the most common cause leading to 6 to 20 million deaths annually worldwide. Early recognition of severity, identification of risk factors and prompt therapeutic strategies are crucial to prevent irreversible organ dysfunction and death.

Physiological factors determining the systemic perfusion (Fig 1)

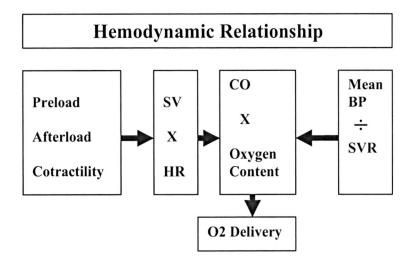

- Clinically the tissue perfusion and oxygen delivery depends on cardiac output (CO), Blood pressure (BP), pulse volume (PV) and arterial oxygen saturation.
- The CO is the product of Stroke Volume (SV) and Heart rate (HR) CO = SV x HR
- Stroke volume (SV) is determined by the pumping function of the ventricles, which is derived from the contractility, preload, afterload, and vascular resistance.
- Net oxygen delivery to the tissue is the product of Cardiac output and oxygen content

Classification of Shock according to eatiology (Table 1)
  1. Hypovolemic Shock
  - Due to the loss of circulating volume which reduces the cardiac output
  2. Distributive Shock
  - Mal distribution of circulating volume due to the leakage of intravascular fluid through the capillary bed into the interstitial space due to endothelial damage, known as "third spacing".
  3. Cardiogenic Shock
  - Occurs due to the Impairment of cardiac contractility secondary to disorders of cardiac muscle, valvular disease or abnormalities in the conduction system.
  4. Extra-cardiac Obstructive Shock
  - There is an impairment of forward blood flow leading to poor circulation

Table 1 Classification of Shock according to aetiology:

	Mechanisms	Causes
1. Hypovolemic	Fluid-electrolyte loss	Diarrhea, vomiting Heat stroke, Burns Excessive renal loss
	Blood loss	Trauma GI bleed Surgery Intracranial bleed
	Endocrine disorders	Diabetes mellitus Diabetes Insipidus Adrenal Insufficiency
	Inborn error of metabolism (IEM)	Hyperammonemia, Organic acidemia
2. Distributive	Sepsis (early phase)	
	Anaphylaxis	Antibiotics Vaccines Blood products Anesthesia Insects Food
	Drugs and toxins	Barbiturates Antihypertensive Phenothiazines, Tranquillizers
	Neurogenic	Head and spinal cord injury General and spinal anesthesia
3. Cardiogenic	Congenital Heart Disease	Hypoplastic Left Heart (HLHS) Pulmonary Atresia (PA) Transposition of Great Vessels (TOGV)
	Ischemic	Perinatal asphyxia Kawasaki Disease
	Arrhythmias	Supraventricular Tachycardia (SVT) Complete Heart Block
	Myocardial depressants	Drugs Electrolyte imbalance
	Sepsis (late Phase)	
	Cardiomyopathy / Myocarditis	
4. Extracardiac (Obstructive)	Outflow tract obstruction	Pulmonary embolism Tension Pneumothorax Cardiac Temponade Coarctation of the Aorta Interrupted aortic Arch

Table 2 Clinical and Cardiovascular signs of Shock

Clinical signs	Hypovolemic	Distributive	Cardiogenic
Pulse pressure	Narrow	Widened	Narrow
Skin perfusion: Color, Temperature, Capillary refill	Pink Cool distally Normal to prolonged	Pink Warm (early) Normal to prolonged	Mottled, gray or blue Cool to cold Prolonged
Level of consciousness	Usually normal unless severe	Lethargic/agitated Coma (late)	Lethargic to coma
Urine output			
Respiratory rate	↑	↑ to ↑↑	↑↑
Breath sounds	Normal	Normal or with crackles	Rales / grunting
Heart Rate	↑	↑ to ↑↑	↑↑
Pulse quality	Thready	Early: bounding Late: thready	Thready

Classification of Shock According to Physiologic Status

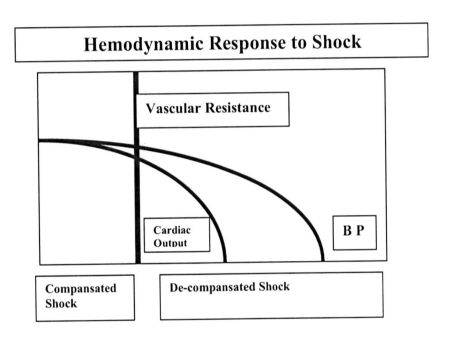

1. Compensated Shock
- Systolic blood pressure is within the normal range.
- Signs and symptoms of inadequate tissue and organ perfusion e.g. lactic acidosis, oliguria and altered level of consciousness are present

The baroreceptors, chemoreceptors and various neuro-humoral mechanisms like epinephrine, vasopressin and rennin angiotensin mechanism act to compansate the circulation and perfusion back to normal.

2. Decompensated Shock (Fig below)

Presence of clear signs of shock and systolic hypotension

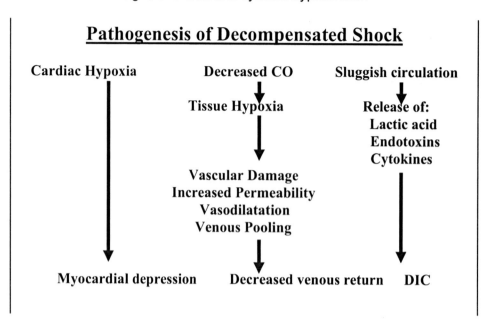

Pathogenesis of Decompensated Shock

Cardiac Hypoxia   Decreased CO   Sluggish circulation

Tissue Hypoxia   Release of:
Lactic acid
Endotoxins
Cytokines

Vascular Damage
Increased Permeability
Vasodilatation
Venous Pooling

Myocardial depression   Decreased venous return   DIC

3. Irreversible Shock

Irreversible circulatory decompensation resulting from profound alteration in vascular tone unresponsive to therapy

Clinical features of Shock in its different stages of progression

System	Low perfusion	Compensated	Decompensated
CNS	-	Restless/ apathy	Confused / Stupor
Respiratory	-	Tachypnea	More of tachypnea
Acid-base	-	Compensated metabolic acidosis	Metabolic acidosis
GIT	-	Decreased motility	Paralytic ileus
Kidney	Oliguria, high urine specific gravity	Oliguria	Oliguria/anuria
Skin	Delayed capillary refill	Cool extremities	Mottled, cyanotic, cold extremities
CVS	Tachycardia	Tachycardia, weak pulses	Tachycardia, absent pulses

Cardiopulmonary failure results if shock remained untreated or inadequately treated

Clinical evaluation of a patient with shock: Rapid Cardiopulmonary Assessment

    A. General Appearance
- Color
- Mental status
- Activity, movements
- Age appropriate response stimuli.

    B. Evaluation of Airway, Breathing and Circulation (ABC)

       1. Airway
- Maintainable, requiring suctioning or bag and mask ventilation
- Not maintainable, requiring intubation and mechanical ventilation

       2. Breathing
- Respiratory rate, Respiratory effort, Air entry / tidal volume
- Skin color

       3. Circulation: Cardiovascular function
- Heart rate
- Pulses, capillary refill time, color of skin
- Systolic/diastolic BP and peripheral pulses

    End organ function
- Brain
- Skin
- Kidneys (normal urine output 1-2 ml/Hg/hr)

Normal Heart Rate:

Age	Awake	Mean	Sleeping
New born – 3 mos	85-205	140	80-160
4 mos - 2 yrs	100-190	130	75-160
3 yrs – 10 yrs	60-140	80	60-90
> 10 yrs	60-100	75	50-90

Fifth Centile (Lowest acceptable limits) of Systolic BP (American Heart Association 2000)

Age	SBP (mmHg)
Term Newborn (0-28 days)	60
1-12 mos	70
1-10 years	70 mmHg + (2 x age in yrs)
> 10 years	90 mmHg

The fifth (5th) centile of the systolic BP is the minimum requirement in a healthy well-perfused child. Five percent (5 %) of normal children have an SBP < 5th centile.

Capillary refill time: Time to return of peripheral perfusion after pressure on heel of the child. Normal capillary time <2 seconds

Recognition of shock and patient monitoring:
1. Early recognition of shock or impending shock requires a high index of suspicion and it is crucial in the life saving therapeutic interventions
2. Appropriate history
3. Repeated and careful examination of the child's physiologic status
4. Monitoring:
   a. Non-invasive monitoring:

   O2 saturation, BP, temperature, respiration, urine output, acid base status
   b. Invasive monitoring:

   CVP estimates left ventricular end diastolic volume, normal CVP 3-5 newborns, and 8-10 in children

   Swan-Ganz catheter pulmonary artery pressure monitoring

   Arterial line for accurate BP measurements

Management
1) **Maintenance of Airway**, Breathing and Circulation (ABC) takes priority

2) **Reliable vascular access** and large bore cannula should be inserted. If peripheral access is not available in 60-90 seconds, one must do intraosseous cannulation.

3) **Monitoring of vital signs** (HR, BP, temperature, RR, oxygen saturation)

4) **Fluid therapy**: Normal saline or Ringer's lactate, 20 ml/kg in 5-10 minutes and can be repeated up to three doses.

5) **Assisted ventilation**
   - Airway control should be based on clinical state of the patient and not only on the blood gas or oxygen saturation (O_2 sat)
   - Child with circulatory failure may appear stable but with decrease in oxygen delivery to muscle including the diaphragm can rapidly fatigue leading to respiratory failure

6) **Inotrope/Vasopressor**:

   a. Dopamine
   Mode of action: α_1 β_1 D_1 simulation
   - Effective vasopressor for fluid refractory hypotensive shock on the setting of low vascular resistance
   - Exerts its action through the release of epinephrine and norepinephrine, both are exhausted in cases of decompensated shock
   Dose: 2-20 microgram /kg/minute

b. Dobutamine
Mode of action: $\alpha_1 \beta_1 \beta_1$
- Useful in cardiogenic shock
- In volume depleted patients it nay cause significant vasodilatation and increase pulmonary shunting.
- It has a potential of decreasing the cardiac output and oxygen delivery
- Best use in the combination of other inotropes.
Dose: 2 – 20 microgram /kg/min

c. Epinephrine (endogenous catecholamines)
Mode of action
- α_1 Increases systemic vascular resistance, BP, coronary pressures
- α_2 Reduces splanchnic, renal, muscular and dermal vascular flow
- β_1 Increase myocardial contractility, HR
- β_2 Relaxes skeletal muscle, vascular bed and bronchial smooth muscles
Dose: 0.05 – 1 microgram /kg/min

d. Norepinephrine
Mode of action: $\alpha_1 \alpha_2 \beta_2$
Dose: 0.05-1 ugm/kg/min

7) **Type 3 phosphodiesterase inhibitors:**
Prevent hydrolysis of cyclic AMP thus potentiating the effect of β receptor stimulation in cardiac and vascular tissue.
Milrinone preferred in the presence of liver dysfunction
Amrinone, in renal dysfunction
These drugs should be discontinued in the presence of tachyarrythmia, hypotension or diminished vascular resistance. Treat with norepinephrine as it stimulates the α receptors.

8) **Corticosteroid** (American College of critical care Guidelines) Reccomonded use of steroids (Hydrocortisone) in
- Catecholamines resistance
- Proven adrenal insufficiency (serum cortisol: < 18 mg/dl)
Dose: Physiologic 12.5 mg/ m²/day, Stress 50-100m/m²/day

Supportive Therapy
1. Fluid resuscitation alone may suffice to correct the metabolic acidosis
2. Severe metabolic acidosis (pH $\leq$ 7.2) may aggravate the cardiovascular and neurologic depression.
3. Correction of electrolyte abnormalities
4. Antibiotic therapy should be initiated at the earliest in patient with septic shock.
5. Acute renal failure: conservative and or peritoneal/hemodialysis
6. Adequate nutritional support to offset the effect of excessive catabolism in shock
7. Stress ulcer is common and can lead to GI bleed or toxic ileus. Treat with antacid and H_2 receptor antagonist.
8. Coagulation abnormalities may complicate hypoperfusion of any etiology.
Blood product replacement may be required.

Summary

- Shock is a clinical syndrome characterized by extreme degree of poor tissue perfusion leading to generalized tissue hypoxia and multiorgan failure
- Hypovolemic shock from fluid loss (Dehydration) is the most common cause in children
- Neuroendocrine mechanism maintains BP and tissue perfusion (compensatory phase of shock) With progression of the disease process, tissue hypoxemia sets in with anaerobic metabolism and release of inflammatory mediators leading to cell injury and without prompt intervention ultimately lead to multiorgan failure.
- Early recognition of impending shock, prompt intervention and appropriate monitoring are essential to successful outcome
- Management directed at maintaining ABC of resuscitation
- In general it is important to recognize that any infant or child with severe or sustained shock regardless of etiology develops some degree of myocardial dysfunction. Many will require fluid administration even in the absence of documented fluid loss and / or pharmacologic drugs to increase the cardiac output.
- Specific treatment directed at the causative factor is essential and the above supportive measures will sustain life and improve outcome until such time the etiology comes under control
- Mortality is high in patients who develop multiorgan failure despite availability of newer treatment modalities.

1.19 Central Venous Access Devices (VAD)

Central venous access devices (VAD) are being increasingly used in patients who require short to long-term IV therapy. VAD ensures the safe delivery of chemotherapeutic agents, other medications, blood and blood products, TPN, IV fluids and allows blood sampling in reliable and relatively safe manner without much discomfort to patients. Unfortunately, complications of these devices are not uncommon and can significantly affect the treatment outcome. It is therefore necessary for medical staff to maintain expertise in care so as to minimize patient morbidity and maximize the life span of these devices.

Types of Central Venous Access device

Long-term venous access catheters: simple central lines can stay in situ for maximum 4-6 weeks while Hickman for 6 months and Port a cath can stay up-to 2-3 years.
They are of two types:
- External catheters
- Implantable catheters

External devices are tunnelled subcutaneously from an exit site. A Dacron cuff on the catheter positioned in the subcutaneous tunnel promotes fibrous in-growth around the catheter thereby reducing the chances of accidental dislodgement.

The devices can be seen in X-ray. They have one to four lumens as per requirement. One should note that more lumens the greater the chances of infection.

A.   External Catheters

Simple central lines
They are used for emergencies like shock or severe dehydration where intravenous access is difficult. They may be used for up-to 4-6 weeks. The disadvantage is that the chances of infection are high and the device can dislodge easily.

Peripherally Inserted central lines (PICC)
PICCs are inserted into an ante-cubital vein and positioned so that the tip resides in the superior vena cava. PICCs are suitable for patients requiring long-term antibiotics, patients with tracheostomy who are unable to tolerate the insertion of a central line. The advantage of PICCs is that it can be inserted at the bedside and it has low rate of complications.

After inserting any central line it is mandatory to have a Chest X-ray to check the position of the catheter tip and to see if Pneumothorax has occurred.

Hickman Catheter
This is an external catheter available in different French sizes and with 1-3 lumens. It needs special surgical skill to insert and remove it. Since there are 2-3 lumens, one lumen can be dedicated for blood collection, one for TPN and one for fluids or chemotherapy administration. The disadvantage is that, as half the catheter is outside the body, the patient cannot be send home with the catheter and needs to take care when bathing etc. It can remain in place for up to 6 months.

B. Implantable Catheters

Are similar to an external catheter except, instead of exiting the skin, a port housing is anchored in a subcutaneous pocket, which can be accessed with a special non-coring Huber needle. Huber needles minimize the coring to the silastic membrane. When these devices are not in use they are safe under the skin and do not need much maintenance. The disadvantages of these devices are that they must be accessed through the skin each time the device is used. These devices need special surgical procedures to insert and remove them.

Port-A-Cath
This is the most frequently used implantable device. Implantable ports are available with single or double lumens. Double lumen ports are large in size and not suitable for Pediatrics populations. They need special surgical skill to insert and remove them. They usually have a single lumen so the use is limited but adequate. The patient can be sent home with the inserted port without risk of dislodgement and precautions during bathing. These can remain in place 2 – 3 years.

Dressing and Maintenance
Skin tunnelled catheters/ Implantable Ports:
After the placement of the catheter, the initial dressing change should be done after 24 hours. The suture needs to be removed after 7 days. The exit site suture should be removed after 14 days when the tissue in-growth has occurred around the Dacron cuff.
Subsequent dressing should be done every 72 hours for Mepore or every 6th to 7th days for a transparent dressings. Dressings must be changed whenever damp, loosened or soiled. The dressing should be checked once every nursing shift.

Implantable ports.
If a patient needs continuous access to the port, the Huber needle is secured by a transparent dressing with a piece of sterile gauze placed under the needle. This will prevent movement of the needle and minimize the possibility of a pressure sore developing on the patient's skin.

Maintaining Patency
The flushing technique is very important in preventing occlusion of all CVADs A rapid push-pause or pulsated flushing technique is recommended. This creates turbulence thereby decreasing the risk of fibrin and platelet adherence in the internal walls of CVADs thus minimizing the risk of occlusion. If the CVADs have more than one lumen, each one should be flushed separately.

Blood Sampling
A strict aseptic technique must be maintained at all times. After collecting blood or infusion of blood products, it is important to flush with at least 15-20 ml of normal saline.

Complications
Insertion Complications
Air embolus, Pneumothorax, hemothorax, arterial puncture, nerve injury, atrial fibrillation, catheter mal-position and thrombosis

Infections

1. Exit Site Complications

An exit site infection is characterized by localized erythema and tenderness at the exit site of an external catheter. Signs of infection may or may not present. The exit site should be cultured and aggressive local wound care undertaken as well as IV or oral antibiotics against gram-positive organisms administered..

2. Tunnel infection

A tunnel infection is an advanced infectious process in which the subcutaneous track of the catheter has developed an infection. Surrounding cellulites along the catheter track is frequently present. Systemic signs of infection are present. The catheter must be removed, cultures sent for testing and antibiotics given.

Pocket Infection

This is a suppurative infectious process around an implantable port and is like a tunnel infection. Cultures must be sent for testing and antibiotics started. The port must be removed.

Line Sepsis

Line sepsis is a potentially serious complication of long-term CVADs. Common organisms are *Staphylococcus epidermidis, Staphylococcus aureus, streptococcus, Pseudomonas, E coli* and *Candida*. Initial treatment of line related infection should include appropriate empiric antibiotic coverage to include both gram-negative and gram-positive organisms. Recurrent infections with the same organisms, persistent positive cultures of the same organisms or a patient with a deteriorating clinical condition in spite of appropriate antibiotics are indication for removal of the catheter. Line sepsis with fungus is very difficult to eradicate and usually requires removal of catheter.

3. Catheter occlusion

Persistent withdrawal occlusion (Inability to aspirate blood)

If it is impossible to aspirate blood from the device make sure the needle is in correct position in the port. Try to irrigate with 10-20 ml of normal saline. Change the patient position to supine, lateral, arms raised etc. Huber needle may need to be changed. IF it is still impossible to aspirate, a chest X-ray to be taken to check the position of the catheter. If the position is correct various thrombolytic agents (Streptokinase, Urokinase) may be used

Complete occlusion of catheter

If the block is complete (neither the blood can be aspirated nor the solution be infused, this may be secondary to presence of clotted blood or that the TPN has formed a calcium-phosphate complex in the line. Maintaining positive pressure within the catheter at all times can prevent this. To prevent this always make sure you flush the catheter with 20 ml normal saline after collecting blood samples or infusing TPN.

If case of block due to a blood clot, then one can dissolve it by filling and leaving the catheter with small dose of heparin (500-1000 units), try and aspirate after few hours. If it is still blocked then try using fibrinolytic agent like Streptokinase or Urokinase.

Instil 1ml of Urokinase into the catheter and wait for 30-60 minutes. If a repeated instillation fails, try Urokinase continuous infusion 200u/kg/ hr for 24 hours. The agent should, if possible, be aspirated from the catheter when patency is restored. If available, a tissue plasminogen activator (t-PA) is more efficient in restoring the patency of clotted catheters.

Indication for removal of catheters

- Bacteraemia and or clinical symptoms persisting beyond 72 hours despite appropriate antibiotics through catheter
- Progressive infection at exit site or subcutaneous tunnel, especially *Pseudomonas* infections
- Bacteraemia due to *Corynebacterium* or *Candida* species.
- Unstable patient and or development of hypotension due to sepsis.
- Evidence of septic emboli or endocarditis.
- As a general rule, when the catheter is no longer functional or not required it should be removed.

Protocol for the Port-a-cath needle insertion and it's maintenance

Port needle insertion or flushing is a delicate procedure. All precautions should be taken with surgical hygiene by using a mask, gloves and gown. The dressing trolley should be prepared with the utmost sterile technique.

Instruments needed
10 ml syringe with Normal saline and 5 ml syringe with 500 units of heparin.
Port needle and three-way connector should be kept ready flushed with N. Saline.
A partly cut swab should be ready.

Procedure:
The skin overlying the port surface must be cleansed, sterilized and a window sheet used to cover the surroundings. Avoid the previously penetrated site on the skin to reinsert the needle. Use only a non-coring type needle. Avoid human traffic in the treatment room while the procedure is underway.

Fix the Port with the finger and insert the needle at the middle till it touches the bottom. Do not push further. Aspirate and make sure there is a free flow of blood, if not, change the position of the patient and try again.

Pack the cut swab underneath the port needle and fix the needle with Tegaderm film. Make a loop of the tube and fix it well.

Connect the three-way adaptor and connect to the IV line. Never leave the hub open.

Check the dressing at least once a day and make sure the needle is changed on every 6th day or earlier if needed.

When removing the needle, stabilize the port with two fingers, slowly push the heparin and gently remove the needle. Once flushed with 500 units of heparin the port can be left for 4-5 weeks. Change the dressing any time when it is loose, soaked or stained

Precautions in using the Port
If no free fluid is going in, do not exert too much pressure as it can break the port connections.

Push heparin using a 2 ml syringe, leave it for sometime and try again
If all attempts fail, take a chest X-ray to visualize the position of the port. Compare the position with the earlier X-ray. If it is still blocked, call for help.

Remember, a little care and precaution and little extra time can save a lot of time, energy, money and even life.

1.20 Safe Prescribing

Current research shows that approximately 60% of medication errors are generated at the prescribing stage. Children are a vulnerable group and medication errors in this age range have an increased potential for fatal out come. The responsibility of the prescribing doctor is to write a safe and correct prescription having considered the clinical circumstances of the patient.

Prescribing information:

The doctor must CLEARLY prescribe and state:

1. The **right drug on the right patient's prescription sheet**
2. The **approved generic name** of the drug to be administered
3. The **dose** of the drug
4. The **route of administration**
5. The **time and frequency**
6. The **infusion fluid** in which the drug should be diluted
7. The **volume** of an infusion fluid
8. The **final concentration** of the drug infusion
9. The **calculated rate** at which the infusion is to be administered i.e. 'ml per minute', 'drops per minute', 'mg per minute' or 'ml per hour'.
10. Which intravenous line to be used for administration of drugs, where more than one line is in use, e.g. **peripheral or central line**.

Where administration of a drug is by continuous intravenous infusion or where the infusion rate is to be adjusted according to patient response, the doctor should record full details.

First dose: (See also individual policies for Specialty areas)
Bolus administration – the first dose must always be given by the doctor, and he/she must sign on the patient prescription sheet.

The doctor must be present in the ward during the first five (5) minutes of the infusion of the first dose of any antibiotic drug.

Note: The doctor should recognize that the nurse if has reasonable grounds to question the accuracy or completeness of a prescription, has a duty to do so, also if the prescription be so written that it is unclear, he/she has a duty to seek clarification from the prescriber and may refuse to give the drug.

Select recommendations and guidelines for safe prescribing:

- Always write legibly.
- Use electronic prescription writing tools when possible.
- Remember that "mental slips" occur frequently in the prescribing process -- focus on the task at hand.
- If interrupted during prescribing-, review process from beginning, then complete.

Provide complete information with orders/prescriptions.

- Patient's first and last name, age,
- Important patient-specific data that influence drug therapy
- Generic and brand name (Do not use abbreviations for drug names)
- Dosage form
- Route (do not use abbreviations that are commonly confused ("au," "ou," "pt," "pr," "sc," "sq," etc.)
- Provide clear, unambiguous, and complete directions for use
- Provide any information needed by patient, family, nursing, or pharmacy to assure effective drug therapy and reduce error risk

Use metric system only.

Prescribe liquid medication doses in weight (i.e., "gm," "mg"), not volume, unless it is the convention (i.e., antacids). If volume is used, include "mg" dose and desired concentration of liquid drug formulation.

- Do **not** use trailing zeros (1.0 mg).
- **Always** use leading zeros - a zero before a decimal point (0.1 mg).
- Spell out "units," never use abbreviation "U."
- Do not use "ug" to abbreviate micrograms.

Always provide dosing equation, patient weight or body surface area, and calculated dose for chemotherapies and pediatric patients.

- Double-check all calculated doses.
- **Always re-read order when finished.**
- Provide indication for medication use with prescriptions.
- Review pertinent patient history/medical records, laboratory and diagnostic results before prescribing.
- Take careful patient medication history, and record effectively.

Always review basic patient characteristics when prescribing -- adjust drug therapy accordingly. Make a note of the following factors:

- Allergies
- Age, Sex, Weight
- Renal and Hepatic functions
- Past medication use
- Concurrent disease states

Review basic drug-related information prior to prescribing.

Reason for and goals of drug therapy

Contraindications/precautions, Potential adverse reactions

Concurrent therapies

Drug interactions

Patient ability to understand and carry out treatment plan

Use verbal orders only when necessary, have the person read your order back to you. Spell out potential sound and look-alikes (PENICILLIN or PENICILLAMINE).

Always write complete orders, don't write orders such as "resume pre-op meds."

Create an environment of communication with patients and caregivers.

Limit number of medications prescribed by consistently prescribing the same drug within a class whenever appropriate.

Read up-to-date drug information prior to prescribing any medication you are   unfamiliar with.

Maintain up-to-date knowledge of potential medication error risks (visit Institute for Safe Medication Practices at www.ismp.org regularly).

1.21 Practicing Evidence Based Medicine (EBM)

Introduction:

Formal medical education is unable to cope up with the rapid advances in medicine. The new diagnostic tests; treatments and literatures are emerging every day. Medical students can face the challenge of the information overload. The principles and practice of EBM is one way of information mastery and can also serve as a life long learning tool. Following example sheds more light on the subject and is very useful in understanding the concept of EBM

Clinical Example/Scenario:

A 7 year old child is brought to the out patients department with a progressively increasing history of pain in the right leg for the past two days and inability to walk. There is no history of injury or fever. On examination the child is afebrile, unable to bear weight on the right leg and pain on passive movements of the hip. The power was grade 4/5 in the flexors of the thigh. There were no inflammatory signs or evidence of soft tissue infection. The white blood count and the erythrocyte sedimentation rate are normal.

At this stage several questions may come to ones mind including
1. Is this a neurological or a problem of the joints?
2. Is this a case of child abuse?
3. What are the possible causes of hip pain in this child?
4. How do we confirm a diagnosis?
5. Should the child be referred to he pediatrician or orthopedic surgeon?

How should one proceed?

In the past the junior doctor would consult his seniors, who would ask him to refer the child to the orthopedics or do a test depending on his knowledge and experience in managing similar cases.

Today the doctor could define his question, go on to the Internet and find the answers from various sources including the National Library of Medicine, determine that the answers have scientific merit and can be relevant to his patient in question, before applying the research results. To do this, they need a certain set of knowledge and skills that have been termed as *"Evidence-based Medicine"*.

Definition:

Evidence-based medicine (EBM) has been defined as "the conscientious, explicit, and judicious use of current best evidence in making decisions about the care of individual patient. The practice of evidence based medicine means integrating individual clinical expertise with the best available external clinical evidence from systematic research[1]

Steps to practice EBM: The practice of EBM involves 5 steps:
1) Assess the patient
2) Ask questions
3) Acquire the evidence
4) Appraise the evidence and
5) Apply the evidence to the individual patient.

1. Assessing the patient

Based on the history, examination and investigations in the above case a diagnosis of irritable hip was made. One of the questions that arose was whether an X Ray or ultrasound is better at detecting a joint effusion.

2. Asking questions

During our assessment we discovered that there are issues about which we need to update our knowledge. To do this, we need to define our questions well so that searches can be done efficiently, thus saving valuable time. The components of a well-articulated question include four aspects (PICO):

- A statement describing the <u>patient</u> or disease process being addressed.
- The <u>intervention</u>, or exposure being considered
- The <u>comparison</u> intervention or exposure, when relevant
- The clinical <u>outcomes</u> of interest.

In this particular situation the question framed was – In a child with an irritable hip is X Ray better than ultrasound in detecting hip effusion.

3. Acquiring the Evidence

In this particular scenario we tried PubMed, SUM Search and TRIP database. The search terms used were "irritable hip and ultrasound and radiography", SUM search found 6 articles, of which 1 was useful[2], PubMed identified 39 articles none of them were relevant, TRIP database identified 2 "Evidence Based synopsis", one of which was an article which briefly summarized six studies.

Other useful sources from where answers could be obtained are

S.No	Information Source	Website
1	Cochrane Library	http://www.update-software.com/publications/cochrane/
2	TRIP database	http://www.tripdatabase.com/index.html
3	Pubmed	http://www.ncbi.nlm.nih.gov/entrez/query.fcgi?DB=pubmed
4	SIGN - Guidelines	http://www.sign.ac.uk/
5	SUM Search	http://sumsearch.uthscsa.edu
6	Up-To-Date	http://www.utdol.com
7	E Medicine	http://www.emedicine.com
8	Best bets	http://www.bestbets.org
9	National Guideline Clearinghouse	http://www.guidelines.gov
10	Clinical evidence	http://www.clinicalevidence.com/ceweb/index.jsp

Table1. Top 10 useful sites for practicing Evidence based Medicine.

4. Appraising the evidence – Critical appraisal

In all the studies found , ultrasonography was found to be gold standard for the detection of hip effusions. Therefore no comment about the sensitivity or specificity of ultrasound itself can be made. Radiography is, however clearly less sensitive than ultrasonography at detecting hip effusions[2].

The evidence obtained can be pre appraised like in the above example or one may have to do the critical appraisal as described below.

There are four issues in critical appraisal; Relevance, Validity, Consistency and Significance of results.

Relevance- of the research paper to your patient can be found by comparing the PICO question formulated in your case scenario with that of the research paper. If they match the study is relevant to you.

Validity – To check whether the study is good or not, we look for three kinds of bias
   a. Selection bias.
   b. Measurement bias.
   c. Bias in analysis

The presence of bias does not disqualify the study but we have to judge how it affects the study in terms of internal validity or external validity. The internal validity is important for any study as it asses the methods and results of the study. External validity is the application of the study done to the patient/population in question. No study is free of bias in terms of internal validity and one has to be assessed individually.

Consistency-
Consistency may be internal or external. Internal consistency looks at the different analysis conducted in the study. For example, in a typically paper there may be an adjusted and unadjusted analysis, certain sensitivity analysis, analysis for subgroups and analysis of primary and secondary outcomes. If these analysis yield the same answer, say in favor of the new treatment, then the results are considered internally consistent. External consistency refers to the consistency of the study's finding with the evidence from biology, from other studies and even with experience of other clinicians.

Significance of the information (results):
This depend on the study PICO and your patients PICO, also you need to answer – how good was the test/treatment in terms of statistical and clinical significance, does it match the patients concerns and expectations besides social and cultural values.

5. **Applying the results to your patient.**
   Having found the relevant information that is on the paper, valid, consistent and important, the question is whether the test or treatment may be useful for your patient/ practice? You need to determine (or best guess) your patient's disease probability or risk of adverse outcome and then consider how these will change with the application of the new test or treatment and what the risk and cost of new interventions is going to be? What does your patient, think about the benefits and risks associated with the new test or treatment? Are these considerations will be good to apply (or not to apply)?

Clinical bottom line in the above case scenario was that ultrasonography is more sensitive than plain X ray in detecting hip effusions. It should be the first imaging investigation for the irritable hip[2].
A practice, which is based on these considerations, is aptly called 'evidence based clinical practice'

2

Neonatology

2.1 Examination of Newborn

Introduction

Complete newborn examination is essential not only for detection of congenital anomalies but also to assess clinical condition soon after birth and prior to discharge. A brief physical examination should be performed in the delivery room to rule out obvious major congenital anomalies, birth injuries and cardio respiratory distress.

Time of Examination:

1. Immediately after birth

2. Before discharge from maternity unit

3. Whenever there is any concern about the infant's progress

Observation of General Condition

- Measurements: Weight, Length, Head circumference.

- Assessment of Gestational age

- General well being, feeding, weight gain.

- Posture: Healthy term infants exhibit flexion posture.

- Activity: Check if the baby is lethargic hypotonic or having asymmetrical movements of arms

- Skin: Observe for dry, peeling skin, rashes, pustules, petechiae, discoloration and pigmentation

- Look for congenital anomalies and body symmetry

- Color: Look for pallor central cyanosis, polycythemia and jaundice. Acrocyanosis may be normal within 24- 48 hours. But may be the result of cold, stress, shock and polycythemia

Systemic examination:

Head & Neck

- Palpate the anterior fontanelle, saggital, coronal and lambdoid sutures and posterior fontanelle. Exclude presence of a third fontanelle, craniotabes and premature fusion (synostosis) of skull sutures.

- Palpate for **caput and cephalhematoma** (former is a boggy swelling present at birth on the presentation part not limited by suture line, while later is fluctuant swelling appearing after 24 hours of birth and bound within the suture lines).

- The eyes are easily examined if opened by the baby spontaneously on rocking motion. Check for **red reflex**. Shine a light from the side to detect cataracts. Note presence of flattened bridge of nose or epicanthic folds.

- Choanal atresia is checked for by seeing if the infant can breathe with mouth closed and then with left and right nostril occluded alternately. If in any doubt check nasal airways with a feeding tube.

- Sternomastoid muscles should be palpated for any hematoma and the range of rotation of head to each side checked.

- A short neck is often significant and webbing should be looked for.

- Ears which are unusual in size or shape, are floppy and lacking in normal cartilage, and especially if low placed, are of significance and may be associated with urinary tract abnormalities.

- The mouth should be fully inspected with a good light and spatula and the palate inspected right back to the uvula to exclude minor degrees of cleft palate

Chest

- Asymmetry, thoracic cage defects and spinal scoliosis should be noted.

- **Apex beat** position should be confirmed to help determine heart size and possible presence of mediastinal shift or rarely dextrocardia.

- Auscultation of the chest may help give additional information.

- Presence of a significant **murmur** in itself in the absence of associated evidence of cardiac failure (i.e. increased respiratory rate, unexplained pallor, cyanosis, sweating, enlarged liver and gallop rhythm), would only be an indication for checking on femoral and peripheral pulses, x-ray of heart, doing an electrocardiograph and watching carefully.

Abdomen

Scaphoid abdomen suggests the presence of a gross diaphragmatic hernia. Slightly Distended abdomen may be normal. Grossly distended abdomen calls for more detailed examination and frequently additional investigations to determine cause.

- The **liver and spleen** should be felt for. Routine palpation of **kidneys** should be carried out to determine whether they are enlarged and if so, their position, size, shape and consistency be elicited.

- Careful inspection of **umbilicus** should include checking on adequacy of cord, tie, or clamp. Presence of single umbilical artery should alert for presence of other associated internal congenital abnormalities.

Genitalia

- Abnormality suggestive of **ambiguous genitalia** should always be checked carefully and where present, the infant referred early for specialist assessment and possible biochemical, hormonal, cytological and chromosomal study.

- In boys the presence of the 'hooded foreskin' strongly suggests the presence of **hypospadias** which strongly contra-indicates carrying out circumcision operation as the skin may be needed to repair the defect.

- Check for the **testis** bilaterally and exclude undescended or retractile testes

- Inguinal **hernias** should be looked for and other things being equal, be excised as soon as possible, preferably before the infant goes home.

- In girls an attempt should be made to separate the vulva. In this way, presence of vaginal cysts and vulval fusion will not be missed.

Anal region (Imperforated Anus)

This can be excluded by routine careful examination of the anus. Any unusual appearance in this warrants careful investigation. It has to be remembered that passage of normal meconium does not preclude the need for careful examination, e.g. imperforate anus with associated recto-vaginal fistula. While routine digital examination of anus is not regarded as necessary, insertion of thermometer in taking temperature is advocated.

Femoral Pulses

Routine palpation of femoral pulses and comparison with the brachial or radial pulses may be the first indication of the Coarctation or of interruption of the thoracic aorta. Presence of normal femoral pulses does not exclude Coarctation.

Developmental dysplasia of hip

Recognition in the early neonatal period is essential for proper treatment to be started early enough to result in the most satisfactory end results. The chances of early diagnosis by demonstration of positive **Ortolani' s sign** are greatest when the examination is carried out immediately after birth. The standard method is **Barlow's test.** (See section on CDH)

Feet

All feet should be examined at birth and for **club feet** (talipes, equino varus or talipes varus) or calcaneo valgus deformities.

Nervous System

The presence of normal activity and limb movements and normal limb tone should be checked. In addition attempts should be made to elicit normal grasp and Moro 'startle' reflex. Inability to do this strongly suggests significant abnormality of central or peripheral nervous system.

Spine

Examine for sinus, pits and meningomyelocele.

Conclusion

Routine physical examination takes only a few minutes and should be carried out in all infants at the earliest possible time after birth, and again before discharge. Routine physical examination excludes obvious abnormalities and helps make possible an earlier diagnosis of many not quite so obvious conditions. Many serious correctable congenital malformations can be detected at birth or within a few days, provided they are thought of and looked for. Early diagnosis greatly increases the chances of successful management and good outcome.

2.2 Prematurity and its complications

Birth weight is often used to define prematurity although it may not always relate well with the gestational age as in cases with small for date or IUGR babies.

Definition of prematurity:
    According to gestational age:

< 37 completed weeks:	Premature
< 32 weeks	Very premature
$\leq$ 28 weeks	Extremely premature

    According to birth weight

Low birth weight (LBW):	< 2500 Gms
Very low birth weight (VLBW):	< 1500 Gms
Extremely low birth weight (ELBW):	< 1000 Gms

Infants <1500 Gms are considered at increased risk for problems associated with prematurity.

Etiology
Predisposing factors for prematurity remain largely unknown.

Risk factors for prematurity based on epidemiologic studies:
1. Low socioeconomic status
2. Mothers < 16 or > 35 years old
3. Acute or chronic maternal illnesses
4. Multiple gestations (Twin/Triplet....)
5. Past H/O premature delivery
6. Obstetric factors
7. Fetal and placental conditions

Major expected complications in premature babies:
1. Temperature dysregulation
2. Respiratory: Respiratory Distress Syndrome (RDS)
3. Neurological: Intraventricular hemorrhage (IVH)
4. Cardiovascular: Patent Ductus Arteriosus (PDA)
5. Gastrointestinal: Necrotizing Enterocolitis (NEC), Hyperbilirubinemia)
6. Metabolic: Hypoglycemia, osteopenia of prematurity
7. Ophthalmologic: Retinopathy of Prematurity (ROP)
8. Infections

I. Temperature dysregulation

Newborns must adapt to their relatively cold environment by the metabolic production of heat as they are not capable to generate shivering response.

Definition of hypothermia: Core body temperature < 36° C.
Premature babies are more prone for hypothermia for the following reasons:
1. A larger skin surface area to weight.

2. Decreased subcutaneous and other fat stores
3. Lack of calories to provide thermogenesis and growth.
4. Limitation of oxygen consumption in some Preterm because of pulmonary problems.

Management to prevent heat loss

1. The infant after birth should be dried immediately and placed in a preheated radiant warmer that are servo controlled or in a double walled incubator.
2. The infant should be covered with warm blanket or dry towel and the head covered with a cap during transport.
3. A semi-permeable, semi-occlusive polyurethane dressing (Tegaderm) layer over the torso and extremities may reduce insensible water loss by 30%   improving fluid-electrolyte balance.
4. A radiant warmer should be used during major procedures.
5. The use of tent made of plastic wrap is effective in preventing both heat loss by convection and insensible water loss.

II. Respiratory Distress Syndrome (RDS)

Definition: The primary cause of RDS or hyaline membrane disease is inadequate pulmonary surfactant due to prematurity leading to poor inflation of lungs (stiff lungs)

History:
Predisposing risk factors for surfactant deficiency
1. Immature lungs: Prematurity, maternal diabetes, pulmonary hypoplasia.
2. Acute impairment of surfactant production, release or function due to: Perinatal asphyxia, cesarean section without labor, pulmonary infection, meconium aspiration syndrome etc.

Clinical signs are usually evident within 4 hours after birth characterized by expiratory grunting, tachypnea, chest recessions, and cyanosis

Characteristic radiographic features are low volume lungs, reticulo-granular or ground glass appearance of lungs fields with air bronchogram.

Differential Diagnoses:
Group B streptococcal Pneumonia,
Persistent Pulmonary Hypertension

Management
1. Temperature control is crucial
2. Indications for mechanical ventilation
   - For surfactant administration (Survanta: 4 ml or 100 mg/ kg/dose, given as maximum of two doses)
   - Increasing respiratory acidosis and hypoxemia despite >50% FIO_2
   - Severe respiratory distress or apnea
   - FiO_2 requirements $> 50\%$

3. Fluids and nutrition
- Careful monitoring of serum electrolytes, weight, and frequent fluid adjustments to avoid complications like PDA dehydration due to increased insensible water loss.
- VLBW in whom poor glucose tolerance and large transcutaneous losses are expected are usually started at 100-120 ml/kg/day
- ELBW maybe started at as high as 120-140 ml/kg/day using 5% dextrose

4. Electrolyte (sodium, potassium, and calcium) are started on the second day as TPN.

5. Circulation and maintenance of BP and perfusion:
- Judicious use of blood products or volume expander (normal saline)
- Inotropic agents may be used to support circulation if BP Is low

6. Infection

Pneumonia may duplicate the clinical signs and radiographic appearance of RDS so septic screen should be obtained and antibiotics started if indicated.

7. Minimal handling

Complications:

Intraventricular Hemorrhage (IVH)

Chronic lung disease (CLD)

Patent ductus Arteriosus (PDA)

Outcome
- Overall 5-10% mortality secondary to infections, IVH, CLD

Prevention
- Antenatal steroid (Dexamathasone, or Betametahsone) given to mother's with premature labor between 24-36 weeks of gestation ± with premature rupture of membranes (PROM)
- Prevention of factors related to prematurity

III. Patent Ductus Arteriosus (PDA)

Definition

PDA represents the persistence of the terminal portion of the 6th branchial arch.

Clinical Features
- Hyperdynamic precordium / bounding pulse especially dorsalis pedis pulse
- Tachypnea / tachycardia
- Murmur audible in only 22-50% of cases. It is harsh systolic ejection murmur heard over the entire precordium but loudest at the left upper sternal border and left infraclavicular area
- Cardiomegaly in 22% of cases
- Plethoric lung fields

Diagnosis: Echocardiogram (M-mode measurements):
- Ratio of LA: AO diameter > 1.5:1 is indicative of significant PDA
- Rule out PDA dependent complex cardiac disease

Complications: CLD, NEC, IVH

Differential Diagnosis
- Arteriovenous fistula
- Aortopulmonary window

Management
1. Fluid restriction: 20-30% from the baseline total fluid requirement
2. Indomethacin: 0.1 mg/kg per dose daily for 6 doses (Caution: Platelet and Renal functions should be normal)

Prevention
1. Antenatal steroid
2. Covering the chest of < 1000 gm baby during phototherapy. The light exerts a photo relaxing effect on the smooth muscle of the ascending aorta, left pulmonary artery and ductus arteriosus.
3. Cautious fluid management to avoid fluid overload.

IV. Chronic Lung Disease (CLD)

Definition
It is the result of baro-trauma produced by the mechanical ventilation with abnormal reparative processes in immature lungs of genetically susceptible infant

Diagnostic criteria
- Infants < 32 weeks gestation and requiring oxygen at 36 weeks of gestation
- Infants born > 32 weeks gestation and requiring oxygen at 28 days postnatal age.

Factors contributing to the Genesis of CLD

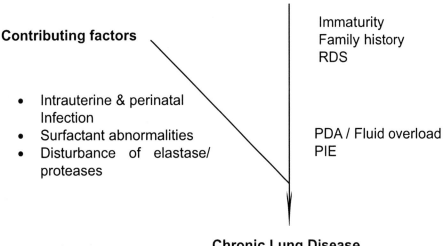

Predisposed infants

Contributing factors

Immaturity
Family history
RDS

- Intrauterine & perinatal Infection
- Surfactant abnormalities
- Disturbance of elastase/ proteases

PDA / Fluid overload
PIE

Chronic Lung Disease

Stages of CLD

Stage I	Similar to RDS
Stage II	Diffuse haziness with increased density & normal to low lung volume
Stage III	Streaky densities with bubbly lucencies (Like sponge)
Stage IV	Hyperinflation with larger lucent areas interspersed with streaky densities

Typical clinical findings

- Tachypnea, Chest recessions,
- Fine rales on auscultation.
- Oxygen dependency

Management

1. Fluid restriction 130-150 ml/kg /day
2. Nutrition is crucial to hasten the healing process. High caloric requirement 150-160 calories/kg/day).
3. A diuretic (Frusemide, spironolactone, and hydrochlorothiazide) as pulmonary edema is the major component of the disease.
4. Bronchodilator as there is a significant increase in airway resistance.
5. Corticosteroids: controversial but may be administered in infants with severe CLD who is ventilator dependent.
6. Gentle ventilation
7. Monitoring for complications like cor pulmonale, hypertension, hearing and vision impairment, and metabolic imbalance secondary to diuretics, neurodevelopmental milestones and growth parameters.

Prognosis

- Mortality: 10 -20% in the first year of life
- Radiographic abnormalities gradually improve and normalized over time but in some infants these findings often persist up to childhood.

Long-term morbidities:

1. Pulmonary: Tachypnea, recessions, wheezes, and cyanosis may last for months to years
2. Neuro-developmental delay / deficits
   - 1/3 to 2/3 of infants with CLD will be normal by 2 years of age and subsequent improvement may occur in the remaining.
   - Motor coordination delays and visio-perceptual impairment
3. Growth Failure
   - Inversely proportional to birth weight / gestational age
   - Influenced by the severity and duration of the CLD
   - Weight is most affected, head circumference the least affected

V. Intraventricular hemorrhage (IVH)

Definition

Hemorrhage into the ventricles originating from the sub-ependymal germinal matrix due to circulatory factors affecting the venous system in a premature infant.

Predisposing factors:
1. RDS, Pneumothorax, asphyxia and high ventilator pressures increasing the CVP
2. Asphyxia, seizures, hypercarbia, endotracheal tube suctioning and handling of the baby increases the cerebral blood flow.
3. Hypocarbia causes deficiency in the regulation of the germinal matrix (GM) blood flow
4. Platelet and coagulation disturbances as a result of early hypocoagulable state in a premature infant lead to increased bleeding tendency.

Staging of IVH
Grade I   Subependymal hemorrhage
Grade II   Definite IVH (< 50%) without ventricular dilatation
Grade III Extensive hemorrhage in lateral ventricles with dilatation
Grade IV   Extension of the hemorrhage into the brain parenchyma.

Clinical features
1. Catastrophic (sudden deterioration within minutes to hours)
   - Sudden increase in oxygen or ventilatory requirement
   - Fall in BP and / peripheral mottling or pallor
   - Acidosis
   - Seizures (generalized tonic) / decerebrate posturing
   - Stupor to coma / flaccid quadriparesis
   - Apnea

2. Saltatory (hours to days)
   - Altered level of consciousness
   - Hypotonia
   - Subtle seizures / abnormal eye movements
   - Abnormal tight popliteal angle

3. Asymptomatic (25-50% of cases)
   - Sudden unexplained deterioration in the general condition

Investigations
1. Cranial ultrasound (US): First scan is usually done routinely in all preterm babies between 3-5 days, the second and the timing of the follow up scan depends upon the initial abnormality and subsequent clinical course.
2. Screening for periventricular leukomalacia is performed at 4-6 weeks age or at 32-34 weeks gestational age.

Management
1. The acute management is mainly supportive and requires control of ventilation, maintenance of metabolic status, optimal nutritional state and seizure control.
2. Systemic blood pressure should be maintained with cautious attention to the fluid therapy.
3. Blood products transfusions if required.

Prognosis

Severity of IVH	Incidence of definite neurologic sequelae (%)
Grade I	5
Grade II	15
Grade III	35
Grade IV	90

Complications
1. Post hemorrhagic Hydrocephalus develops in 1/3 cases
   - Usually develops in 10-20 days following IVH
   - May arrest or spontaneously resolve in 50-65% of cases.
2. Periventricular leukomalacia leading to cerebral palsy CP

VI. Sepsis (see chapter 2.4)

VII. Hyperbilirubinemia (see chapter 2.5)

VIII. Necrotizing Enterocolitis (NEC)

Definition
Acute intestinal necrosis syndrome of unknown etiology

Risk factors
1. Prematurity is the greatest risk factor due to
   - Compromised immune system and abnormal IgA function
   - Immature intestinal mucosa
   - Suppressed GIT enzymes and humoral activity
   - Altered auto regulation of GIT blood flow

2. Maternal disorders (toxemia, abruption placentae)
3. Neonatal course   (asphyxia, PDA, rapid increase in feeds, sepsis)
4. Neonatal intervention: UAC/ UVC catheters, exchange transfusion

Interaction of main factors in the genesis of NEC

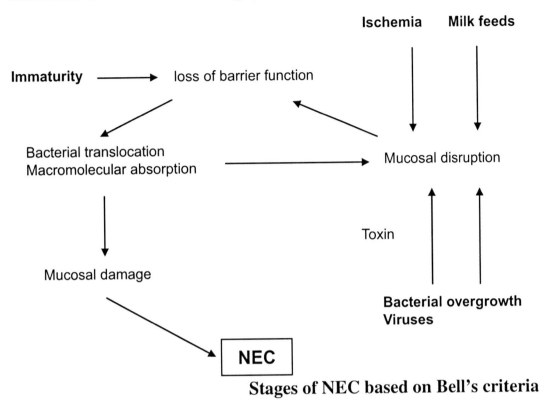

Stages of NEC based on Bell's criteria

Stage I: Suspected NEC
- History of perinatal stress
- Systemic signs: respiratory distress, temperature instability, lethargy, apnea
- GIT: Poor feeding, gastric stasis, vomiting, abdominal distension
- X-ray: distended bowel loops (non-diagnostic)

Stage II: NEC confirmed
- Any features of stage 1 plus
- Gross GI bleed, marked abdominal distention
- X-ray: distended bowel loops, pneumatosis intestinalis, fixed bowel loops

Stage III: Advanced NEC
- Any features stages I or II plus
- Deterioration of vital signs, evidence of shock and marked GI hemorrhage
- X-ray features: any features in Stage II plus pneumoperitoneum

Radiographic hallmark of NEC
1. Pneumatosis Intestinalis: air within the subserosal bowel wall and or diffuse bubbly pattern within dilated bowel loops
2. Large immobile loop suggestive of gangrenous bowel loop
3. Indications of bowel perforations
   - Pneumoperitoneum
   - Gasless abdomen

Management:
   Medical
     1. Maintenance of airway and ventilation
     2. Monitoring of vital signs
     3. NPO and gastric drainage to decompress the abdomen to prevent further gut ischemia.
     4. Volume replacements to correct losses from the circulation into the gut or peritoneum.
     5. Triple antimicrobial regimen to cover gm +ve and gm –ve and the anaerobes
     6. Maintenance of normal urea, electrolytes, calcium and hydration (Hypokalemia is common).
     7. Blood product transfusions when required
     8. Abdominal x-ray in left lateral decubitus every 6 to 12 hourly depending upon the severity.
     9. Involve the pediatric surgeon

   Surgical:
   20-50 % of Infants with NEC require surgery. Common indications for surgery are:
     1. Intestinal perforation seen 40-70% of cases
     2. Abdominal signs including fixed dilated bowel loops on serial x-rays, or abdominal erythema or the development of an inflammatory mass.
     3. Failure of intra-abdominal signs to resolve.

Outcome
     1. Relapse occurs in 10% of cases, usually within a month of initial presentation.
     2. Overall survival rate is 70-80%
     3. Mortality very high in less than 28 weeks of gestation and birth weight less than 1000 gms or the presence of extensive disease, bacteremia, DIC, or persistent ascites
     4. Long term Neuro-developmental disability in survivors with severe NEC
     5. In the absence of short bowel syndrome, the outcome is good

IX. Retinopathy of Prematurity (ROP)

Definition
ROP is the cessation of normal retinal vascular proliferation with subsequent hyper-proliferative neovascularization due to retinal ischemia and its disfigurement.

Risk factors
     1. Low gestational age, Low birth weight
     2. Duration of mechanical ventilation
     3. Hyperoxia (Oxygen toxicity)

Stages of ROP
   Stage I: Demarcation line between the vascularized and non-vascularized retina
   Stage II: The line is replaced by a ridge, which projects anteriorly into the vitreous
   Stage III: Neovascularization projecting from the ridge forwards into the vitreous
   Stage IV a) Retina is partially detached with vascular tortuosity and engorgement.
       b) Retina partially detached, macula involved
   Stage V: Retinal detachment

Management
Routine screening for ROP should be performed by an ophthalmologist on all infants with birth weight <1500 gms or <32 weeks gestation at 4-6 weeks age.

Specific treatment requires
1. Laser photocoagulation therapy to destroy the peripheral zone of avascular retina to decrease the Vaso proliferative process.
2. Correction of refractive errors

Prognosis
1. Stage I and II, most show regression
2. Stage III, show good response to treatment
3. Stage IV, functional vision is greater if macula is not involved
4. Stage V, no useful vision even with surgery and 30% develop glaucoma

Currently no proven methods are available to prevent ROP

Different Stages of ROP:

Stage I ROP

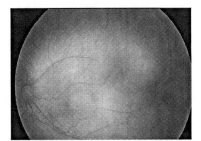

Pre-retinal detachment

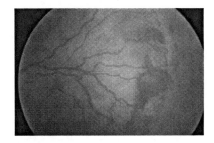

Stage II ROP

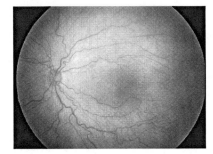

Stage III ROP

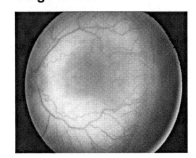

X. Osteopenia of prematurity

Definition: Under mineralization of bones

Etiology
1. Deficiency of calcium and phosphate
   - Low calcium and phosphate stores, most mineral is transferred to baby in the last trimester, which is missed due to preterm delivery.
   - Diet low in calcium and phosphorus
   - Use of diuretics esp. Frusemide

- Renal phosphorus loss

2. Vitamin D deficiency

Clinical features

Signs of rickets are evident by 2-4 months or at term corrected age

- Respiratory insufficiency or failure to wean from the ventilator
- Hypotonia
- Pain on handling due to pathological fracture
- Decreased linear growth with, frontal bossing, enlarged fontanell and sutures, craniotabes.

Radiographs

- Loss of 40% of bone mineralization can occur without x-ray changes
- X-ray changes: Osteopenia, or rachitic changes

Photon density (bone density) more reliable in detecting Osteopenia

Biochemical findings

1. Calcium or phosphate level may be normal or slightly decreased
2. Solitary elevation of the alkaline phosphatase.
3. Low 1, 25(OH) or D3 or high PTH done in refractory cases.

Management

1. Calcium and phosphate supplement, mineral fortified milk
2. Ensure vitamin D stores (150 – 400 IU/ day)

Prevention

1. Frusemide induced renal wasting
   Combine with or change to thiazides or by giving it alternate day
2. Avoid non-essential handling instead passive physical activity for 5-10 minutes may enhance growth and bone mineralization
3. In the ELBW, repeat rickets screen at 4-8 weeks post discharge.

Counseling of parents on Prematurity and its complications:

This is based on the following factors:

1. The degree of prematurity and severity of illness.
2. Growth and nutritional milestone
   - Infants with numerous complications during hospitalization may have periods of growth delays related to the medical / nutritional consequences of their illness
   - In general, infants with chronic medical conditions may not exhibit "catch up growth" until early childhood or school age and some former preterm infants may remain small throughout life.
3. Evidence of disabilities
   - Minor disabilities e.g. learning problems, poor coordination or short attention span can be overcome by early intervention
   - Severe disabilities e.g. brain damage, blindness, chronic lung disease require on going multidisciplinary care
4. Long-term outcome may be difficult to predict as in some the consequences may not be evident until the child is of school going age.

2.3 Perinatal Asphyxia

Definition
Lack of oxygen **(hypoxia)** and / or lack of perfusion **(ischemia)** of sufficient magnitude and duration prior to or during delivery causing multiorgan anoxic insult in a newborn.

Mechanisms of asphyxia during labor, delivery and immediate postnatal period:
1. Interruption of the umbilical circulation (cord compression or accidents)
2. Altered placental gas exchange (Early placental abruption)
3. Inadequate perfusion of the maternal side of the placenta (maternal hypotension / hypertension from any cause or abnormal uterine contractions)
4. Impaired maternal oxygenation (cardiopulmonary disease, anemia)
5. Failure of the neonate to accomplish lung inflation and successful transition from fetal to neonatal circulation

American Academy of Pediatrics (AAP) and American College of Obstetric and Gynecology **(ACOG) 1992** guidelines to establish diagnosis of perinatal anoxia:
1. Profound metabolic or mixed acidemia (pH < 7.00) in an umbilical artery sample
2. Persistence of an APGAR score of 0-3 for longer than 5 minutes
3. Seizures, hypotonia or coma
4. Multi organ involvement (kidneys, lungs, heart, liver and intestines)

Affected target organs: Kidneys 50%, CNS 28%, Heart 25%, Lungs 23%

Clinical manifestations (based on the Sarnat and Sarnat's 1972) staging of Hypoxic Ischemic Encephalopathy (HIE):

	Stage 1	Stage II	Stage III
Level of consciousness	Hyper alert or irritable	Lethargic or obtunded	Stuporous/comatose
Neuromuscular Control	Overactive	Diminished movements	Absent spontaneous movements
Muscle tone	Normal	Mild hypotonia	Flaccid
Posture	Mild distal flexion	Strong distal flexion	Intermittent decerebration
Stretch reflexes	Overactive	Overactive	Decreased or absent
Neonatal reflexes	Normal	Suppressed	Absent
Autonomic Function	Generalized Sympathetic	Generalized Parasympathetic	Both systems depressed
Pupils	Mydriasis	Miosis	Variable, often unequal
Respirations	Spontaneous	Spontaneous, occasional apnea	Periodic, apnea
Seizures	None	Common (24 hours of age)	Decerebration

EEG	Normal (awake)	Early: Gen.slowing Later: periodic pattern	Early: periodic pattern, Late: total isopotential
Duration of symptoms	<24 hours	2-14 days	Hours to weeks
Outcome	100% normal	80% normal; Abnormal if symp persist >5-7 days	About 50% die, remainder develop severe sequel

Differential Diagnosis

The following problems may be the cause or the result of asphyxia.

1. Effect of maternal drugs or anesthesia
2. Acute blood loss
3. Acute intracranial bleeding
4. CNS malformation
5. Neuromuscular disease
6. Cardiopulmonary disease
7. Mechanical impediments to ventilation (airway obstruction, hydrops, diaphragmatic hernia, pleural effusion, pneumothorax)
8. Infection

Complications

- Intracerebral hemorrhage
- Hypoglycemia, hypocalcemia, hyponatremia
- "Shock Lungs", Persistent Pulmonary Hypertension (PPHN)
- Transient myocardial ischemia
- Acute Tubular Necrosis (ATN)
- Necrotizing Enterocolitis (NEC)
- Liver dysfunction: consumption of clotting factors, hypoalbuminemia
- Thrombocytopenia

Investigations

1. Blood gas: Mixed acidosis / metabolic acidosis with hypoxemia
2. High lactate indicative of systemic hypoperfusion
3. Blood glucose: Hyperglycemia initially due to release of catecholamines followed within 2-3 hours by hypoglycemia that can aggravate the brain insult.
4. Hypocalcemia may compromise cardiac contractility and may cause seizures
5. CBC: thrombocytopenia
6. Renal profile indicating renal insufficiency or Hyponatremia due to SIADH
7. Septic screen to rule out associated infection as a cause
8. ECG may show sign of transient myocardial ischemia (ST depression in the mid precordium and T-wave inversion in the left precordial leads.
9. EEG: see table on Sarnat and Sarnat's HIE staging and / or to monitor sub- clinical seizures
10. Liver function tests: enzymes may be raised / albumin low.
11. Coagulation profile: PT and APPT may be prolonged
12. Urine dipstick for specific gravity, presence of hematuria
13. Fractional excretion of sodium to confirm renal ischemia

Imaging:
1. Magnetic resonance imaging (MRI) + diffusion weighted images (DWI)
   - Is the modality of choice
   - Often show abnormalities within the first few hours and prognostically useful if persistent
2. Cranial Ultrasound may reveal hemorrhage or periventricular changes in preterm babies
3. CT scan of brain
   - Assesses the degree of cerebral edema
   - Not useful in predicting sequelae in premature because of excess water and lower myelin content obscuring the gray-white matter differentiation.
   - Useful in demonstrating focal ischemic lesion in the middle cerebral artery.
4. Echocardiogram may show PPHN, decreased left ventricular contraction and to rule out cardiac anomaly

Management:
Monitoring of multi-organ function
1. Adequate airway and ventilation
   Oxygen and PCO_2 level should be maintained normal.
   - Hyperoxia may cause decrease in cerebral blood flow or exacerbate free-radical damage
   - Hypercapnia causes cerebral acidosis and cerebral vasodilatation causing more flow to the uninjured areas with relative ischemia to damaged areas ("steal phenomenon") and extension of infarct size. Also increase flow is associated with intra-cerebral hemorrhage due to loss of cerebrovascular autoregulation.
   - Hypocapnia (< 3.5 KPA) may decrease Cerebral blood flow

2. Replace volume slowly preferably guided by central venous pressure (CVP) keeping 5-8 mmHg in term and 3-5 mmHg in prematures

3. Maintain cerebral perfusion by maintaining the mean arterial pressure (MAP) 45-50 mm Hg in term infants, 35 - 40 mmHg in 1000 -2000 gms and 30 -35 mmHg in < 1000 gms babies

4. Electrolytes, glucose, and calcium should be maintained normal.

5. Control of seizures (Phenobarbitone, Phenytoin, midazolam) to limit further compromise of the neurologic status

6. Blood products transfusion if required

7. To avoid fluid overload and the exacerbation of cerebral edema, both SIADH and ATN (acute tubular necrosis) should be managed by limitation of free water administration, Give only replacement of insensible losses plus urine output, usually 60 ml /kg /day

Counseling:
1. The outcome of HIE depends on the severity of the injury and the degree of brain damage. The Sarnat scores are commonly used indicator of HIE predictive ability for which infants are at risk for sequelae. Long-term outcome may be difficult to predict as in some the

consequences may not be evident until the child is school aged.

2. Indicators of poor outcome
   - Severe prolonged asphyxia
   - HIE stage III
   - Early onset Seizures < 12 hours that are difficult to control
   - Presentation of abnormal neurological signs at discharge (usually >1-2 weeks of age) esp. the absence of Moro's reflex
   - Persistent Oliguria < 1 ml kg/hr for 36 hours
   - MRI showing abnormal signal in Diffusion Weighted study
   - Elevated intracranial pressure (ICP) > 10 mmHg

3. Management of disabilities
   - Minor disabilities, learning problems, poor coordination or short attention span or visual impairment maybe improved by early intervention.
   - Severe disabilities e.g. brain damage, blindness; chronic lung disease will obviously require multi disciplinary approach to the care of major and minor needs of these babies.
   - 3-13% of cerebral palsy are associated with intrapartum asphyxia
   - Physio / occupational therapy

4. Regular follow up by Pediatrician

2.4 Neonatal Sepsis

Introduction:

Despite advances in perinatal care in the past decades, sepsis and its complications still continue to be a significant cause of morbidity and mortality in hospitalized and non-hospitalized preterm and mature babies. Early recognition, diagnosis and treatment are essential as the progression from mild symptoms to death can occur in less than 24 hours.

History: Enquire about risk factors
1. **Maternal factors**
   a. Premature onset of labor
   b. Prolonged rupture of membranes (PROM) > 18 hours
   c. Maternal peripartum infection (WBC > 15000, fever > 100.4°F or 38.4°c during or within 24 hours of labor, maternal tachycardia, fetal tachycardia, uterine tenderness and foul smelling amniotic fluid)
   d. Vaginal discharge
   e. Prolonged labor
   f. Difficult / instrumental delivery
   g. Poor socioeconomic status
   h. Maternal substance abuse
   i. Maternal urinary tract infection
   j. More than six per vaginal examinations
   k. Sustained fetal tachycardia (> 160/min)
   l. Unhygienic delivery

2. **Neonatal risk factors**
   a. Prematurity (< 37 weeks)
   b. Low birth weight (rate of sepsis is 10 times higher in infant < 1000 gms and 8 x higher in 1000-1500gms compared with infants weighing 2000-2500gms. The rate of meningitis is 3-17 x more in infant < 2500gms.
   c. Male sex
   d. Black race
   e. Multiple congenital anomalies
   f. Low APGAR scores (< 6 at 1 or 5 minutes)
   g. Infants >7 days who required intensive care (degree of prematurity, presence of central venous or arterial catheter and poor skin integrity)

Why newborns are more susceptible for sepsis?
1. Host immunity
   a) Neutrophils:
   - Defective chemotaxis and opsonization
   - Less deformable, less able to move to the site of inflammation.
   - Neutrophils reserves are easily depleted because of the diminished response of the bone marrow esp. in premature babies.
   - Decrease adherence and less ability to marginate
   - Failure to deaggregate in response to chemotactic factors
   b) Macrophages / monocytes
   - The chemotactic and bactericidal activity and antigen presentation by these cells are not fully competent

c) T-cells
  • Don't effectively produce the cytokines that assist with B cells stimulation and differentiation

d) Immunoglobulin
  • IgM low, IgE trace, IgG deficient, IgA absent

e) Complement
  • Deficiency in the alternative > classic pathway.

2. Prematurity
  • Inadequate amount of transferred maternal immunoglobulin
  • Low complement
  • Poor skin cornification

3. Portal of Entry
  • Abrasions and cuts, mucosal injury, cannula, catheters and endotracheal tube placements open the way for bacterial invasion

4. Indiscriminate use of antibiotics

Classification and Characteristics of Neonatal Sepsis:

Characteristics	1. Early onset (EOS)	2. Late onset (LOS)
Onset	90% presents within 24 hours, 5% between 24-48 hours, rest up to 6 days of age.	7-28 days
Risk	Prematurity, chorioamnionitis, PROM > 18 hrs	Prematurity, Poor hygiene NICU interventions
Presentation	Respiratory	Fever, CNS changes
Transmission	Vertical, maternal genital tract	Postnatal environment
Course	Fulminant esp. in premature with multisystem involvement. Pneumonia common	Insidious, focal infection. Meningitis common
Organisms	Group B streptococci (GBS), E. Coli Listeria Monocytogenes	Staphylococci, E, Coli, Enterobacter, Candida, Pseudomonas, Serratia, Acinetobacter, Anaerobes (10 -15 %)
Mortality	15-50 %	10-15 %

Clinical presentations of early onset of sepsis:
  • Can manifest as asymptomatic bacteremia, generalized sepsis, pneumonia and / or meningitis.
  • Clinical signs usually apparent in the first hours of life. 90% are symptomatic by 24 hours of age.
  • Respiratory distress is the most common presenting symptoms (mild tachypnea and grunting with or without supplemental oxygen requirement to respiratory failure.
  • Gastrointestinal symptoms: poor feeding, vomiting, and ileus

- Less common presentations are: Irritability, lethargy, temperature instability, poor perfusion and hypotension.
- Persistent pulmonary hypertension (PPHN) can accompany sepsis.
- DIC with purpura and petechiae can occur with more severe septic shock
- Meningitis may presents as seizure, apnea and depressed sensorium but there may not be any neurological features

Clinical manifestations of late onset sepsis:
- Range from mild increase in apnea to fulminant sepsis
- Lethargy
- Increase in number and severity of apnea
- Feeding intolerance
- Temperature instability
- Increase in Ventilatory support or dependency

Investigations:
No single laboratory test has been found to have acceptable sensitivity and specificity for predicting infection. The approach to newborn suspected of sepsis must start with review of risk factors, evaluation of clinical manifestations with interpretation of laboratory studies.

Most importantly one must have a high index of suspicion, low threshold for performing septic screen and starting the antibiotics for any presumed sepsis until proven otherwise.

1. Cultures
  a) Blood culture
- Aerobic cultures are appropriate for most of the bacterial causes of neonatal sepsis.
- Anaerobic cultures are indicated in neonates with abscesses, bowel involvement, refractory pneumonia and massive hemolysis
- Fungal cultures should be sent whenever clinically suspected

Blood should be obtained from peripheral vein or from umbilical vessel right after placement. Blood sample should not be less than 0.5 ml.

  b) CSF cultures   including cell count, protein, glucose and gram stain
  c) Urine culture has little value in the immediate postnatal period but of value in late onset sepsis
  d) Culture of abscesses and / or discharge
  e) Gram stain for preliminary identification of the organism.

2. Complete blood and differential counts should be ordered in all high-risk   infants. Serial results may be more useful to determine changes associated with infection. Normal counts have been seen in 50% of culture positive sepsis. Thrombocytopenia is an indicator to sepsis.

3. C-reactive protein (CRP), an acute phase protein associated with tissue injury is elevated in 50- 90% of infants with systemic bacterial infections. It rises within 24 hours of infection, peaks within 2-3days and remains elevated until infection is resolved. It may be an indicator used as to show response to antibiotics and/ or relapse of infection.

4. Coagulation profile: PT, APTT, fibrinogen, FDP levels

5. Imaging
- Chest x-ray may reveal presence of infiltrates / or consolidation, Atelectasis or granular pattern
- Abdominal x-ray in suspected necrotizing enterocolitis
- Head ultrasound to demonstrate the progression of complications
- Abdominal ultrasound may show fungal balls in the kidneys or bladder
- CT scan to document complications of meningeal infection.
- Bone scan for suspected osteomyelitis

6. Biochemical studies
- Acid-base parameters
- Serum electrolytes, glucose, calcium
- Liver function test

Management of neonatal sepsis:
1. Maintenance of airway and ventilation
2. Reliable vascular access and monitoring of vital signs (Temperature, HR, RR, BP)
3. Fluid and electrolyte balance. Treatment of shock if present with fluids and inotropes
4. Antimicrobial therapy should be instituted earliest.
5. Blood products (PRBC, platelet, FFP) transfusions when required.
6. Nutrition to offset the effect of excessive catabolism.

Choice of antimicrobial regimen for sepsis and meningitis:
The initial choice of antibiotics prior to results of culture depends on local knowledge of predominance of micro-organism and their sensitivity pattern. Ampicillin plus Gentamycin is usual combination in EOS and cloxacillin plus Cefotaxime in LOS. Antibiotic can later be changed according to the culture results.

Organisms	Antibiotic	Sepsis	Meningitis
GBS	Ampicillin or Penicillin G	10-14days	21 days
E. Coli	Cefotaxime or ampicillin and Gentamicin	14 days	21 days
Coagulase Negative Staph.	Vancomycin	7 days	
Enterobacter Klebsiella	Cefotaxime, or Cefipime or Meropenem Plus Gentamycin	14 days	21 days
Enterococcus	Ampicilline or Vancomycin Plus Gentamicin	10 days	21 days
Listeria	Ampicilline or Penicillin Plus Gentamycin.	10-14 days	21 days

Pseudomonas	Ceftazidime or Piperacillin/Tazobactam Plus Gentamicin or Tobramycin	14 days	21 days
Staph Aureus	Nafcillin	10-14 days	21 days

Complications:

    Early:

        Hypoglycemia

        Bleeding abnormalities

        Hypotension, shock and multi-organ failure

    Late:

        Neurological complications in meningitis (Hydrocephalus, Cerebral palsy, Mental retardation)

        Chronic lung disease

        Renal failure

        NEC

Prognosis

- With early diagnosis and treatment, long-term complications can be prevented.
- Related directly to the early recognition and prompt treatment. Residual neurological damage can occur in 15-30%.

Counseling based on the following

1. Outcome depending on the gestational age and disease acuity, prevention remains the cornerstone in the management of sepsis.
2. Hygiene and routine practices such as hand washing,
3. Umbilical Cord care and breastfeeding to prevent infection
4. Updating immunizations

2.5 Neonatal Hyperbilirubinemia

Definition:
Jaundice is visible yellow discoloration of skin and sclera due to elevated serum bilirubin. In neonates clinical jaundice may appear when the serum total bilirubin (STB) levels exceed 120 micro mol/L. Chemical Hyperbilirubinemia is defined as an STB level of >2.0 mg/dl (34 u mol/L).

Since all new born babies do get jaundice in initial few days of life, a distinction has to be made between benign **Physiological jaundice** and **Pathological Hyperbilirubinemia** that requires further evaluation and intervention.

Types of Neonatal Jaundice:
1. Physiologic v/s Pathologic Hyperbilirubinemia
2. Unconjugated v/s Conjugated Hyperbilirubinemia

Physiologic Jaundice
Definition:
> **Healthy term baby:** Unconjugated bilirubin level <200 u mol/L by day 3-4 falling gradually in 2-3 d reaching normal level before 2 wks of age

> **Preterm:** Unconjugated bilirubin 170-204 u mol/L by 5-6 days falling gradually, persisting for up-to 2-4 wks.

Causes: It is caused due to multiple factors:
1. Short life span and Increase breakdown of fetal RBC
2. Higher erythrocyte mass (Physiological polycythemia) in the neonate
3. Decrease albumin, ligandin, UDPG
4. Liver immaturity leading to decreased conjugation of bilirubin
5. Sterile gut

Clinical evaluation of a newborn with jaundice:
History:
- Time of onset of jaundice
- Gestational age and birth weight
- Family history of jaundice, anemia, splenectomy
- Family history of liver disease
- History of significant jaundice in previous sibling
- Maternal history: TORCH Infection, Rh or ABO incompatibility
- L & D: oxytocin use, delayed cord clamping, perinatal asphyxia & trauma
- History of meconium passage, Cephalhematoma
- Feeding history

Physical Examination
- Assess the extant or depth of jaundice (Light or deep)
- Presence of pallor, plethora, petechiae, edema/hydrops
- Bruises, Cephalhematoma or enclosed hemorrhage
- Hepato-splenomegaly
- Signs of sepsis
- Chorioretinitis
- Evidence of hypothyroidism

Pathological Neonatal Jaundice

Occurs when additional factors are superimposed over the basic ones described above

Features of Pathologic Jaundice

- Clinical jaundice in the first 24 hours of life
- Jaundice in sick New-born
- Total Bilirubin level above physiologic limits
  - ➢ 250 u mol/L on Day 2
  - ➢ 300 u mol/L thereafter
- Direct serum bilirubin concentration >1.5-2 mg/dl or >20% of total bilirubin
- Serum total Bilirubin concentration increasing by more than 5 u mol/L per hour or 5 mg/dl (85 u mol/L) per day
- Jaundice persisting for >2 weeks in a full-term infant and 3 weeks in pre-term infants
- Pale stool and dark urine color

Causes of Unconjugated Hyperbilirubinemia

1. Increased hemolysis (Excessive production of bilirubin)
   - A. Blood group incompatibilities
     - a. Rh Isoimmunization
     - b. ABO Incompatibility
     - c. Minor blood group incompatibility
   - B. RBC enzyme abnormalities
     - a. G6PD Deficiency
     - b. Pyruvate kinase deficiency
   - C. Sepsis
   - D. RBC membrane defects
     - a. Spherocytosis
     - b. Elliptocytosis
     - c. Poikilocytosis
2. Non-hemolytic processes
   - A. Accumulation of blood in extra vascular compartments
     - a. Cephalhematoma
     - b. Bruising
     - c. Occult bleeding
   - B. Increased bilirubin production
     - a. Polycythemia
     - b. IDM (Infant of Diabetic Mother)
3. Impaired conjugation or excretion
   - A. Increased/enhanced entero-hepatic circulation
     - a. Bowel obstruction
     - b. Ileus
     - c. Infant not fed
   - B. Hormonal deficiency/ decreased clearance
     - a. IEM (Inborn Error of Metabolism)
     - b. Hypothyroidism
     - c. Hypopituitarism
     - d. Breast Milk Jaundice

     C. Disorders of bilirubin metabolism
        a. Crigler-Najjar syndrome
        b. Gilbert Disease
        c. Lucey-Driscoll syndrome

Causes of Conjugated Hyperbilirubinemia
1. Extra hepatic Obstructed bile flow with or without hepato-cellular injury
    A. Biliary Atresia
    B. Choledochal cyst
2. Hepatocyte injury with normal bile ducts
    A. Iatrogenic (Use of TPN)
    B. Infections (Viral, bacterial, parasitic)
    C. Metabolic
    D. Storage diseases
    E. Part of syndromes

Investigations:

Early-onset Jaundice:
- Total and Direct Bilirubin
- Blood Group and DCT
- CBC. Reticulocyte count
- Infection screen: viral/ bacterial
- Serology for congenital (STORCH) infections, Urine for CMV
- G6PD

Prolonged Jaundice
- Total and Direct Bilirubin
- Thyroid Function Test
- Urine for reducing substance: Clinistix and clinitest (Galactosemia)
- LFT's
- Alpha 1 antitrypsin assay
- Screen for Cystic Fibrosis
- Serum amino acid screen

Management Unconjugated Hyperbilirubinemia in the Newborn Infant
- Adequate hydration
- Phototherapy
- Exchange Transfusion
- Pharmacological agents
  - inhibition of heme oxygenase
  - Liver enzyme induction by use of Phenobarbitone
  - suppression of isoimmune hemolysis
  - inhibition of enterohepatic circulation by urso-deoxycholic acid
  - Bile acid binding with choles tyramine

Mechanism of Phototherapy action
1. Photoisomerization of un-conjugated bilirubin
2. Structural isomerization
3. Photo-oxidation

Side effects of Phototherapy
1. Increase insensible water loss
2. Watery diarrhea
3. Low Ca in premature
4. Mutations, sister chromatid exchange & DNA breaks
5. Bronze baby syndrome
6. Prolonged ductal patency in ELBW (PDA)
7. Disturbed bonding of mother and baby

Exchange Transfusion
Indications
- When Phototherapy fails to prevent rise in bilirubin to toxic levels
- Severe in utero hemolysis
- Bilirubin level in excess of the Phototherapy levels
- Signs and symptoms of acute bilirubin encephalopathy

Complications of Exchange Transfusion
- Electrolyte and acid base disturbances: Hypocalcaemia, Hypomagnesaemia, Hypoglycemia, Hyperkalemia, Metabolic acidosis
- Circulatory overload
- Infections
- Bleeding
- Hypothermia / Hyperthermia
- NEC
- Complications of Umbilical catheters

Complications of Hyperbilirubinemia
1. **Acute Bilirubin Encephalopathy**
   A. Early phase: Lethargy, Hypotonia, Poor sucking and feeding
   B. Intermediate phase: Moderate stupor, Irritability and Hypertonia
   C. Advanced phase
      a. Deep stupor to coma
      b. Pronounced retrocollis-opisthotonos
      c. High pitch shrill cry
      d. Poor feeding
      e. Apnea, seizures/ death
2. **Chronic bilirubin encephalopathy (Kernicterus)**
   A. athetoid cerebral palsy
   B. Hearing dysfunction
   C. Upward gaze palsy of eyes
   D. Intellectual handicap

Long Term Follow up of a New born with Jaundice
- BAEP for hearing check
- Neurodevelopment (Assessment of milestones) up to school age
- Evaluation for Neuro-deficits.

2.6 Prolonged Neonatal Jaundice

Definition: Any jaundice that still present after 10 days of age in term and 14 days in pre-term

Causes of prolonged Jaundice in New born babies:
- Persistent Hemolysis:
  - RBC enzyme deficiency- G6PD, and others
  - RBC morphology defects-Spherocytosis,
- Liver diseases. - Neonatal hepatitis, Biliary atresia
- Metabolic liver diseases: Galactosemia, Tyrosinemia, Fructosemia, Urea Cycle Disease, lipid storage dis., Defects of bile acid metabolism, Alfa1Anti trypsin def.
- Inspissated bile syndrome secondary to Hemolytic Disease of Newborn, Total Parenteral Nutrition
- Cystic fibrosis
- Inherited defect of bilirubin transport- Dubin Johnson and Rotor syndrome
- Inherited defect of bilirubin conjugation- Criggler Najjar syndrome 1&2, Gilbert disease
- Hypothyroidism
- Infection esp. Low grade UTI
- Pyloric stenosis
- Breast milk jaundice

Scheme of Investigations and Differential diagnosis of Prolonged Neonatal Jaundice:

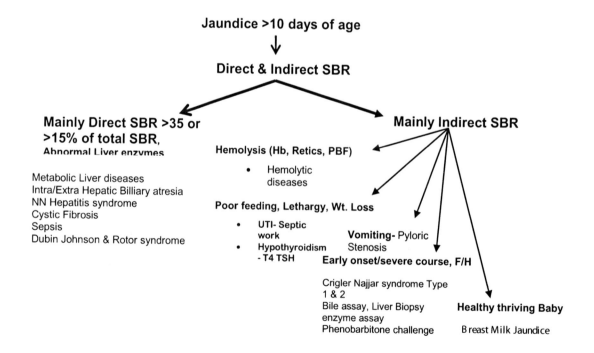

2.7 Neonatal Parenteral Nutrition

Introduction:
- Many sick and/or pre-term newborns cannot obtain adequate nutrition via the GI tract and, thus, require parenteral nutrition (**PN**) support.
- In some, GI function is adequate to allow partial feedings (**Partial PN**)
- In others, the GI tract may not function for days to weeks (e.g., necrotizing enterocolitis), so the infant receives total nutrition parenterally (**TPN**).

General Guidelines
- Sick newborns usually have increased caloric requirements.
- Minimal caloric requirements to prevent catabolism are at least 30-50 kcal/kg/d.
- For growth, minimal requirements are 80 kcal/kg/d and protein intake of >2 gm/kg/d. For adequate growth, aim for 100 kcal/kg/d and protein intake of 3 g/kg/d for term infants and 3.5 g/kg/d for pre-term infants.
- Providing parenteral amino acids at a rate of 1.5 to 2 g/kg/d as soon as possible after birth (within hours) can preserve limited body protein stores in sick premature.
- Although growth can be obtained with PN, **Enteral feedings should be initiated as soon as feasible**, because of risks associated with PN.

Infusion routes:
1. **Peripheral** route is used for partial PN and short-term use. Peripheral PN solutions cannot exceed 12.5% dextrose or 3.5 % amino acids due to the risk of thrombophlebitis and should not contain calcium because of the serious complications resulting from extravasations of calcium and consequent tissue necrosis.
2. **A central venous catheter delivers Central PN.** This route is used for patients who require long-term nutritional support, usually TPN.

Composition of Parenteral Nutrition
1. Fluid requirements:

60 – 75 ml/kg	1st day of life
75 – 85 ml/kg	2nd day
80 – 100 ml/kg	3rd day
100 -125 ml/kg	4th day
125 – 150 ml/kg	5th day and thereafter

This requirement may be increased if losses are increased, e.g., very low birth weight (< 1 kg), gastroschisis, omphalocele and phototherapy.

2. Fluid requirements in Infants and Children age one month or older

Weight	Fluid
1 – 10 kg	100 ml/kg/d
10 – 20 kg	1000 ml + 50 ml/each kg over 10
>20 kg	1500 ml + 20 ml/each kg over 20

3. **Protein:**
   - Start amino acids at 1 g/kg/d. Advance by 0.5 gm/kg/d in pre-term infants and by 0.5 – 1 gm/kg/d in term infants.
   - Recommended maximum is 3 g/kg/d in term infants and 3.5 g/kg/d in pre-term infants and 4 g/kg/d for Extremely LBW infants.
   - Include protein in your caloric count. Protein yields 4 kcal/g
   - Potential complications/risks include:
     - Acidosis
     - Hyper-ammonemia
     - Elevated BUN
     - Cholestasis with prolonged administration

4. **Carbohydrate: is administered as dextrose**
   - Begin usually with 4-6 mg/kg/min using D10 – D12.5 % solution. Alternatively, calculate the glucose infusion rate that the infant is already receiving and advance from there.
   - Very pre-term infants may not tolerate that much dextrose and may even need small dose of insulin as an infusion to achieve adequate caloric intake without hyperglycemia.
   - Advance by 1-3 mg/kg/min daily to a maximum of 12 to 15 mg/kg/min
   - Dextrose yields 3.4 kcal/g.
   - Potential complications/risks include:
     - Hyperglycemia or hypoglycemia
     - Glycosuria and potential osmotic diuresis
     - Cholestasis and/or hepatic steatosis with high caloric intake usually from long-term high concentration infusion.

5. **Fat**
   - Intravenous lipid emulsions are essential components of TPN. They provide essential fatty acids and are a concentrated energy source critical for growth and development of infants not receiving enteral feedings.
   - There are potential safety concerns regarding administration of lipid emulsions to very low birth weight infants and infants with Hyperbilirubinemia, pulmonary hypertension and serious pulmonary disease.
   - To minimize the adverse effects of lipids, use the following guidelines:
     - Provide sufficient lipids to prevent essential fatty acid deficiency
     - Monitor for evidence of lipid intolerance
     - Adjust lipid dose based on clinical status
   - A lipid intake of 0.25 – 0.5 g/kg/d is required to prevent essential fatty acid deficiency.
   - Include lipid emulsion in calculations of total fluid intake.
   - Lipids yield 9 kcal/g
   - IV lipid preparations are available as a 20% soybean emulsion that yields 2 kcal/ml
   - Deliver IV lipids over 20 hours (Keeping 4 Hours off)
   - Do not allow lipids to exceed 60% of total caloric intake.
   - Potential complications/risks include:
     - Hyperlipidemia
     - Potential risk of kernicterus at low levels of unconjugated bilirubin because of displacement of bilirubin from albumin binding sites by free fatty acids.

> Potential increased risk or exacerbation of chronic lung disease
> Potential exacerbation of Persistent Pulmonary Hypertension
> Lipid overload syndrome with coagulopathy and liver failure.
> Sepsis: Lipids are good medium for bacterial growth

Guidelines for initiating and increasing I V lipid emulsions according to clinical status:

Gestation	Weight / Diagnosis	Initiate at 0.5 g/kg/d by:	Advance by 0.5 g/kg/d by:	Reaching to 3 g/kg/d by:
Pre-term	<1,500 g/ stable	3rd Day of life	7th day of life	11th day life
	> 1,500 g/ stable	3rd day of life	4th day of life	9th day of life
	Very unstable	3rd day of life	When status improve	When status improve
Term	No Pulm. disease	3rd day of life	4th day of life	9th day of life
	Severe pulmonary disease	Consider at 7th day of life	When status improves	When status improves

6. **Electrolytes and Minerals**
   - Electrolyte requirements are adjusted according to serum values and clinical conditions

Sodium	2-4 mmol/kg/d
Potassium	2-3 mmol/kg/d
Chloride	2-4 mmol/kg/d
Calcium	50-90 mg/kg/d
Phosphate	40-70 mg/kg/d
Magnesium	0.5-1 mmol/kg/d

   - Acetate is metabolized to HCO_3 and is used to adjust acid-base status.

7. **Trace Elements**
   - Trace elements are recommended as 0.2 ml/kg/d of trace element solution containing zinc, manganese, copper and chromium.
   - Pre-term infants need additional zinc (300 mcg/kg/d) and selenium (2 mcg/kg/d).
   - Term infants on TPN >4 weeks also need selenium (2 mcg/kg/d)
   - In infants with cholestasis, discontinue the trace element solution and give

Zinc	100 mcg/kg/d for term infants, 400 mcg/d total for pre-term infants
Chromium	0.17 mcg kg/d
Selenium	2.0 mcg/kg/d

8. **Vitamins**
   - Pediatric multivitamins are recommended as 2 to 5 ml/kg/d.

9. Heparin

- I unit per ml is added to all central venous lines and to all peripheral infusions running at < 2 ml/hr in order to maintain catheter patency.

Suggested Monitoring during Parenteral Nutrition

Parameter	Frequency
Weight	Daily
Length and OFC	Weekly
Serum glucose	Every shift during week 1, then daily
Serum electrolytes, Mg, Ca, P, Hct	2-3 times in first week then weekly
Alkaline phosphatase, LFT	Weekly

Discontinuation of Parenteral Nutrition

- PN may be stopped when the infant is tolerating > 100 cc/kg of enteral feeding or is receiving < 25 cc/kg/d of PN, The rate of dextrose administration should be tapered to prevent rebound hypoglycemia while Lipids may be stopped without tapering.

2.8 Neonatal Seizures

Neonatal period is limited to the first 28 days of life in a term infant. For premature infants, this goes from birth until 44 weeks from conception.
Most neonatal seizures occur in the first 10 days of life.

Incidence: 3/1000 in full term infants to 60/1000 in premature infants.

Neonatal seizures markedly increases long-term morbidity & mortality. Presence of neonatal seizures is an important predictor of long-term physical and cognitive deficits.

Types of seizures:

1. **Subtle seizures:** Are the most common type of seizures seen in neonates, comprising about half of all seizures in term & preterm newborns. It includes a broad spectrum of behavioral phenomena, occurring in isolation or in combination like horizontal eye deviation, chewing, sucking or lip smacking movements, drooling, and limb movements like cycling, boxing, rowing or swinging movements. Autonomic phenomena with or without motor manifestations.
2. **Clonic:** Stereotypic and repetitive biphasic movements with a fast contraction and slow relaxation phase. Most commonly unifocal may be multifocal or generalized.
3. **Tonic:** Sustained period of muscle contraction without repetitive features. It may be generalized or focal. Prognosis is poor.
4. **Myoclonic:** Fast contractions and non-rhythmic character. May occur in multifocal or generalized pattern. Usually associated with a poor long term outcome.

Difference between true and pseudo seizures:
   True seizures are rarely stimulus-sensitive, cannot be abolished by passive restraint or repositioning of the baby, are associated with autonomic changes or ocular phenomenon.

Causes of Neonatal seizures:

   1. **Asphyxia, Hypoxic ischemic encephalopathy.**
   2. **Hemorrhage**, IVH, neonatal arterial stroke,
   3. **Cerebral vein thrombosis.**
   4. **Infections**, like TORCH infection, Bacterial, e.g. E. Coli, GBS Sepsis, Viral.
   5. **Electrolytes imbalance,**
      Hypoglycemia
      Hypocalcaemia
      Hyper / hyponatremia
      Hypomagnesaemia
   6. **Inborn Error of Metabolism**
      Nonketotic hyperglycinemia, Urea cycle defects, MSUD and Organic acidemia.
   7. **Pyridoxine deficiency / dependency.**
   8. **Narcotic drugs withdrawal.**
   9. **Cerebral Dysgenesis like Agyria/pachygyria, polymicrogyria.**
   10. **Benign familial neonatal seizures.**
   11. **Benign idiopathic neonatal seizures**

Evaluation of Neonatal Seizures:

History: Clinical history provides important clues to the likely etiology
    Family history: of neonatal seizures, bleeding disorder.
    Antenatal: H/o TORCH infections, fetal distress, PIH, drugs.
    Natal: Events of second stage of labor, type of delivery, h/o fetal distress, resuscitation, Apgar score, Gestation, etc.
    Postnatal: Onset of seizures, h/o feeding, temperature instability etc.

Physical Examination:

Infants with neonatal seizures are frequently lethargic between seizures often appear sick. Look for underlying cause (Sepsis, Intracranial bleeding, Dysmorphic syndrome, Hepatomegaly, Micro or macrocephaly etc.)
Neurological exam may be essentially normal in between the seizures.

Lab studies
    CBC, CRP,
    Full septic work up including blood, urine & CSF culture
    Serum electrolytes, blood sugar, Ca, Mg and blood gases
    Coagulation profile
    TORCH screen
    Tandem MS, Urine organic acids

Imaging
    Cranial ultrasound
    Cranial CT scan or
    Cranial MRI

Other tests:
    EEG
    Video EEG
    Echocardiography

Management of NN seizures:

Step 1 Stabilize vital signs like heart rate, respiration, blood pressure, hydration etc.

Step 2 Correct transient metabolic disturbances.
    a. Hypoglycemia: target blood sugar 4 to 6 mmol/L
    10% dextrose water I.V. bolus dose 2-4 ml/kg, Followed by infusion to provide glucose @ 6-8 mg/kg/min, tapering off gradually
    b. Hypocalcaemia: 10% Ca. Gluconate IV at 2 ml/kg slow push under cardiac monitoring.
    c. Hypomagnesemia, 50% Magnesium sulphate I/M at 0.2 ml/kg.

Step 3 First line drug, **Phenobarbital** 20 mg/kg I/V loading dose followed by maintenance dose 5-8 mg/kg/day.

Step 4 Second line drug, **Phenytoin** 20 mg/kg, IV, not faster than 1 mg/kg/mint, Maintenance dose 5-8 mg/kg/day.

Step 5 Benzodiazepines
   a. **Lorazepam**, 0.05-0.1 mg/kg IV slow push, onset within 2-3 mints.
   b. **Diazepam**, 0.1-0.3 mg/kg IV, slowly.
   c. **Midazolam:** bolus 0.02 –0.1 mg/kg may be followed by Continuous infusion of 0.06-0.4 mg/kg/hr

Other steps:
   Pyridoxine trial: In refractory cases Pyridoxine 50-100 mg IV may be used under continuous EEG monitoring, if baby respond, maintenance dose 10-100 mg/day is then continued. If I.V. preparation is not available, oral dose of 50 mg bid can be used.

   Intubation /Ventilation if indicated

Further inpatient care:
   Patients with seizures resulting from intracranial hemorrhage should have head circumference measurement daily, rapid increase in head circumference indicate hydrocephalus.
   Anticonvulsants medication's concentration should be monitored during initial periods.
   A general recommendation is to use anticonvulsants for 6-12 wks, if baby remain seizure free then medication may be tapered gradually or the dose not increased thereby letting the baby grow out of anticonvulsant treatment.
   If baby on 2 anticonvulsants than one should be tapered first before considering withdrawing the other, if seizures recur, then restart original anticonvulsants.

Follow-up care:
   Neurology out patient evaluation and follow up are needed. Developmental evaluation is required for early identification of physical or cognitive deficits.
   Complications:
         Cerebral palsy Spasticity.
         Hydrocephalus
         Mental retardation
         Epilepsy
         Feeding difficulties
         Deafness

Prognosis and counseling:
   Major predictors of long-term outcome:
         1) Etiology
         2) EEG
         3) Gestational age.
         4) Others- Neurological exam & neuroimaging findings

If EEG background is normal, the prognosis is excellent for seizures to resolve and normal development is likely. Severe EEG background abnormalities indicate poor prognosis, such babies frequently develop cerebral palsy and epilepsy. The presence of spikes on EEG is associated with a 30% risk of developing future epilepsy.

The prognosis following neonatal seizures that result from isolated subarachnoid hemorrhage is excellent, with 90% of children not having neurological deficit.

Gestational age has prognostic significance, seizures in preterm babies have more adverse neurological outcome as compared to term infants.

Benign familial neonatal seizures typically occur in first 48-72 hrs; disappear by 2-6 months of age. A family history of seizure is usual and baby's development is normal.

Benign idiopathic neonatal seizures typically present at 5th day of life and are often unifocal.

Benign sleep Myoclonus is a benign condition, occurring only during sleep. EEG is normal.

Prognosis of NN seizure according to etiology

Etiology	Normal Outcome
Hypoxia-ischemia	**50%**
Meningitis	50%
Hypoglycemia	50%
Subarachnoid Hemorrhage	90%
Early hypocalcaemia	50%
Late Hypocalcaemia	100%
Intraventricular hemorrhage	10%
Cerebral Dysgenesis	0 %
Unknown etiology	75%

Genetics

3.1 Approach to a Dysmorphic Child

Syndromes represent a recognizable pattern of congenital anomalies. One should consider the possibility of a syndrome in a dysmorphic child if a child has:

> 3 minor anomalies or
> 1 major anomaly or
One major and two minor anomalies.

Definitions:

1. **Malformations:** are defects due to developmental anomalies of body parts. Examples are cleft lip/palate, Polydactyly or Holoprosencephaly. They can be major or minor, isolated or multiple.

   Major malformations are severe, cause functional defects and may need surgical intervention. The frequency at birth is 2-3%. e.g. Cleft lip/Palate, CHD's etc.

   Minor malformations are primarily cosmetic, e.g. small ear, ear tag or Polydactyly. If only one minor anomaly is present, the chance of finding an associated major anomaly is 3%. While it is almost 90% if 3 or more minor anomalies are there.

2. **Deformations** are secondary defects in a normally formed structure caused by mechanical pressure. They have good prognosis with low risk of recurrence. Example is clubfoot due to oligohydramnios.

3. **Disruptions** are morphological defects caused by external forces that lead to destruction of a tissue e.g. amniotic bands causing amputation of a limb.

4. **Dysplasia** is due to abnormal cellular organization or function. Only one tissue type is affected e.g. ectodermal dysplasia or skeletal dysplasia.

Clinical Evaluation:

- **History**: Detailed 3 generations pedigree analysis, parental age at conception, consanguinity, abortions or stillbirths, exposure to drugs, teratogens, maternal disorders and infections.

- **Examination:**Describe all abnormal external and than internal features from top to bottom. Good observation, anthropometric measurements, compare bilateral features to identify asymmetry, look for anomalies of external genitalia, signs of delayed puberty, growth or mental retardation, speech delay, presence of hearing loss or eye abnormalities.

- **Investigations**: Depend upon the anomalies encountered. If strong suspicion of a chromosomal disorder is present then **Karyotyping** is essential for diagnosis. In case it is normal and still a chromosomal disorder is suspected then molecular cytogenetic techniques such as Fluorescence in Situ Hybridization (**FISH**) can be used to detect **micro deletion syndromes**, examples are William syndrome, Prader Willi syndrome and Miller Dieker syndrome.
  Imaging such as skeletal survey, CT or MRI, Echocardiography or Ultrasound scan may be needed to look for internal anomalies. **Metabolic screen** may be needed in some cases.

3.2 Common Genetic Disorders

Definition: Genetic disorders are diseases caused partly or completely by a defect in genes.

Estimated frequency: Between 3.5-5 %.

Type of Genetic Disease	Frequency per 1000 people
Single gene diseases (total)	4.5-15
Autosomal dominant	2 - 2.9
Autosomal recessive	2 - 3.5
X-linked	0.5 - 2
Chromosomal aberrations	5 - 7
Multi-factorial disorders	70 - 90
Congenital malformations	19 - 22

(Weatherall, 1991)

Classification:
1. Single gene disorder
    1. Autosomal dominant.
    2. Autosomal recessive.
    3. Sex-linked recessive.
    4. Sex linked dominant.
2. Multi factorial inheritance.
3. Chromosomal abnormalities:
    * Numerical anomalies.
    * Structural anomalies.
4. Mitochondrial inheritance.

A.   Autosomal Dominant Inheritance:
For a dominant disorder, only one copy of abnormal gene is necessary to develop the disease. Vertical pattern of transmission (Disease occurring in successive generations)

* Patients usually have an affected parent (except in cases of new mutations or incomplete penetrance).
* Males and females are equally likely to be affected.
* Recurrence risk for each child of an affected parent is 50%
* Normal siblings do not pass the trait on to their offspring.

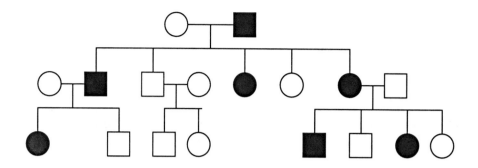

Examples:

Neuro cutaneous syndromes like Tuberous sclerosis, Neurofibromatosis
Spherocytosis, Von willibrands disease
Familial hypercholesterolemia,
Huntington's disease, Achondroplasia and Marfan's syndrome.

There are several phenomenons that are associated with Autosomal dominant inheritance:

1. **Variable expressivity**: Different individuals with the same mutation may develop different phenotype due to difference in environment and the modifying effects of other genes.

2. **Late onset:** when a disease has an onset later in life, affected individuals may have passed the gene to their offspring before they even knew they carried it themselves e.g. Huntington's disease.

3. **New Mutations:** When parent is not affected nor had the abnormal gene, the disease in offspring is caused due to spontaneous mutation for that child only. In such situation there is no increased risk of recurrence. It is therefore essential to examine both parents for even minor signs of the disease in question before giving genetic counseling. 85% of cases of Achondroplasia are the result of new mutations.

4. **Incomplete penetrance:** A phenomenon where some individuals with a disease-associated genotype do not develop the disease. For example if only 30 people out of 50 who have a disease-associated mutation actually develop the disease, it is incompletely penetrant.

B. Autosomal Recessive Inheritance

- Horizontal pattern of inheritance (Disease is found in siblings or in one generation alone, parents are a-symptomatic carriers).
- Either sex can be affected, on average in equal numbers.
- Recurrence risk is 25% for siblings
- Consanguinity is common.
- All offspring of an affected person are obligate carriers.
- Carrier probability is 50%

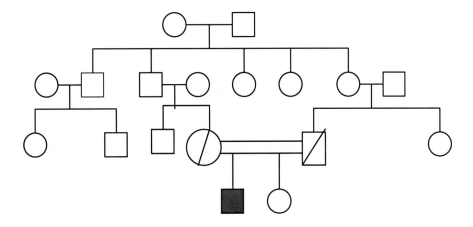

Examples:

Most IEM (Galactosemia, Tay-Sachs disease, Mucopolysaccharidoses and PKU)
Cystic fibrosis
Sickle cell anemia, Thalassemia,
Congenital adrenal hyperplasia

C.   Sex- Linked Recessive Inheritance

As the X chromosome in a male child is always inherited from the mother therefore, father never transmit the disease to his son (No Male to male transmission), affected males always get the disease from their mothers.

- All daughters of affected father are obligate carriers.
- Sons of heterozygous mother have a 50% chance of being affected
- Maternal uncles are more likely found to be affected
- These diseases are usually inherited from affected grandfather to grandsons.

Examples:

Color blindness
Hemophilia, G6PD deficiency
Duchenne muscular dystrophy
Most IEM are autosomal recessive, only a few IEM are X linked e.g. OTC deficiency causing a urea cycle disease, Hunter syndrome (MPS-II), Leish Nyhan syndrome and Fabry's disease.

D.   Sex linked Dominant inheritance

- Affects both sexes, but females are only mildly affected due to presence of extra X chromosome
- No father to son transmission, but all daughters of affected father have the disease
- No skip generation

Examples:
Vitamin D dependent Hypophosphatemic rickets
Incontinentia pigmenti

Diagnosis of Monogenic diseases:
Single gene disorders are usually diagnosed by DNA mutation analysis using gel electrophoresis.

Chromosomal Abnormalities

Are caused either due to defect in number or structure of a chromosome

A. Numerical Abnormalities: Normal human cells contain 46 chromosomes, one pair each of the 22 autosomes plus 1 pair of sex chromosomes. **Euploidy** refers to exact multiple of the number of chromosomes found in a normal haploid gamete (egg or sperm cell). In humans, the euploid number is 23.

Polyploidy refers to any multiple of the Euploid number. In humans, **diploidy** is 46 (2x23) and **triploidy** is 69 (3x23). Polyploidy can arise due to errors in meiosis during gamete formation, problems during fertilization, or errors in mitosis during early stages of embryo formation.

Aneuploidy is any number of chromosomes that is not an exact multiple of the Euploid number. In humans, this is most often due to the gain or loss of a single chromosome. **Monosomy** has 45 chromosomes; **trisomy** is when there are three copies of a single chromosome with 47 total chromosomes. All monosomy and trisomies (except for trisomy 13, 18, and 21) result in early spontaneous abortion. An abnormal phenotype is the result of excess or deficiency of the genes carried on the affected chromosomes.

Autosomal Aneuploidy:

Those who survive to term are trisomy 13, 18, and 21. Signs and symptoms of these disorders include cleft lip and palate, limb deformities, severe malformations of the nervous system, heart malformations, and mental retardation. Trisomy 13 and 18 are usually lethal within early infancy. It is therefore important to understand to avoid any surgery or intensive life support measures (ventilation and TPN etc.) to such babies. All they need is tender loving care.

Down syndrome

Down syndrome is a chromosomal condition that is associated with mental retardation, a characteristic facial appearance and hypotonia in infancy. People with Down syndrome are at an increased risk for heart defects, gastro esophageal reflux or celiac disease, and hearing loss. Some children may develop hypothyroidism and rarely leukemia or Alzheimer's disease.

Incidence is 1 in 800 to 1,000 births, and is increased by increasing maternal age.

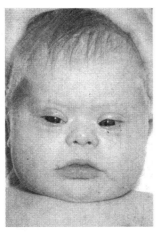
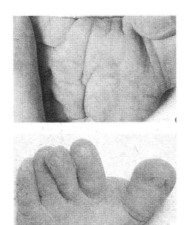

Risk for Down syndrome in relation to maternal age at conception	
Maternal Age	Incidence
20 Years	1:2000
30 Years	1:1000
40 Years	1:100
45 Years	1:32
50 Years	1:12

Types of Down syndrome: Based on the chromosomal pattern three genetic variations of Down syndrome are described.

1. Classical Trisomy: (95% cases) Extra chromosome 21 is found in all cells. This results from Non-disjunction or non-separation of two 21 chromosomes and is mostly associated with advanced maternal age.

2. Translocation type: (3-4% of cases)

3. Mosaic Trisomy: (1% of case), Here the extra chromosome 21 is present in some, but not all, cells of the individual as a result the phenotype is mild.

Clinical Features:

- Muscle hypotonia, hyper flexibility of the joints
- Microcephaly, Brachycephaly and flat occiput
- Fine silky straight hair
- Flat facial profile, depressed nasal bridge
- Almond shaped, Upward slant of the eyes, Epicanthic folds (Lunar shaped fold of skin at the medial end of eyes)
- Dysplastic small and low set ears (Normally 1/3 of ear lies above the line drawn backward from the lateral part of the eye)
- Protruded tongue (Not large tongue but due to small oral cavity)
- Simian crease (Single transverse palmer crease)
- Large space between big and second toe
- Mental retardation
- CHD: Mostly Ostium primum or common A-V canal defect, VSD, PDA
- Atlanto-axial subluxation is rare but serious defect due to hypoplasia of odontoid process causing sudden death if neck is excessively retracted during surgery for Intubation under anesthesia leading to sudden compression of cervical spinal cord.
- Duodenal atresia and imperforate anus.

Diagnosis is made clinically at birth and confirmed by karyotyping

Recurrence risk of Down syndrome in subsequent pregnancies: This depends upon the type of anomaly that baby has:

Karyotype	Recurrence risk
1. Regular Trisomy	1% above the age risk
2. Translocation	
Both parents normal	2-3%
Carrier mother	12%
Carrier father	3%
Either parent with t(21q:21Q)	100%
3. Mosaic	1%

Useful websites:
1. The Down Syndrome Medical Interest Group (UK): **www.dsmig.org.uk**
2. Down syndrome: Health Issues (up to date health information for professionals and parents): **www.ds-health.com**
3. Growth charts for children with Down syndrome: **www.growthcharts.com**
4. Educational issues: **www.downsed.org**

T u r n e r Syndrome

A disorder caused by the partial or complete loss of genetic material from one of the X chromosomes in a female.

If a spermatocyte missing an X chromosome fertilizes a normal egg containing a single X, the fetus will have X Monosomy (e.g. having only a single X-chromosome in all cells).

Incidence is 1 in 8000 live births (1 in 4000 females) and is sporadic in nature.

Clinical Features: Depends on age of presentation:

A. New born: Mostly present as lymph-edema of hands and feet (Non pitting type swelling) with low posterior hairline and redundant skin folds on the back of neck.

B. Children: Mostly present with short stature with combination of following features:

- Webbed neck
- Shield chest with wide spaced nipples
- Low posterior hair line
- Wide carrying angle (Cubitus verum)
- Coarctation of aorta with High blood pressure in arm esp. right arm, weak femoral pulse and radio-femoral delay
- Complications like Hypothyroidism, Diabetes and Renal anomalies.

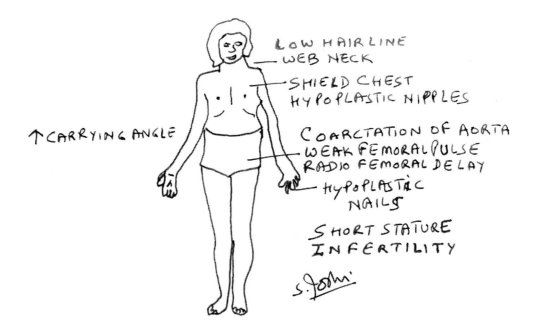

LOW HAIRLINE
WEB NECK
SHIELD CHEST
HYPOPLASTIC NIPPLES
↑CARRYING ANGLE
COARCTATION OF AORTA
WEAK FEMORAL PULSE
RADIO FEMORAL DELAY
HYPOPLASTIC NAILS
SHORT STATURE
INFERTILITY
S.John

C. Adolescent Girls:

- Delayed puberty due to ovarian failure

- Hypergonadotropic hypogonadism

D. Adults:

- Infertility due to ovarian dysgenesis

- Osteoporosis

Diagnosis is by karyotyping and clinical features.

Management: Growth hormone for the height gain and cyclical sex hormone therapy for initiation of puberty.

Trisomy 18 (Edward's Syndrome)

Trisomy 18 is a relatively common syndrome affecting approximately 1 out of 6,000 live births, and affecting girls more than three times as often as boys. It is caused by the presence of an extra number 18 chromosome, which leads to multiple abnormalities. Many of these abnormalities make it hard for infants to live longer than a few months.

Clinical Features:

- Antenatal: Unusually large uterus (Polyhydramnios), Small placenta

- Low birth weight infant, Hypertonic posture prominent occiput

- Clenched hands (Overlapped finger, see figure)

- Rockerbottom feet (Convex feet like a wooden rocking horse)

- Low-set ears, Small jaw (micrognathia), Microcephaly

- Hypoplastic (underdeveloped) fingernails

- Umbilical hernia or inguinal hernia, Diastasis recti, Cryptorchidism

- Crossed legs (preferred position)

- Congenital heart disease: VSD, ASD, PDA

- Renal anomalies: Horseshoe kidney, Hydronephrosis, Polycystic kidney

- Coloboma of iris

- Severe developmental failure

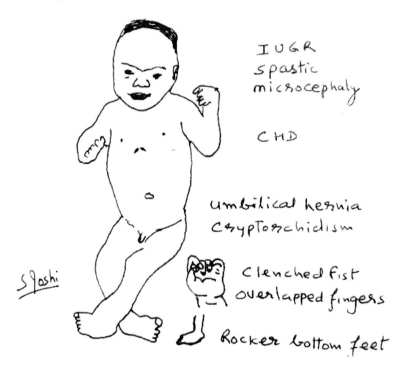

Diagnosis:

Physical examination may show an excess of arched type finger print patterns. X-rays may reveal a short sternum. Chromosome studies show trisomy 18, partial trisomy, or translocation.

Prognosis:

The abnormalities of trisomy 18 are generally not compatible with more than a few months of life. Fifty percent of the affected infants do not survive beyond the first week of life. And most of remaining die by first birthday.

Prevention:

Prenatal diagnosis of trisomy 18 is possible with an amniocentesis and chromosome studies on amniotic cells. Parents who have a child with translocational trisomy 18 and want additional children should have chromosome studies.

Trisomy 13 (Patau Syndrome)

Trisomy 13 occurs in about 1 out of every 10,000 live births. It causes multiple lethal abnormalities therefore more than 80% of children die within the first month of life. Trisomy 13 is associated with severe defects of the brain and mid face dysmorphia that lead to seizures, apnea, and breathing irregularities. The eyes are small with defects in the iris (coloboma). Most infants have a severe cleft lip cleft palate, and low-set ears. Congenital heart disease is present in approximately 80% of affected infants. Hernia and genital abnormalities are common.

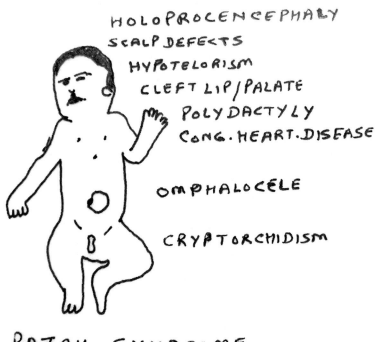

Clinical Features:

- Severe mental retardation, Seizures, microcephaly, multiple scalp defects (absent skin)
- Small eyes (microphthalmia), hypotelorism -- eyes may actually fuse together into one cyclops eye, Iris defects (coloboma)
- Large cleft lip and/or palate, Micrognathia
- Pinna abnormalities and low set ears
- Simian crease
- Extra digits (polydactyly)
- Hernias: umbilical hernia, inguinal hernia
- Undescended testicle (cryptorchidism)
- Hypotonia

Diagnosis:

The infant may have a single umbilical artery at birth. There are often signs of severe congenital heart disease: VSD, ASD, PDA or Dextroversion of the heart

Gastrointestinal x-rays or ultrasound may reveal malrotation of the internal organs.

MRI or CT scans of the head may reveal holoprosencephaly, where the 2 cerebral hemispheres are fused and are filled with a bag of CSF.

Chromosome study confirms the diagnosis by showing trisomy 13, partial trisomy, trisomy 13 mosaic, or translocation.

Prognosis: Extremely short survival time (few weeks to months only).

Prevention:

Trisomy 13 can be diagnosed prenatally by amniocentesis with chromosome studies of the amniotic cells. Trisomy 13 mosaicism and partial trisomy 13 also occur. Parents of infants with trisomy 13 caused by a translocation should have genetic testing and counseling, which may help them prevent recurrence.

Klinefelter Syndrome

Klinefelter syndrome occurs in male as a result of an extra X chromosome (XXY). The most common symptom is feminine look and infertility.

It is found in about 1 out of every 1,000 newborn males. Older age women > 35 years at conception are slightly more likely to have a boy with this syndrome.

XXY males can occur due to non-disjunction of X-chromosomes during prophase of meiosis I in females. One of the eggs from such meiosis could receive both X-chromosomes, and the other would receive no X-chromosomes, if these eggs were subsequently fertilized with normal sperm, various sex chromosome aneuploidies could occur:

Non-disjunction during sperm production can also result in aneuploidy of sex chromosomes.

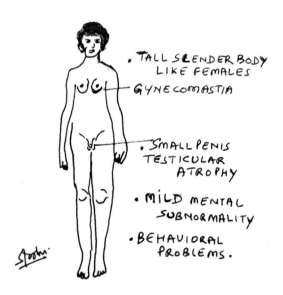

Clinical Features:
- Small, firm testicles, Small penis,
- Sparse pubic, armpit, and facial hair
- Sexual problems
- Enlarged breasts (called gynecomastia)
- Tall stature: Abnormal body proportions (long legs, short trunk)

- Learning difficulty
- Infertility

Diagnosis:

- Karyotyping -- 47 XXY
- Sperm count -- Low
- Serum testosterone -- Low
- Hypergonadotropic hypogonadism (High FSH, LH and estrogen levels)

Treatment: Testosterone therapy can achieve the following:

- Increase strength, improve concentration, mood, self esteem and sex drive
- Improve appearance of muscles, grow body hair

Prognosis:

Most patients can expect a normal, productive life. Social and educational supports can help patients reach their potential.

Complications:

The syndrome is associated with an increased risk of breast cancer, extragonadal germ cell tumor (a rare tumor), lung disease, varicose veins, and osteoporosis. There is also an increased risk for autoimmune disorder such as lupus, rheumatoid arthritis, and Sjogren's syndrome.

Despite normal or high IQ, learning disabilities are common. The risks of dyslexia, attention deficient hyperactivity disorder, and depression may be higher.

Fragile X Syndrome

It is the most common cause of mental retardation and developmental disabilities in boys. The incidence is between 1:2500 and 1:4000 births. It is a single gene disorder transmitted on the X chromosome. It is found both in males and females but males are typically affected more severely.

Clinical Features: External appearance may be normal. Most cases are detected on screening due to positive family history or because a school age boy who is referred for investigation of his mental sub normality or abnormal behavior with autistic features. As the children grow older they may show some characteristic facial features like long face with large mandible and long prominent ears. At puberty characteristic macro-orchadism (large testis) may appear.

Behavioral problems:

- Attention Deficit Hyperactivity Disorder, Anxiety and impulsivity
- Autistic behavior: Poor eye contact, Poor adaptation to changes in routine, Resistance to being touched or held, Hand flapping, Pervasive Developmental Disorder

Childhood Development

- Wide spectrum of cognitive functional and developmental disabilities
- Fine and gross motor delays, sensor motor problems, speech and language dysfunction, IQ may decline during childhood
- Visual learners (majority), relatively strong imitation skills
- Autistic (up to 15 percent)

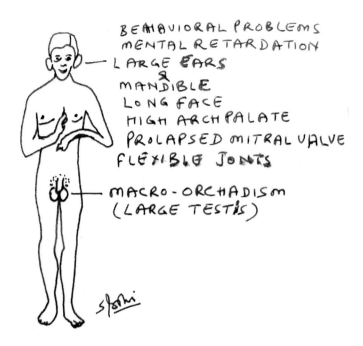

BEHAVIORAL PROBLEMS
MENTAL RETARDATION
LARGE EARS
&
MANDIBLE
LONG FACE
HIGH ARCH PALATE
PROLAPSED MITRAL VALVE
FLEXIBLE JOINTS

MACRO-ORCHADISM
(LARGE TESTIS)

Genetic aspects of Fragile X Syndrome:

- FMR-1 gene is located on the X chromosome. This gene makes a protein essential for normal brain functioning. **Normally**, the genetic code for the FMR-1 gene contains 5-50 repetition of CGG sequences.

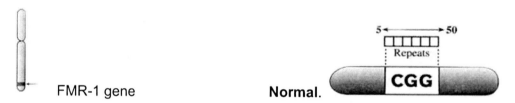

FMR-1 gene   **Normal.**

- **Pre-mutation carrier** of fragile X syndrome has 50-200 repeats and he or she will not be affected but act as carriers with risk of having affected children.

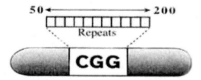

- If the number of repeats increase to >200 then the individual will be **affected**. This number will disrupt the code and prevents the production of the FMR protein.

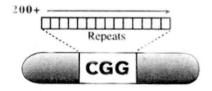

Family members who have fewer repeats in the FMR1 gene may not have mental retardation, but may have other problems. Women may have premature menopause or difficulty in getting pregnant. Both men and women may have problems with tremors and poor coordination.

Diagnosis: Molecular DNA analysis using PCR to look for the number of CGG triplet repeats.

Treatment: There is no specific treatment. Instead, effort is directed toward training and education so that affected children can function as high level as is possible.

Structural Chromosomal Abnormalities

- *Deletions* involve loss of material from a single chromosome. The effects are typically severe since there is a loss of genetic material. There are many deletion syndromes causing severe neurological disease, mental retardation and structural Dysmorphic features in various combinations e.g. Williams syndrome, Prader Willi syndrome etc.

- *Inversions* occur when there are two breaks within a single chromosome and the broken segment flips 180° (inverts) and reattaches to form a chromosome that is structurally out-of-sequence. There is usually no risk for problems to an individual if the inversion is of *familial* origin but if it is a *de novo* (new) mutation then there is slightly increased risk due possibly to an interruption of a key gene sequence.

- *Translocations* involve exchange of material between two or more chromosomes. If a translocation is *reciprocal* (balanced) the risk for problems to an individual is similar to that with inversions: usually none if *familial* and slightly increased if *de novo*.

Multi-factorial Inheritance

This is caused due to interplay between Polygenetic and Environmental factors.
- Several genes are involved in the ultimate expression of the trait.
- No single gene is shown to be dominant or recessive.
- All of the genes act in an additive manner - each "adds" or "removes" a small amount from the overall phenotype.
- The genotype and environment interact to produce the final phenotype
- The effects of this inheritance varies:

    1. Most affected children have normal parents

    2. Recurrence risk increases with the closeness of individual to the affected individual (i.e. how many genes are shared) The monozygotic twins usually share most genes and are at highest risk., followed by di-zygotic twin, normal sibling, cousins and so on.

        As the degree of relatedness decreases, so does the likelihood that relatives share the same combination of genes over multiple loci. Parents and their children have 1/2 of their genes in common. An uncle and his niece will only have 1/8 of their genes in common.

155

3. Recurrence risk increases with the severity of the condition in the parents

Examples: Congenital heart disease, Cleft lip and palate, Pyloric stenosis, Congenital dislocated hips, Diabetes, Cancer, Obesity, Hypertension etc.

Mitochondrial Inheritance

Mitochondria are not governed by our genome, they possess their own. The mitochondrial genes are responsible for production of enzymes required for energy production. Mitochondrial diseases usually lead to myopathy, cardiomyopathy and/ or encephalopathy.

The diseases are fortunately rare.

They are always maternally transmitted because every individual inherits the mitochondria from mother through the ovum (Sperms don't contain mitochondria).

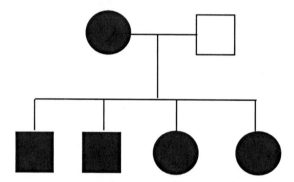

Characteristics of Mitochondrial diseases:

1. Children of affected father will never inherit the disease.

2. All children of affected mother will inherit it but in different combinations of severity. Some may be severely affected while others only minimally, depending on the number of abnormal mitochondria present in a particular ovum.

Examples: Mitochondrial encephalopathies (MERRF and MELAS Syndrome), Hepatopathies, Myopathies etc.

3.3 Genetic Counseling

Genetic Counseling: Is a process of family education for not just telling the risk of reoccurrence but educating them about all the aspects of a genetic disease in question including: how it is caused, its course, complications, prognosis, its management and prevention of its recurrence in the family. The information is to be transmitted to those requesting it in a sensitive, culturally appropriate and understandable way. Family need to be supported in the decision making process in a non-directive way (i.e. giving the options without telling them what they are supposed to do).

Prerequisites for Genetic Counseling:
A. Detailed family history and 3-generation family tree
B. Accurate Diagnosis
C. Understanding of the medical aspects of the disorder (etiology, natural history, treatment, prognosis, burden)
D. Understanding the inheritance pattern (recurrence risk)
E. Understanding the psycho-social impact of the information

Indications for Genetic Counseling:

- Children with significant malformations.
- Children with common birth defects (neural tube defects, congenital heart disease, cleft lip/palate, clubfoot, CDH, multiple vertebral anomalies, atresia or stenosis of GI tract).
- Families who have had a fatally malformed infant (stillborn or neonatal death).
- Idiopathic mental retardation especially when:
  o The child has evidence of a metabolic disturbance,
  o Multiple sibs are affected or a parent and child are similarly affected
  o Multiple males in a family are affected
- Newborns with suspected IEM:
- Children with loss of milestones or/and organomegaly beginning at several months to several years of age who were previously apparently thriving.
- Cases of abnormal sexual development, primary amenorrhea or aspermia.
- Cases of early complete or partial hearing loss or blindness, neurodegenerative disorders, short stature, premature heart disease, immune deficiency, abnormalities of the skin, hair or bones and sickle cell anemia/Thalassemia, other blood disorder or coagulopathy.
- Mothers desiring more children who:
  o Are on chronic medications (anticonvulsants, antimetabolites, thyroid antagonists, steroids, etc.)
  o Are "on drugs" (including alcohol)
  o Have had recurrent pregnancy losses
  o Are over 35 or have husbands over 55
  o Have a previous retarded or malformed child
  o Have questions about prenatal diagnosis for any disorder.

Genetic counseling may be required before conception, during pregnancy, after birth or even later when the disease manifests.

Prenatal Diagnosis: Use of following techniques to determine the health of an unborn fetus:

- Ultrasonography
- Amniocentesis
- Chorionic villus sampling
- Identifying Fetal blood cells in the maternal blood
- Maternal serum alpha-fetoprotein (MSAFP), beta-HCG and estriol (uE3) levels

Amniocentesis:

Removing a small amount (10 – 20ml) of the fluid that surrounds the fetus. The fluid contains cells belonging to the fetus. These cells are used for chromosome, genetic or both tests. The fluid itself may be tested for the level of Alfa Feto-protein or other biochemical metabolites. Most amniocenteses are performed between 14 and 20 weeks gestation. Risks with amniocentesis include fetal loss (0.5%) and maternal Rh sensitization.

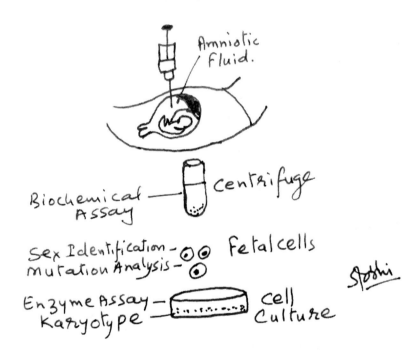

Chorionic villus sampling (CVS): The advantage of this technique is that it can be performed much earlier (beginning of 10th to 13th week gestation) thus permitting a safe termination if indicated prior to age of viability. CVS involves removal of a small amount of chorionic villi tissue located on the outside of the fetal gestational sac. As this tissue is part of fetus therefore it gives genetic information about baby. CVS has the disadvantage of small but still a significant risk of fetal loss (0.5 to 1% higher than amniocentesis). The tissue obtained is used for biochemical, enzyme analysis or for genetic testing.

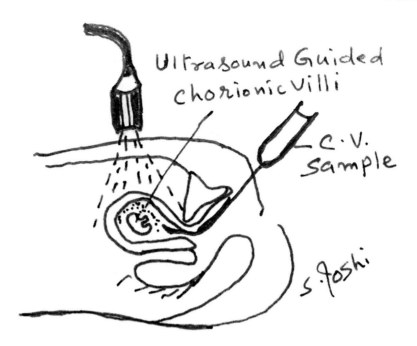

Triple Screen: This includes testing for the 1. Maternal serum – alfa fetoprotein (MS-AFP), 2. Beta human chorionic gonadotrophin (HCG) and 3. Conjugated estriol (uE3). The test help in the increased detection of fetal abnormalities such as listed in the table below

Condition	MS-AFP	uE3	Beta HCG
Neural tube defect	High	Normal	Normal
Trisomy 21	Low	Low	High
Trisomy 18	Low	Low	Low
Molar pregnancy	Low	Low	Very High
Twin/Triplet pregnancy	High	Normal	High
Intrauterine death	High	Low	Low

The test gives 95% prediction for the Down syndrome that must be confirmed on chromosomal analysis on fetal cells obtained by amniocentesis or CVS biopsy.

Preimplantation Genetic Diagnosis (PGD):

PGD is a technique used to identify genetic defects in embryos created through In Vitro Fertilization (IVF) before transferring them into the uterus to ensure birth of a normal baby.

The process starts with a basic IVF. When the embryo is at the 8-cell stage, 1-2 cells (blastomeres) are removed and sent to the genetic laboratory for diagnosis using either polymerase chain reaction (PCR) or fluorescence in situ hybridization (FISH) techniques, depending on which disease is being sought. The unaffected embryos are then transferred into the mother's uterus for continuation of pregnancy.

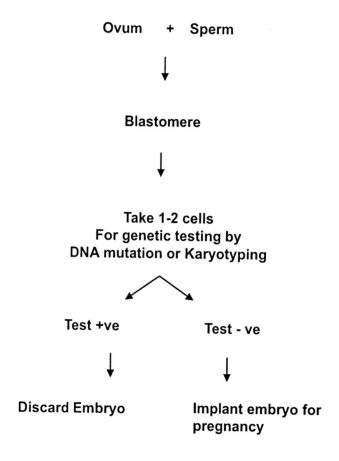

Ovum   +   Sperm

↓

Blastomere

↓

Take 1-2 cells
For genetic testing by
DNA mutation or Karyotyping

Test +ve   **Test - ve**

↓   ↓

Discard Embryo   **Implant embryo for**
                 pregnancy

Indications for PGD:

- Couples in whom at least one partner has a family history of inheritable genetic disease, carries such a disease, or is otherwise affected by such a disease
- Women 35 years or older (to test for aneuploidy due to maternal age)
- Women with recurrent pregnancy losses, which could be caused by an abnormal chromosomal set coming from either the male or female partner
- Couples with chromosome translocations, which can cause implantation failure, recurrent pregnancy loss, or mental or physical problems in offspring
- Couples with repeated IVF failure
- Men with infertility requiring intracytoplasmic sperm injection (ICSI)

Ethical issues about PGD:

- Some people fear that the examination of an embryo may be misused for discrimination. Some worry that PGD can be used to design the "perfect baby."
- Some people are concerned that the single removed cell could have developed into a fetus but was destroyed by the test. Some consider this murder.
- Fertilized cells found to carry a genetic defect are not implanted and are allowed to die in the dish.
- Some genetic diseases manifest when the host is aged 30-40 years or even older. Critics argue that a cure might be found during the interim period.
- Some people consider the use of PGD for sex selection for social and personal reasons to be inappropriate interference with the natural selection of progeny.

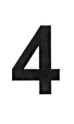

Metabolic Diseases

4.1 Introduction to Inborn Errors of Metabolism

IEM in Oman:
- Fairly new specialty in Oman, Started from June 1998
- Before this, late diagnosis or Non diagnosis caused severe morbidity & Mortality
- Family history of children dying of similar disease in the past was not uncommon
- All sorts of diseases do exist in Oman, till now we have identified >250 children with IEM
- Diagnostic and treatment facilities are now available in Oman.
- Our treatment results are quite comparable to any other center

What are the Inborn Errors of Metabolism (I.E.M.)?

In 1908, *Sir Archibald Garrod first* identified four such disorders and noted some similarities in them:
- Diseases were caused by a point defect in metabolism of simple intermediary metabolites like amino acids or carbohydrates
- The defect was Life long & permanent
- Transmitted as a recessive trait in the families
- Not significantly affected by treatment

1934, *Folling* discovered **Phenyl-Ketonuria (PKU).**
This disease resembled the description of Garrod,
It was caused by defect in conversion of Phenyl Alanine to Tyrosine
It caused severe mental retardation in children which was preventable by dietary restriction of Phenyl-Alanine

Definition and characteristics of IEM:

As the name suggests, these diseases are inborn or hereditary, caused due to genetic mutation leading to **point defect** in the metabolic pathway of Proteins, Fats, Carbohydrates, Vitamins, Minerals or other Complex organic compounds

Currently **>400** such disorders are known
>100 diseases manifest in Neonatal period
>100 diseases affect CNS with a danger of brain damage if treated poorly

Early and pre-symptomatic recognition by **screening program** is therefore highly desirable. Due to the genetic nature they are recurrent, especially in consanguineous families. Treatment requires life long commitment and **Genetic counseling** is highly important to prevent recurrence

Incidence:

Individually IEM are quite rare but collectively are quite common.
Incidence is variable depending upon Gene frequency in the population (PKU in USA is the commonest disease in Caucasians with incidence of 1:10,000 while MSUD is quite rare, 1:300,000). Exact incidence can only be found by nationwide screening program
Collective incidence of IEM in western countries is 1:5000 while in Oman from our estimate is likely to be <1:1700 (three times more common)

Causes of High incidence of IEM in Oman:
- High consanguinity with high gene frequency in certain tribes
- Large Family size leading to more likelihood of disease manifestation
- Lack of proper Genetic counseling

Classification of IEM: IEM Can be classified in many ways

A. Biochemical classification: Is an easy way to classify but is not clinically useful
-Diseases of **Protein** metabolism
-Diseases of **Lipid** metabolism
-Diseases of **Carbohydrates** metabolism
-Diseases of **Complex Substances** metabolism

B. Small V/S Large Molecule Diseases (Sinclair classification)-
- Small Molecule diseases: Involving Protein, Lipids & Carbohydrates
- Large or complex Molecule diseases: Mucopolysaccharides, Mucolipids, Sphingolipids

C. Clinical classification (Saudubray)-
- Intoxication type diseases
- Energy Deficiency diseases
- Storage Diseases.

Biochemical Classification

1) Defects of Amino Acid Metabolism

- Phenylalanine	Phenylketonuria
- Tyrosine	Tyrosinemia
- Methionine	Homocystinuria

- Branch Chain Amino Acid (Leucine, Isoleucine, Valine):
    Maple Syrup Urine Disease
    Organic Acidemia:
        Propionic Acidemia
        Methylmalonic Acidemia
        Isovaleric Acidemia

-Ammonia Detoxification. Diseases: Urea Cycle Diseases

2) Lipid Metabolic Dis.
Fatty Acid Oxidation Disorders
Hyperlipidemia

3) Carbohydrate Meta. Dis.

- Galactose	Galactosemia
- Fructose	Fructosemia
- Pyruvate	Congenital Lactic Acidosis

- Glycogen   Glycogen Storage diseases

4)   **Diseases due to Complex Molecule storage**

-Mucopolysaccharide storage   Mucopolysaccharidosis

-Mucolipids   Mucolipidosis

-Sphingolipidosis   Gaucher disease, Sandhoff disease

Pathogenesis of IEM

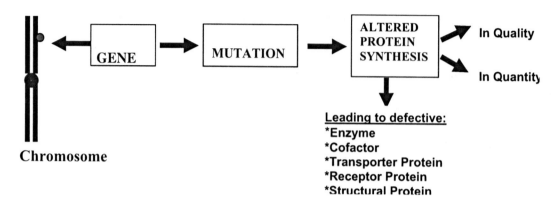

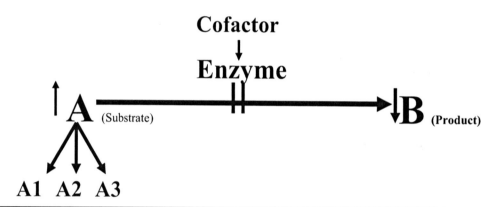

- TOXIC EFFECTS ON METABOLICALLY ACTIVE ORGANS: CNS, LIVER, KIDNEY, HEART, MUSCLES
- STORAGE IN R.E.SYSTEM: LIVER, SPLEEN, BONE MARROW
- ENERGY DEF.: ENCEPHALOPATHY, MYOPATHY, CARDIO MYOPATHY

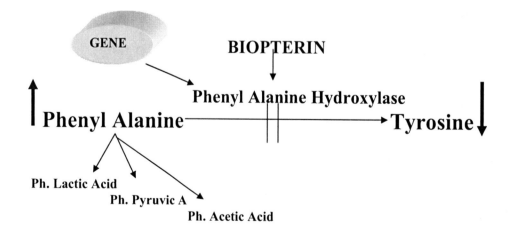

164

Clinical Presentation of IEM Diseases

Clinical symptoms are often nonspecific and often confused with severe overwhelming diseases like septicemia, Meningitis, cardiac failure and sequel of birth asphyxia. The specific manifestations depend on the organs involved
Clinical presentation also depends on type of molecule involved:

Small molecules will produce **Intoxication type diseases**
Defect in Energy production pathway will produce **Energy deficiency disease**
Complex molecules will produce **Storage disease**

1)   Intoxication type Diseases

A. Presentation in the Neonatal period:

This is the most common mode of presentation of IEM in the neonatal period. The scenario is that new born is usually born full term with uneventful perinatal period (differentiating IEM from Asphyxia and overwhelming diseases in preterm babies) Within a few days of normal life and feeding (window period: time taken to accumulate toxic metabolic products) the new born becomes progressively sick, first developing poor feeding, lethargy and vomiting, leading to semi-coma, coma, seizures and respiratory difficulty or apnea requiring artificial ventilation (Toxic Metabolic Encephalopathy). The disease if still not recognized will lead to shock, DIC and multi-organ failure and death.
Delay in treatment is the commonest cause for brain damage with eventual poor prognosis despite offering adequate treatment.

B. Presentation in older children:

If the enzyme deficiency is milder (3-10%) or the neonate is rescued from the initial presentation then the disease will present in the later childhood as *recurrent acute toxic encephalopathy.*
In the state of normal health the metabolism is quite balanced, but during the time of Stress, catabolic process predominates leading to acute de-compensation.

The stress catabolism in the child could be due to:
Acute infections: URTI, Acute Gastro-enteritis
Vomiting, fasting or poor feeding due to various reasons
Overfeeding of offending substance (high protein or fat diet)
Trauma or Surgery

During this time child will develop:
Acute persistent vomiting with severe dehydration or shock
Abdominal Pain (can be confused with abdominal emergency)
Altered sensorium (Encephalopathy)
Hypoglycemia
Unusual smell
Abnormal biochemical profile (severe metabolic acidosis with high anion gap, Ketosis, Lactic acidosis, Hyperammonemia)
Rey's syndrome like picture

Aetiology of toxic encephalopathic diseases:
- Aminoacidopathies - MSUD
- Organic Acidemia – Isovaleric, Propionic or Methyl Malonic acidemia
- Urea Cycle Diseases

2)   Energy Deficient Type diseases

Energy production is a catabolic process. Glucose is the primary source of immediate energy needs, fats are used when glucose stores are exhausted, and Neo-glucogenesis is used for glucose production from protein and fats sources. Most energy deficient disorders present with Hypoglycemia, lack of energy leading to poor activity, hypotonia, poor feeding and growth, dysfunction of organs that rely heavily on energy: Encephalopathy, Myopathy, Cardiomyopathy, liver and kidney dysfunction.

Etiology:

Disorders of pyruvate utilization:
- Congenital Lactic Acidosis
- Disorders of Krebs cycle
- Mitochondrial Respiratory chain disorders

Fatty Acid Oxidation Disorders

Defects of Gluco-neogenesis

Clinical Manifestations:
- Hypotonia
- Progressive Encephalopathies
- Myopathy
- Cardiomyopathy-CHF, Shock
- Dysmorphia
- Poor feeding, NG Feeding & FTT despite adequate nutrition
- SIDS

Biochemistry
- Hypoglycemia
- Severe lactic acidosis with high Anion Gap
- Ketosis (Except in Fatty Acid Oxidation Diseases)

3) Lysosomal Storage Diseases (LSD)

These diseases are caused by deficiency of Lysosomal enzymes required for breakdown and recycling of complex substances

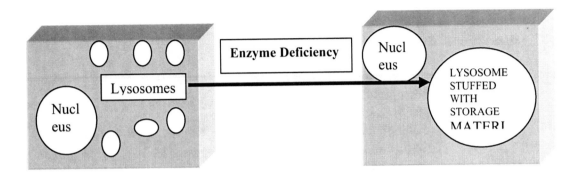

Depending on site of involvement, the diseases are of 3 types:

A. **CNS** Storage: Grey matter, White matter or combined (Neuronopathic) diseases

B. **PERIPHERAL** organ storage (Non Neuronopathic): Reticulo Endothelial system (Liver, spleen, Bone marrow)

C. **MIXED** TYPE Depending upon onset of disease which is again determined by type of mutation, severity of the enzyme deficiency & duration of symptom free interval the diseases can be of various Subtypes:
- Infantile
- Juvenile
- Adult types

A) Clinical presentation of CNS Storage diseases

Grey matter disease presentation:
Mental retardation
Developmental regression
Seizures
Retinitis Pigmentosa
Cherry red Macula
Loss of Vision & Hearing

White matter disease presentation:
Paralysis with long tract signs: Spasticity
Movement disorders: Ataxia, Choreo-athetosis
Optic Atrophy

B) Clinical picture of peripheral storage diseases:

Hepato-Splenomegaly
Dysmorphic or coarse Facies
Bone marrow involvement: Pancytopenia
Dysostosis multiplex (Multiple bone dysplasia), Joint stiffness
Failure to thrive & Short stature

C) Mixed types: Combination of above two types

Etiology of storage diseases:

Mucopolysaccharidosis
Muco Lipidosis
Sphingolipidosis: Gaucher disease, Neiman Pick disease,
Gangliosidosis (Sandhoff disease)
Leukodystrophies

Diagnosis:

Normal Biochemistry
Peripheral blood film may show storage vacuolated lymphocytes
Enzyme assay: on Plasma, Lymphocyte or Skin Fibroblast culture
Mutation Analysis for carrier identification or prenatal diagnosis

Treatment:

No treatment available for neuropathic form of diseases
Bone Marrow Transplant
Enzyme replacement therapy: In Gaucher dis., MPS-1, 6
Gene therapy: Still experimental

Investigations in a suspected IEM case:

A: **Primary level tests:** Needed in all cases for initial evaluation.
  1. Blood Glucose & Electrolytes
  2. Blood Gas, Anion Gap (Na + K - Cl + HCO_3) = <15 meq/L
  3. Urine Ketones
  4. Blood Lactate / Pyruvate levels
  5. Plasma Ammonia
  6. General tests like CBC, LFT, CK, Uric acid

B: **Secondary tests (Specific tests):** Ordered for confirmation according to the diagnosis suspected on initial evaluation.
  1. Blood Tandem Mass Spectrometery **(TMS)** for Amino Acid & Acyl Carnitine levels
  2. Blood & Urine Amino Acid levels by HPLC or Chromatography (When TMS is not available)
  3. Urine Organic Acids analysis by GCMS
  4. Urine MPS, Oligosaccharides, Reducing substance

C: *Tertiary level tests:* These tests are difficult to perform, time consuming and available only at selected laboratory, therefore ordered only in special situation like prenatal diagnosis, carrier detection, prior to BMT or liver transplantation or when diagnosis is not possible by primary or secondary level testing as in storage diseases.
  1. Enzyme Assay on blood cells, skin fibroblast or biopsy of organs.

2. Molecular testing for mutations analysis

Interpretation of test results:

DISORDER	ROUTINE LAB TESTS				SPECIAL TESTS		ENZYME ASSAY		
	Blood Gas	Ketones	Lactic Acid	NH4	ORG. ACID	AMINO ACIDS	WBC	Skin	Tissue
MSUD		+				+	+	+	
ORGANIC ACIDEMIA	Acidosis +++	+ +	+	+	+ +		+	+	
CONG. LACTIC ACIDOSIS	Acidosis ±	±	+ + +	+	±		+	+	
UREA CYCLE DISEASES	Resp. Alkalosis	+		+ + +		+			+ Liver
N K H						+	+	+	
STORAGE DISEASES							+	+	

+ (Present), ± (May be present), NKH (Non Ketotic Hyperglycinemia)

Difficulties in diagnosing IEM:
- Lack of awareness
- Non consideration
- Lack of availability of tests
- Lack of postmortem facilities

Important diagnostic clues to suggest IEM:
- History of Consanguinity
- Sudden severe illness in a well new born
- Biochemical abnormalities
- Unusual smell
- Family History of similar disease (Alive or dead child)
- Non response to usual treatment
- Recurrent episodes
- Progressive Neuro regression
- Unexplained multi-system disease

Emergency management of IEM:
- Immediate Treatment - Do not wait for diagnosis
- Collect all necessary tests
- Stop all oral feeds - Especially Proteins
- Prevent catabolism: Start IV (10%) Glucose & electrolytes fluids
- Treat associated sepsis to avoid catabolism
- Correct metabolic acidosis by IV sodium Bicarbonate
- Treat Hyperammonemia - Drugs or Dialysis
- Monitor- Vital & Neuro status, Glucose, pH, Electrolytes, NH4 & Lactate
- Removal of toxic metabolites

* Carnitine or Glycine in Organic Acidemia
* Penicillamine in Wilson Dis.
* Betaine in HCU
- Stimulation of Residual enzyme by cofactor treatment:
  * Biotin   Propionic acidemia
  * Thiamin   MSUD
  * Pyridoxine   Homocystinuria
  * B12   Methyl Malonic Acidemia
  * Riboflavin   GA II, FAOXD
  * Biopterin   Malignant PKU
- Specific diet-after diagnosis- to cut down supply of offending agent
  * PKU   - Lo Fenalac, Phenyl free
  * MSUD   - Ketonex (BCAA free)
  * Homocystinuria   - Low methionine
  * Urea Cycle Dis.   - Cyclinex (essential AA)
  * Organic Aciduria   - Propimex (Isoleucine and Valine free)
  * Galactosemia   - Lactose free
  * Fructosemia   - Fructose & sucrose free
  * Tyrosinemia   - Tyrosine & Phenyl Alanine free

4.2   Recognition of Metabolic disease in a Newborn

Most treatable metabolic disorders in neonates present as acute toxic encephalopathies with one or more following characteristic features:

1)   Consanguineous parents with previous history of death of a baby due to similar presentation.

2)   Mostly a full term baby born after an uneventful perinatal period

3)   Asymptomatic phase of first few days after birth

4)   Acute onset with progressive course – starting with some subtle symptoms like lethargy, poor feeding vomiting that soon progress to coma, seizures, breathing difficulty, multi system organ failure and death.

5)   Presence of certain biochemical abnormalities (See later)

6)   Unusual smell – maple syrup urine disease and isovaleric acidemia have a smell like burnt sugar and sweaty feet smell respectively.

7)   Uncontrolled seizures in neonatal period indicate following disorders
          •Non Ketotic Hyperglycinemia
          •Peroxisomal Disorders
          •Sulfite oxidase Deficiency
          •Pyridoxine Dependency

Laboratory diagnosis of a suspected IEM

Five primary laboratory tests are most useful in differentiating common treatable groups of disorders -
          ▪   Blood Gas and Anion Gap
          ▪   Blood Glucose
          ▪   Urine Ketones
          ▪   Blood Lactic Acid, Pyruvic Acid and Lactate Pyruvate Ratio
          ▪   Serum Ammonia

To avoid conflicting results the tests should be drawn early in the course of disease before starting any therapeutic measures. On the basis of these tests a specific **group** of disorder may be identified (see the table below). This is usually enough to decide the kind of emergency treatment required.

Further confirmation of the diagnosis and the use specific treatment modalities require secondary level tests like blood spot Tandem Mass Spectrometry (for amino acid and acylcarnitine levels) and urine GCMS (gas chromatography and mass spectrometry) for organic acid analysis. These tests may only be done at reference laboratories abroad and need special approval.

Interpretation of Lab tests for IEM:

Disorders	Screening Lab Tests				Confirmatory Tests	
	Blood Gas Anion Gap	Urine Ketones	Lactic Acid	Serum Ammonia	Blood TMS (AA & Acyl-carnitines)	Urine GCMS (Organic Acids)
MSUD	-	+	-	-	+	Not indicated
Organic Acidemia	Severe Acidosis	++	+	+	+	+
Pri. Lactic Acidosis	Severe Acidosis	+/-	+++	+	+	+
Urea Cycle Dis.	Resp. Alkalosis	-	-	+++	+	Not indicated
Non Ketonic Hyperglycinemia	-	-	-	-	+	Not indicated

(+) abnormal test **(-)** Normal test **AA** = Amino Acids, **MSUD** = Maple Syrup Urine Dis.

Emergency Management of a Newborn with suspected IEM

General Principals:
- Collect all necessary tests before starting any treatment
- Stop all oral protein containing feeds
- Monitor vital signs and biochemical parameters periodically
- Collect 3 drops of blood on filter paper (Guthrie card) for Tandem MS.
- Collect 10 ml urine and deep freeze immediately for organic acids analysis by GCMS
- Treat sepsis if indicated
- Prevent dehydration and catabolism by giving full maintenance fluid requirement as 10 to 15% glucose with electrolytes (providing up to 10 mg/kg of glucose, intralipids and a small amount of Amino Acid Mixtures (maximum 0.25 to 0.5 gm/kg/day).

- *Insulin may be used in cases of "hyperglycemia" due to poor tolerance of high glucose infusion as well as for promoting Anabolism.*

- **Formula Feeding:** Until diagnosis is proven, proteins are given in only small amount (0.25- 1.0 gm/kg/d). This can be achieved by feeding Profree Milk Powder with small calculated amount of added Similac or S26 Formula.

- **Correction Metabolic Acidosis:** Metabolic Acidosis is treated only if pH <7.2. Sodium Bicarbonate 8.4% is diluted 1:2 with distilled water and given slowly IV over 20 - 30 minutes as per following formula:

  ml of 8.4% NaHCO3 required = 0.3 x weight x bicarb deficit.

  Since in organic aciduria and primary lactic acidosis there is an ongoing production of organic acids, therefore, subsequent bicarbonate treatment is planned by giving continuous infusion of diluted sodium bicarbonate as IV infusion @ 0.5 to 1 meq/kg/hr.

- **Hyperammonemia – (Ammonia >150 μmol/L)**

Severe hyperammonemia is seen in urea cycle disorders but to a lesser degree is also associated with organic acidemia and congenital lactic acidosis. Hyperammonemia always warrants urgent treatment because every minutes delay causes neuronal damage and bad future prognosis. Management of hyperammonemia is same irrespective of the cause except that **Arginine is used for urea cycle disorders only**.

Sodium Benzoate conjugates with glycine to form easily excretable hippuric acid while **Phenyl butyrate** conjugates with glutamine and excreted as Phenyl acetyl Glutamine, thus leading to a net loss of ammonia producing amino acid pool.

Arginine acts by excreting nitrogen waste by restarting the blocked urea cycle.

The drugs to lower hyperammonemia are given as:

A. Priming (stat) Dose

- Arginine 660 mg/kg (in Urea Cycle Disease cases only)
- Sodium Benzoate 250 mg/kg
- Phenylabutyrate 250 mg/kg
- Diluted in 25 ml/kg of 10% Dextrose, Infused over 90 mts.

B. Maintenance Dose

- Same doses and dilution infused over 24 hours.

Organic Aciduria and use of IV Carnitine

Carnitine helps in restoring mitochondrial functions by removing toxic organic acids. Dose: 200 – 300 mg/kg/d in 3-4 divided doses IV slowly over 2-3 mts.

4.3 Common Metabolic Diseases

Phenylketonuria (PKU):

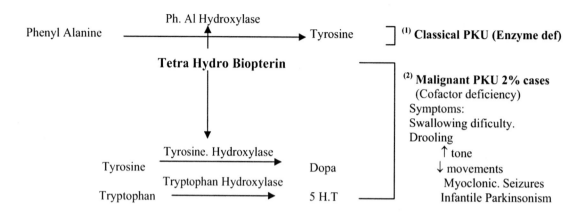

Baby is normal at birth

Progressive severe mental retardation starts in mid infancy, IQ <30

Blonde or fair skin, rash, Light or blue eyes

Mousy odor due to Phenyl pyruvic & acetic Acid

Infantile myoclonic seizures in 25 % cases

Microcephaly

Diagnosis: TMS after 72 hours of normal milk feeding

Plasma Amino Acid:
Phenyl Alanine - >240 micromole/L (Normal = 35-150),
Tyrosine level – Low/N (< 130 micromole/L)
High Ph. Alanine to Tyrosine ratio >3 (N=1-1.5)
No response to BH4 loading test

Treatment – Low phenylalanine milk and diet – to be continued throughout brain growth period (12 Years), and again during pregnancy in females to protect fetus.
Monitoring: - To Prevent Mental retardation – Keep Phenyl Alanine levels 300-400 (<600) micromole/L, <250 micromole/L during pregnancy)

Malignant Phenylketonuria

Phenyl Alanine levels are mildly raised, Symptoms are more severe due to associated deficiency of Neurotransmitters (Dopamine and serotonin)

Diagnosis: Biopterin loading test: by giving 50-100 mg of Biopterin will normalize the Phenyl Alanine within 8 Hrs, differentiating this dis. from classical PKU.

Treatment: Biopterin, DOPA & Carbidopa, 5- hydroxy tryptophane

Branch chain Amino Acid Disorders: MSUD & Organic Acidemia:

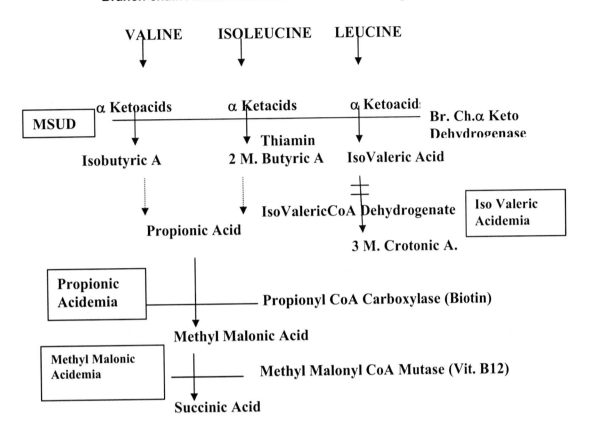

Maple syrup Urine Disease (MSUD)

1) Classical-   <2% Enzyme, Severe Neonatal intoxication Encephalopathy
2) Intermediate- 2-8% Enzyme, Late Onset, Mild Dis.
3) Intermittent- 8-16% Enzyme, Ataxia, Intermittent Intoxication episodes
4) Thiamin Responsive- Mild, Intermittent Type

Classical type –
Presents with early Neonatal (< One week age) Intoxication Encephalopathy
1) Coma, Seizures, Periodic muscle tone changes
2) Maple syrup smell (Like smell of burnt sugar)
3) Hypoglycemia & Ketonuria, Normal blood gas, Lactate & Ammonia Untreated or delay in treatment causes severe sequel
Treatment - Glucose, Dialysis, BCAA restricted diet, Thiamine as cofactor,

Organic Acidemia (Propionic, Methyl malonic & Isovaleric acidemia)
Present as Intoxication type disease onset at 1- 2 wks of life, leading to severe keto-acidosis with high anion gap, High NH4 and Lactate, ↑ Glycine, Neutropenia, thrombocytopenia, neurologic sequel.
Treatment- Hydration, NaHCO3, Diet, Carnitine / Glycine as cofactor.

Urea Cycle Diseases

Urea is synthesized from the waste amino acids to get rid of Nitrogen from the body through the urea cycle. The cycle requires six different enzymes; deficiency of each enzyme can produce a different disease. The clinical manifestations are due to accumulation of ammonia that causes severe toxic encephalopathy. More proximal the defect more severe the manifestations are. Except Ornithine Trans carbamylase deficiency, which is X linked recessive; all other diseases are inherited as Autosomal recessive.

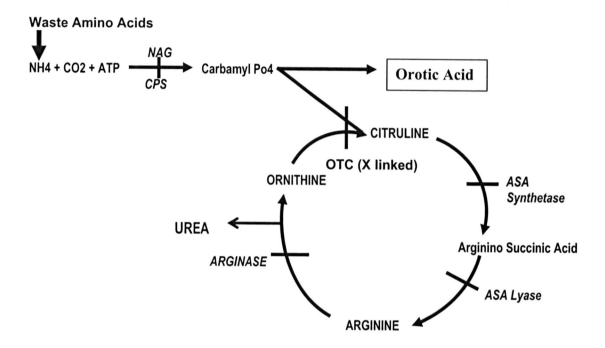

(NAG=N Acetyl Glutamate, CPS= Carbamyl Phosphate synthetase, ASA=Arginino succinic acid, OTC= Ornithine Trans Carbamylase)

Clinical presentation: Onset of disease is mostly with acute Neonatal Encephalopathy, appearing after few days of protein feeding untreated cases develop neurological sequel due to severe hyperammonemia.

Diagnosis: Severe hyperammonemia, Respiratory alkalosis due to stimulation of respiratory centers by high ammonia, Very low blood urea levels.
Diagnosis confirmed by Amino Acid Profile/ TMS showing high citrulline, Arginino succinic acid, ornithine or arginine levels depending on type of disease.

Treatment
- Hydration
- Reduction of Catabolism – High glucose, Essential AA (0.5-1 g/kg), Lipids.
- Removal of high NH4 by drugs using alternate pathway of excretion of waste amino acids by:
    - Sodium Benzoate + Glycine → Hippuric Acid. (Excretes 1 mol NH4)
    - Phenyl Acetate + Glutamine → Phenyl Acetyl Glutamate (2 mol NH4)
- Provide deficient product   -
    - Arginine (Except in Arginase Deficiency)

   o Citrulline (IN OTC) + Aspartate → Arginine (1 mol)
- Peritoneal or Hemo Dialysis in acute resistant cases
- Long term Low protein diet to provide only essential amino acids

Differential Diagnosis of Hyperammonemia in Neonatal Period:
- Urea cycle diseases.
- Organic Acidemia
- Lysinuric Protein Intolerance
- Transient hyperammonemia of new born – Preterm baby, onset at 2-3 day age, ↑ Citrulline leading to variable degree of NH4 → Intensive Rx

Galactosemia

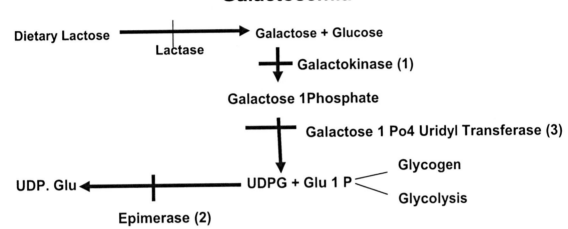

1) **Galactokinase Deficiency-**
  1:40,000
  RBC Enzyme
  Leads to Galactosuria & Cataract due to Galactitol
  Treatment: Early elimination of lactose from diet to prevent cataract

2) **Gen Epimerase Deficiency-**
  Very rare, (RBC + Fibroblast enzyme) Benign – if RBC only
  Produces Classical Galactosemia like picture

3) **G1PUT deficiency: Classical Galactosemia-**
  1:50,000
  Clincal Presentation: Presents with Cerebro- Hepato-Renal involvement
  * Cerebro - Mental Retardation
  * Hepato - Hepatitis like syndrome, Cirrhosis, Hypoglycaemia,
  * Renal   - Aminoaciduria, Proximal RTA (Fanconi's syndrome)
  * Cataract
  * Failure to thrive

  Diagnosis:
  Screening: Positive Clinitest but negative clinistix test on normal milk feeds, type of
      sugar is then confirmed by Urine chromatogram for Galactose
  RBC – Gal IP levels, G1PUT enzyme assay,
  Treatment: Strict Galactose free diet (Lactose free milk and other diet)

Glycogen Storage Diseases (GSD)

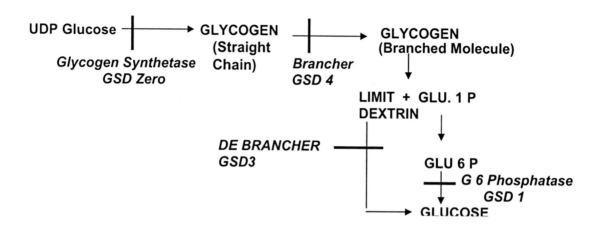

Enzymology:

> **0,1,3,4** – See the diagram
> **2** - Lysosomal α Glycosidase
> **5** - Muscle Phosphorylase
> **6** - Liver Phosphorylase
> **7** - Phospho Fructokinase
> **8** - Phosphorylase Kinase
> **9** - Liver Phosphorylase
> **10** - Muscle Kinase
> **11** - No enzyme identified yet

Clinical features:	Seen in GSD type:
Hepatomegaly	GSD -1,3,6,8,9,10
Hypoglycaemia	GSD -0,1,3,8 (6)
Hepato-splenomegaly-	GSD -3, 4
Myopathy	GSD -5, 7
Cardiomyopathy	GSD -2, (3)
Cirrhosis	GSD -4, (3)
Mental Retardation	GSD -8
Rickets (Fanconi syndrome)	GSD -11
Benign Disease	GSD -6,9,10
Gout	GSD -1

Diagnosis

- Biochemistry: Early morning/Fasting hypoglycaemia, Hypertriglyceridemia, Hyperuricemia, Ketosis, Lactic acidosis
- Abdominal Ultrasound for Liver and spleen
  - Glucagon Test
  - Enzyme Assay for confirmation

Treatment

Prevent hypoglycemia by frequent feeding, Continuous nocturnal intragastric feeding – giving ½ gm Glucose/kg/hr.

Uncooked cornstarch & frequent feeding for long-term Euglycemia

Mucopolysaccharidoses (MPS)

MPS or **Glycosaminoglycans (GAG)** are the substances produced from connective tissues, cartilage & blood vessels. They are recycled in the Lysosomes with the help of lysosomal hydrolase enzymes, deficiency of enzymes lead to storage of complex molecules producing various types of MPS depending upon enzymes involved and clinical phenotypes

Partially degraded GAG are excreted in urine detected as screening test

Only **type 2 is inherited as X linked recessive** all others are Autosomal recessive

General clinical features of MPS: Children are normal at birth, Onset around 6-12 months age

- CNS- Mental retardation
- Skin- Coarse facies, large tongue (Gargoylism)
- Bones- Short stature, multiple skeletal deformities (Dysostosis Multiplex),
- Heart- Valvular heart diseases
- Eyes- Cloudy cornea
- Organs- Hepato-splenomegaly
- Soft tissues- Upper airway obstruction, Stiff Joints
- Death in second decade- except in type 4 which has normal life span

Types & Characteristics of MPS:

Name	Urine MPS	Enzyme	Clinical Features
MPS-1- (Hurler/ Shie	Dermatan, Heparan	L-Iduronidase	CNS, Bone, Eye, Heart, liver, Spleen
MPS 2- Hunter (X-Link dis.)	Dermatan, Heparan	Iduronate sulfatase	Clear cornea
MPS 3- Sanfilippo	Heparan	Heparan N sulfatase	Severe MR, Mild-somatic features
MPS 4- Morquio	Keratan	Galactose 6 sulfatase	severe skeletal, No Mental retardation
MPS 6 Maroteaux Lamy	Dermatan	N-Ac Galactosamine 4 sulfatase	Same as MPS-1 but normal mentality
MPS 7 Sly dis	Dermatan, Heparan	Beta Glucuronidase	Severe type 1 dis.
MPS 9	Hyaluronidase	Hyaluronan	Dwarf, soft tissue masses

Note: There is no type 5 or 8 disease

Diagnosis:
- Urine Mucopolysaccharides analysis (screening test)
- Enzyme assay- WBC, Skin fibroblasts for confirmation

Treatment: *General supportive care & treatment of complications*

BMT: For type-1 disease, before CNS manifestations occur, preferably <2 Years. This corrects most somatic features but not bone & eye manifestations.

Enzyme replacement therapy: For type-1 & type 6 diseases before appearance of mental retardation.

4.4 Counselling of Parents of a child with IEM

As for any chronic illness, parents understanding and co-operation in disease management is utmost important, additionally parents and family should also receive genetic counselling
The counselling for IEM is based on following points:

1. **What are the metabolic diseases?**

    Metabolic diseases are inherited diseases resulting from absence or deficiency in one of important substances called enzymes (fermenters).
    Enzymes play an important role in regulating body metabolism as they convert harmful substances (that accumulate from breakdown of ingested food and milk) into non-harmful or useful substances. The accumulation of the harmful substances in the body could affect brain, liver, kidney and other important organs, thereby producing different clinical symptoms.

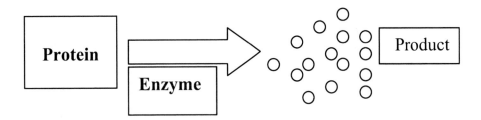

2. **How they are caused?**
    The enzymes in the human being are inherited by two hereditary factors (called genes) one of that comes from father and the other from mother. Since each parent carry one abnormal and one normal gene therefore they do not show the disease but because the affected child inherits both abnormal genes (one from each parent), therefore develops the disease.

    With each pregnancy there are three possibilities: (1) 25% chance of having an affected child (2) 25% chance of having normal child and (3) 50% chance of having a carrier child.

3. **How common are they?**
    The metabolic diseases are in general rare diseases, but they tend to occur more commonly in certain families or tribes especially after a marriage between two cousins. This is because individuals from same family or tribe are more likely to carry similar genes and passing them to their children as shown above.

4. What are the effects of these diseases?

The symptoms of metabolic diseases differ according to the affected organs.

In its most severe form the picture is usually of a normal newborn who within few days after birth on normal milk feeding starts to have excessive sleep, irritability, poor feeding and vomiting, if not treated at this time, it will progress to breathing difficulty, fits, unconsciousness or even death. Even if child survives he is very likely to suffer from a permanent brain damage. Therefore it is vitally important to diagnose and treat these diseases as early as possible.

Sometimes the symptoms may be delayed for few weeks to months if the deficiency of enzyme is partial.

It is also important to know that there are some other types of metabolic diseases that appear later in the childhood and this is because the toxic substances take longer time to accumulate to produce symptoms.

5. How they are diagnosed?

The diagnosis is usually suspected from the symptoms and the clinical examination and is strongly supported if there is a family history of the same disease in the past.

To establish the diagnosis we use blood and/or urine investigations. These investigations depend on measuring the levels of accumulated harmful substances or the depleted useful ones. Sometimes measuring the activity of the missing enzyme is needed for establishing the diagnosis.

Some of these investigations are done in our hospital laboratory and some are sent abroad so the results of these may take long time (up to few weeks). Even when waiting for the results, the treatment is started to prevent further damage.

6. How are they treated?
A.   Immediate treatment :

As soon as a metabolic disease in a newborn baby is suspected, the baby is transferred to the intensive care unit where his condition is stabilized and monitored closely and appropriate medications are offered. When the baby is stabilized, he/she is shifted to the children ward under the care of the metabolic team.

We then design long term plans about the medications and special milk.

Before discharge from the Hospital the parents are involved in the day to day care, administration of medication and preparation of milk for feeding until they are confident in fully managing the baby at home.

B.   Long term management :

i. **Special diet:** is very essential because the patient can not digest the ordinary food especially the normal milk, milk products and animal meat and these should be avoided at all the times. Consumption of Milk or food that is not recommended can make your child sick very easily. Therefore these children are only allowed to eat a special diet and Milk formula that is prescribed by their doctor and the dietician.

ii. **Special drugs: In** most cases life-long special drugs are required. The drugs help either by stimulating the deficient enzyme, or substituting the useful compounds, or getting rid of the harmful substances. The parents must follow carefully the instructions of their doctor and pharmacist in doses, methods of administration and preservation of these medications. The drugs are available in various forms (capsules, Tablets, Powder, Liquids etc.), the preparation and quantity of these drugs should be followed exactly as informed to you by the Pharmacist. Certain drugs need to be stored in refrigerator.

iii. **Management of intercurrent childhood illnesses:** Any illness in the child could cause sudden decompensation and serious health risk therefore a prompt medical attention is required.

C.   Emergency treatment:
If the child is having infection, diarrhea, vomiting, or refusing to eat, he will need more calories (sugar) to prevent excessive breakdown of body proteins and its toxicity. For this purpose, you should start the child on following special drink. This can be made as follows:

To a small bottle of water (500 ml) add:
2 sachets of ORS (Rehydration salt Mixture) or Water
10 – 15 spoons of Maxijule (a special sugar powder)

To feed this solution as much as child likes to drink.
If the child refuses to drink this mixture or vomits, then seek medical attention immediately for IV hydration.

7.   Important points to remember :

i. Always attend the doctor's and dietician's clinic appointments.

ii. Never to stop or change the special milk and drugs without doctor's permission, always keep some extra supply of medications and special milk powder at home.

iii. Seek early medical help either at your local hospital or at SQUH for any illness. You may visit the children ward at SQUH without appointment in any emergency or first call telephone 515745 to talk to the doctor or nurse in charge for advice.

iv. Keep your discharge summary and medical reports handy to show to the treating physician.

v. Never allow the child to fast for more then 6 hours.

vi. Do not expose the child to people with infections and flu illness.

vii. Have regular immunization.

viii. Book your next pregnancy and delivery only at SQU Hospital obstetrics department, so that your next baby is screened and treated without delay if found affected.

4.5 Approach to a Child with Hypoglycemia

Defined as Blood Glucose < 2.5 mmol/L (45 mg %) that complies with Whipple triad:
1. Low Blood Glucose <2.5 mmol/L
2. Presence of symptoms of hypoglycemia
3. Response to Glucose infusion

Etiology

In the Neo Natal period:

1)   ↑ **Insulin:** IDDM, Rh iso immunization, Beckwith syndrome, Pancreatic diseases (Nesidioblastosis)
2)   ↓ **Substrate:** Prematurity, IUGR and Any severe neonatal disease.

In the pediatric age roup:

1)   ↑ **Insulin**: Pancreatic diseases, Beckwith syndrome

2)   **Endocrine disorders**
        ↓ **Anti Insulin Hormone** (Growth hormone, Cortisol, ACTH) Hypo pituitarism, GH def., ACTH def., Addison's disease, Congenital Adrenal Hyperplasia

3)   **Metabolic Diseases**
     * Decreased Substrate – Ketotic hypoglycemia, MSUD
     * Glycogen Storage Dis. – Types 0, 1, 3, 8
     * Gluconeogenesis Defect – Alcohol, Aspirin, Fructose 16, Diphosphatase and Pyruvate Carboxylase deficiency
     * Liver Disease – Galactosemia, Fructosemia, Tyrosinemia
     * FAOXD, Carnitine Cycle Dis, HMG CoA Lyase deficiency. Organic Acidemia

4)   **Miscellaneous causes.**
     * Sepsis, PEM, Malabsorption syndrome, Shock, Burns, Liver dis., Rey's syndrome

Clinical evaluation:

History: Check about the time since last meal, Check if symptoms occur in early morning, postprandial or on fasting. History of any drugs intake.

Examination:
        Hepatomegaly, liver failure, or cirrhosis
        Small genitalia
        Hyperpigmentation
        Short stature
        Glucose requirement: > 10 mg/kg/min indicates hyperinsulinism unless there is marked loss of glucose in urine
     Rule out: Septicemia, severe systemic illness, small for gestation age, maternal diabetes

Laboratory tests during symptomatic hypoglycemia:

Battery of lab tests are needed to ascertain diagnosis. Samples must be taken before correcting the hypoglycemia.

Essential Tests

- Blood glucose for lab confirmation of hypoglycemia if detected on gluco Stix
- Blood gas, Anion Gap,
- Urine or serum Ketones: normal or low indicate fatty acid oxidation defects
- Lactate – may be elevated in any sick child with poor circulation (commonest cause), liver damage, impaired glycogenosis/gluconeogenesis, after seizures, difficult sampling
- Free fatty acids (if available)
- Tandem MS for amino acid and acyl Carnitine diagnostic of amino acidopathies, fatty acid oxidation defects or organic academia
- Urine organic acids by GCMS - diagnostic of Organic acidemia
- Serum insulin and cortisol levels
- Extra serum or plasma kept frozen and saved

Tests needed according to clinical situation:

- CBC, CRP, LFT, CK
- Uric acid, cholesterol/triglyceride in suspected Glycogen Storage Diseases
- Growth hormone
- Ammonia (liver damage)

Treatment:

- **Glucose**: For symptomatic hypoglycemia, give a **bolus** dose of 0.5 G/Kg Glucose intravenously (= 5 ml /Kg of 10% Glucose) stat followed by **Maintenance** Glucose therapy: 7 to 10 mg/kg/min (= 10% glucose 110-150 ml/ kg/day), keeping blood sugar >5.5 mmol/L
- **Monitor** hourly blood sugar until the level is normalized
- Await results of special investigations mentioned above
- **Consult** metabolic specialist or endocrinologist if necessary
- Hypoglycemia due to hyperinsulinism is persistent and is difficult to control requiring **other form of treatment** such as:
  o **Glucagon**: 1 mg/day or 5 to 10 mcg/kg/hour, i.v. over 2 to 3 days,
  o **Diazoxide**: 15 mg/kg/day in 3 doses, may take up to 5 days to work, may cause cardiac failure
  o **Somatostatin**: 1 to 5 mcg/kg/hour i.v.,
  o **Octreotide**: 3 to 20 mcg/kg/day in 3 to 4 does) for long term treatment

Differential Diagnosis: First Rule out sepsis, IUGR, IDM baby, Drugs

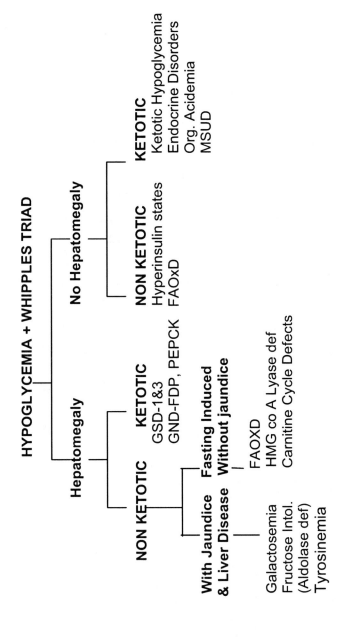

HYPOGLYCEMIA + WHIPPLES TRIAD

Hepatomegaly

No Hepatomegaly

NON KETOTIC

KETOTIC
GSD-1&3
GND-FDP, PEPCK

With Jaundice & Liver Disease

Fasting Induced Without jaundice

Galactosemia
Fructose Intol.
(Aldolase def)
Tyrosinemia

FAOXD
HMG co A Lyase def
Carnitine Cycle Defects

NON KETOTIC
Hyperinsulin states
FAOxD

KETOTIC
Ketotic Hypoglycemia
Endocrine Disorders
Org. Acidemia
MSUD

GSD: Glycogen storage disease, GND: Gluconeogensis defect,
FDP: Fructose Di phosphatase deficiency, FAOxD: Fatty acid oxidation disorders,
PEPCK: Phospho enoyl pyruvic carboxy co kinase deficiency,

4.6   Neonatal Screening

Criteria for screening a disease: The diseases should be:
- Fairly common
- Detectable in Pre-symptomatic phase
- Treatable cost effectively
- Screening test should be easily available, cost effective and have minimal false – ve. results
- Follow up, recall, confirmation and treatment of positive cases should be possible

Diseases amenable to screening in Neonatal period:

Diseases	Tests available
Phenylketonuria	- Ph. Alanine Levels by TMS
MSUD	- Plasma branch chain amino acid levels by TMS
Homocystinuria	- Plasma Methionine Levels by TMS
Fatty acid oxidation disorders	- Acyl Carnitine levels by TMS
Galactosemia	- Galactose & Gal.1-Phosphate assay
Biotinidase Assay	- Colorimetry enzyme assay
Hypothyroidism	- T4 → TSH (if T4 is low) by RIA
Congenital Adrenal hyperplasia	- 17 OH Progesterone ELISA / RIA
Hemoglobinopathies	- Hemoglobin gel electrophoresis
Wilson's Dis	- Plasma Ceruloplasmin Assay by ELISA
Cystic Fibrosis	- Plasma Immuno reactive trypsin assay
Neuroblastoma	- Plasma Vanilo Mandellic acid (VMA) assay
Other diseases-	- Fragile X syndrome, Duchenne muscular dystrophy

The hypothyroid screen is universally recommended, other diseases can be selected for screening depending on the prevalence in the local community. For Oman Hemoglobinopathies and G6PD screen are considered for screening. A pilot program is also undergoing to evaluate IEM screening.

Guthrie Test

Robert Guthrie 1961 designed a bacterial Inhibition test using- Bacillus Subtilis on a culture medium. On the culture plate a bacterial inhibitor (β_2 Thienyalanine) is added. A dry blood spot is then put in the culture media. If the Amino acid levels are high in the blood sample the bacteria will be stimulated to grow around the sample (+Ve test). While there will not be any growth around a normal blood spot.

Agar gel in a Petri dish + Bacillus Subtilis + Bacterial inhibitor + Filter Paper blood (Dry Blood Spot)

↑ Phenyl Alanine will block inhibition causing bacterial growth around blood disk in positive cases.

The positive screened cases are recalled for confirmation of disease by amino acid analysis by HPLC test. The Guthrie test is now a days replaced by more reliable test like Tandem MS

Tandem MS based screening for IEM:

Tandem MS is being utilized for screening neonatal metabolic diseases in the last decade. This technique is very robust, highly reliable and can detect up-to 30 different Inborn errors of metabolism (Amino-acidopathies, Urea cycle diseases, organic Aciduria and fatty acid oxidation disorders) by measuring amino acids and Acyl Carnitine values on one drop of blood collected as dry blood spot on the Guthrie card. The ideal time for performing this test is 72 hours after normal milk feeds as the metabolites need to accumulate in order the test to become positive.

The Guthrie card blood spot sample can be collected even at peripheral hospital and be sent in an envelop to the reference lab by ordinary post thus simplifying the transport procedure and avoiding the difficulties of broken bottles or leaked or clotted samples and the need of special courier service to transport the sample.

4.7 Protocol for the management of intercurrent Hyperammonemia in Urea Cycle Disorders

Any child with known urea cycle disorder when present with sepsis, vomiting, fever, poor feeding, lethargy, irritability, ataxia or abnormal behavior should have blood gases, renal profile and ammonia determination as an emergency. **If ammonia level is >150 μmol/L,** start treatment using the following treatment protocol:

1) Feeding:
Stop all oral protein intake including Cyclinex feeds
If tolerated, give PO/NGT Maxijule formula until ammonia is normal
Start Cyclinex feeds when ammonia level drops to normal

2) IV fluids: if vomiting or altered sensorium
Deficit + Maintenance fluid minus (-) fluids given as drugs infusion
Use 10 to 15 % dextrose in 1/5 saline as IV fluid to increase calorie intake.
Potassium must be added due to extra losses of K+ in urine. Monitor serum **Chloride** as Arginine Hcl. may cause hyper-chloremic acidosis

3) Drugs –
3A) For Citrullinemia cases-
Arginine Hcl 660 mg/kg
Sodium Benzoate & Phenyl Butyrate 250 mg/kg of each
Added together in 25 ml/kg of 10% dextrose & infused **over 90 minutes as bolus** then same doses repeated over 24 hours

3B) For Arginino Succinic Aciduria cases-
Use Arginine Hcl. 660 mg /kg and Phenyl butyrate 250 mg/ Kg mixed in 25 ml/kg 10% dextrose given over 90 minutes then same dose repeated over 24 hours
Persistent vomiting due to above drugs can be treated by Ondancetron (Zofran) 0.15 mg/kg IV.

4) Monitor – Ammonia, Urine ketone & Renal Profile every 8-12 hourly

5) Resumption of oral feeding and medications: When ammonia level is <100μmol/L, start Cyclinex feeds – if tolerated, stop IV medications and re-start oral medications as follows: Arginine 400-700 mg/kg/day,
Sodium Phenyl butyrate 250 mg/kg/day in 4 divided doses.

Immunology

5.1 Recurrent Infections and Immunodeficiency

Normal host immune defence is accomplished by:

1. Non-specific responses that do not involve the production of immunologic memory for their function like naturally occurring barriers, mucociliary clearance, peristalsis, secretions, cells and protein enzymes etc.
2. Specific immune responses from humoral and cellular mechanisms that depend upon immunologic memory for antigen recognition.

Classification
The immunodeficiency states can be classified into:

1. Primary immunodeficiency (PID): Results from defects in the four major host defence mechanisms: T-cell immunity, B-Cell immunity, Phagocyte functions and C o m p l e m e n t system. These defects are mostly genetic in origin leading to quantitative or qualitative defects like:

    a. Failure to produce specific proteins e.g. immunoglobulin in X-linked agammaglobulinemia
    b. Production of altered proteins: Truncated common gamma chain of the interleukin-2 receptor as in X-linked severe combined immunodeficiency.
    c. Enzyme deficiency as seen in adenosine deaminase deficiency.
    d. Defective gp91 as in chronic granulomatous disease

2. Secondary immunodeficiency states: due to an underlying primary cause: e.g.
    a. Infection: e.g. HIV
    b. Drugs e.g. cytotoxic agents, steroids
    c. Protein losing states: Nephrotic syndrome, Protein losing enteropathy, Lymphoreticular malignancy.

Clinical features of primary immunodeficiency

The main clinical feature of PID is recurrent infections, otitis media, pneumonia, sinusitis, bacteremia, osteomyelitis, meningitis, bacterial adenitis and skin abscesses. These infections may respond poorly to routine anti-microbial treatment and require longer duration of treatment. Pathognomonic organisms may include regular organisms like *Strep. pneumoniae* and *H. influenza* or rare organisms such as mycobacterial species. Complications of infection may occur in the form of an abscess that is difficult to drain such as the liver abscess in chronic granulomatous disease; Mastoiditis secondary to ear infections or Bronchiectasis secondary to recurrent chest infection as seen in common variable immunodeficiency.

Complications of live viral vaccination, such as the BCG vaccination, may lead to BCG adenitis or disseminated mycobacterium infection as in severe combined immunodeficiency, chronic granulomatous disease or interferon gamma – Interleukin 12 pathway defect. Oral polio vaccine may lead to paralytic polio in a child with X-linked agammaglobulinemia.

Together with recurrent infections patients with immunodeficiency may present with autoimmune diseases such as hemolytic anemia, thrombocytopenia and neutropenia as in common variable immunodeficiency.

The age of presentation can also give clue to the diagnosis: T-cells defects typically present in early infancy, while B-cells defects are usually delayed until the 2nd half of infancy and onward   due to the passive transfer of maternal antibodies. Phagocytic and complement defects could present at any age. Family history is very important as these diseases are mostly inherited. A history of consanguinity and infantile death may give clues to the nature of the immunodeficiency

Warning signs for suspecting an underlying immunodeficiency:
- Family history of immunodeficiency disease
- 8 new ear infections within 1 year
- 2 serious sinus infections within 1 year
- 2 months on antibiotics with little effect
- 2 episodes of pneumonia within 1 year
- 2 deep-seated infections, such as meningitis, sepsis or osteomyelitis
- Recurrent, deep skin or organ abscesses
- Failure to thrive
- Persistent thrush

Physical examination may include:
- Growth failure
- Absent tonsils and lymph nodes
- Lymphadenopathy
- Hepatomegaly
- Splenomegaly
- Eczematous skin rash

Laboratory Investigations

When immunodeficiency is suspected, the following screening tests should be performed. They may be tailored according to the history with respect to the immune system arm likely to be involved. All of these tests are high-yield and can serve as the screening test followed by more detailed testing when abnormal.
- B- Cell Immunity
  - Quantitative immunoglobulins (IgG, A, M, E)
  - Isohemagglutinins: IgM antibodies.
  - Specific antibodies, response to immunization e.g. Diphtheria and Tetanus titers.
- T-cell immunity
  - Total lymphocyte count
  - T and B cells numbers
  - Delayed hypersensitivity skin tests (individuals >2 years of age)
  - Lymphocyte proliferation assay
  - Lateral chest x-ray in infants to see for thymus size
- Neutrophil
  - Absolute neutrophil count
  - Nitro Blue Test (NBT), or Dihydrorodamine 1,2,3 test (DHR 123) to test for the Oxidative burst.
- Complement
  - Total hemolytic complement test
  - C3 and C4 concentration

More detailed testing of the patient with immunodeficiency can be performed as indicated guided by the results of the screening tests. Specialized testing of the immune system is technically more difficult and expensive. It is performed only at certain laboratories worldwide.

Therapy of primary immunodeficiency diseases may include:
- Intravenous Immunoglobulin therapy in B-cell and T-cell diseases
- Avoidance of live vaccines
- Frequent and judicious use of antibiotics, preferably bactericidal types
- Prophylactic antibiotics and antifungal drugs (Co-Trimoxazole or Itraconazol) as indicated
- Use of irradiated blood products to avoid graft versus host disease
- Gamma interferon in chronic granulomatous disease
- Stem cell transplantation in T-Cell defects
- Hyperimmunizations with bacterial polysaccharide vaccines (e.g. Pneumococcal vaccines) in complement deficiency
- Enzyme replacement or Gene therapy in adenosine deaminase deficiency.

Common Immunodeficiency diseases

1. X-Linked Agammaglobulinemia

X-Linked agammaglobulinemia is a humoral immunodeficiency characterized by recurrent pyogenic infections usually beginning by 5-6 months age due to abnormally very low immunoglobulins level. The B-cells are absent in the blood while T-cells are intact. The disease was first described by Ogden Bruton in 1952, named after him as **Bruton's agammaglobulinemia.**

The disease is inherited by an **X-Linked mode**, the gene has been identified on long arm of X chromosome at Xq22. It encodes an enzyme called Bruton tyrosine kinase (BTK) a B-cell progenitor kinase that is essential for B-cell differentiation.

Infants usually present with recurrent otitis media, pneumonia, meningitis, dermatitis and occasionally arthritis and malabsorption leading to FTT. The organisms most commonly involved are *Streptococcus Pneumonia* and *Haemophilus influenzae*; occasionally other organisms might be involved. Viral infections are usually tolerated however meningoencephalitis due to echoviruses and paralysis related to live virus vaccination has been reported.

Physical examinations usually relate to the repeated infections but X-Linked agammaglobulinemia is characterized by absence of lymph nodes and tonsils; the spleen is of normal size. The diagnosis is usually based on absence or marked deficiency of all five immunoglobulins classes with absence of B-cell in the circulation. Molecular diagnosis for BTK is possible.

Treatment involves aggressive antibiotic therapy for acute episodes and replacement therapy with periodic gamma globulin infusion at doses that will achieve adequate levels to prevent recurrence of infections. Some patients may require prophylactic broad-spectrum antibiotic therapy.

2. Common variable immunodeficiency (CVID)

Is a heterogeneous immunodeficiency syndrome characterized by hypogammaglobulinemia, recurrent bacterial infections and various immunological abnormalities. Familial inheritance is seen in 25% of cases. The genetic defect has not yet been clearly identified, but it could be due to dys-regulation of the genes expression involved in immunoglobulins production. In addition to B-Cell defect, variable degrees of T-Cell dysfunction have been frequently noted.

The incidence of infections shows two peaks: one around 1-5 years and other at 16-20 years of age. Common presentations include recurrent upper respiratory infections, pneumonia, sinusitis, otitis media and bronchiectasis. The **organisms** commonly involved are encapsulated organisms like *Streptococcus Pneumonia* and *Haemophilus Influenzae* however, in patients with bronchiectasis, *Pseudomonas aeruginosa* and *Staphylococcus Aureus* account for the majority of cases.

Physical signs may include marked lymphadenopathy and splenomegaly. Diagnosis of CVID can be made when the level of serum immunoglobulins is decreased with IgG being < 3.0 g/L. IgA is also markedly reduced and in half of the patients IgM is also reduced. Production of specific antibodies is reduced.

Treatment of CVID is with replacement therapy with gamma globulins. Although there is some evidence that it does not halt the progression of lung changes, it certainly does reduce the incidence of pneumonias. The aim of the replacement therapy has not been clearly identified, but it seems that a trough level maintained above 5 g/l significantly reduces the incidence of pneumonia. Patients with CVID may require prophylactic antibiotics therapy in addition to monthly gamma globulins. CVID have increased incidence of autoimmune diseases and malignancies.

3. Severe Combined Immune deficiency (SCID)

Severe combined immunodeficiency has many genetic causes even though the phenotype is fairly uniform. Affected infants present in early infancy with persistent thrush or an extensive Candida diaper rash. They may have intractable diarrhea failure to thrive or a persistent pertussis like cough due to interstitial pneumonia caused by *Pneumocystis Carinii infection.* They may have a morbilliform rash shortly after birth, due to transplacental passage of maternal lymphocytes, which mount a graft-versus-host reaction. Death could result from viral infections.

Diagnosis of severe combined immunodeficiency represents a medical emergency; infants could die rapidly if correction by bone marrow transplantation is not performed. Infants with SCID almost invariably have profound lymphopenia but normal lymphocyte count does not exclude it. Lymphocytes phenotype by flow cytometry reveals marked reduction of T-cells in the presence or absence of B and NK cells according to the underlying molecular defect causing SCID. On stimulation of patient lymphocytes with various mitogens they fail to proliferate. The thymic shadow cannot be seen on a chest film because the thymus fails to become a lymphoid organ. The serum immunoglobulin concentrations are all low, except IgG may be maternal in early infancy.

X-Linked SCID is the commonest form of SCID; the gene is mapped to Xq13 encoding the gamma chain of the interleukin-2 receptor. Autosomal recessive SCID can be the result of defects of JAK-3, RAG 1 & 2 deficiency, or adenosine deaminase deficiency. Many patients with adenosine deaminase deficiency have benefited from regular injections of adenosine deaminase conjugated to polyethylene glycol. Adenosine deaminase deficiency was also the underlying problem treated in the first successful gene therapy.

Treatment of SCID is a stem cells transplant; it should be performed as quickly as possible, since SCID is invariably fatal. In families with a previously affected infant, prenatal diagnosis is now possible so that preparations for transplantation can be made in advance of the birth.

4. Chronic Granulomatous Disease (CGD)

CGD is characterized by recurrent life-threatening infections caused by catalase-positive bacteria and fungi and granuloma formation. Overwhelming infections are commonly caused by *Staphylococcus aureus, Burkholderia cepacia, Serratia marcescens, Nocardia* species, and *Aspergillus* species. The gram-negative organisms usually cause pneumonia and cellulitis. Bacteremia is usually caused by *B cepacia, S marcescens*. The diagnosis of a staphylococcal liver abscess is pathognomonic for CGD and should always prompt screening for CGD. Mycobacterial infection may also occur. Granuloma formation may affect the gastrointestinal and urinary tract presenting with symptoms of obstructions.

Defects are in the reduced nicotinamide adenine dinucleotide phosphate (NADPH) oxidase, the enzyme complex responsible for the generation of hydrogen peroxide and oxygen radicals required for bacterial killing by phagocytes. CGD can be caused by mutations in any of the 4 structural genes of the NADPH oxidase, inherited as X-Linked or in an autosomal recessive manner.

Diagnosis of CGD is made by **Nitro blue tetrazolium test** or the Dihydrorodamine flow cytometry based test.

Trimethoprim-sulfamethoxazole prophylaxis has reduced the frequency of bacterial infections and staphylococcal infections, *Aspergillus* infections are now the leading cause of mortality. Prophylaxis with itraconazol reduces the risk of fungal infections in patients with CGD. In clinical trials, IFN-g therapy reduced infections by 70% in patients with CGD compared to a placebo. HLA-matched bone marrow transplantations have been performed in patients with CGD with very good success.

5.2 Anaphylaxis

Anaphylaxis is a multi-system syndrome resulting from release of mast cell mediators; it may vary from mild and self-limited form to a severe and fatal reaction.

Causes:
- Food allergy: Common in children than in adults
- Insect stings
- Medications
- Radiocontrast media
- Allergen testing or desensitization immunotherapy injections
- Latex allergy
- Idiopathic

Clinical manifestations of anaphylaxis:
- Urticaria and/or angioedema occur in 90% of episodes
- Upper airway edema in 56%,
- Dyspnea and/or bronchospasm in 47%,
- Flushing in 51%,
- Tachycardia, lightheadedness or syncope (hypotension) in 33%
- Gastrointestinal manifestations in 30%.

Anaphylaxis may present as a **biphasic reaction** with recurrence several hours after apparent resolution of the initial signs and symptoms. Biphasic anaphylaxis has been reported in 4 to 20% of cases. Since life-threatening manifestations may recur during the second phase, it is necessary to observe patients for up to 12 hours after apparent recovery from an initial episode of anaphylaxis.

Patho-physiology:
Anaphylaxis via an IgE mechanism requires initial exposure to an antigen. This may result in the production of specific IgE antibodies in susceptible individuals, which bind to the receptors on mast cells. The bound IgE molecules will recognize subsequent exposure to the same antigen. Anaphylaxis is caused by cross-linking of mast cell surface receptor-bound IgE molecules leading to release of chemical mediators of anaphylaxis.

Mediators from mast cells and basophils account for most of the signs and symptoms of anaphylaxis. Histamine is a bronchoconstrictor and causes vasodilatation and increased vascular permeability. The cardiovascular effects of histamine occur through action on both H1 and H2 receptors. Leukotriene possibly cause bronchoconstriction and increased vascular permeability. Tumor necrosis factor released from mast cells also induces nitric oxide production. Nitric oxide production may be responsible for vasopressor-resistant cases of anaphylactic hypotension.

Allergens causing IgE-mediated anaphylaxis are mostly proteins, although most drug allergens are haptens (Incomplete antigens). The most common drug allergens are the beta-lactams (Penicillins and Cephalosporin) and the sulfonamides but virtually any antibiotic can cause anaphylaxis.

The most common food allergens are peanuts, shellfish and fish, and sometimes milk, eggs, seeds and even some fruits and vegetables (e.g. kiwi, avocado). Fatal food anaphylaxis has occurred because of delayed use of epinephrine often due to delayed recognition of the reaction and insidious progression of symptoms to a severe and refractory level. Food allergy has also been noted to disappear more commonly when there is strict avoidance.

Iodinated radiocontrast media are associated with non-IgE-mediated activation of mast cells and basophils. Prior exposure (sensitization), therefore, is not required. Anti-IgA antibodies may cause anaphylactoid reactions when intravenous immunoglobulin is administered to a patient with selective IgA deficiency. Similarly, blood or plasma transfused into IgA deficient patients who possess anti-IgA antibodies of the IgG class may form circulating immune complexes, activate complement, and cause an anaphylactoid reaction.

Atopy is present in an estimated 36-49% of patients with anaphylaxis, whereas an estimated 10-20% of the general population has atopy.

Allergen immunotherapy injections may cause systemic reactions that can be mild, moderate or severe in nature. Fatal reactions have been reported. It is very important to be aware of the risk factors, to institute appropriate precautions, and to be prepared at all times to recognize reactions early and institute promote treatment. Most systemic reactions begin within 20 minutes of injection, but some will occur after 30-60 minutes. Asthma is a significant risk factor for severe reactions to immunotherapy; Reactions have been most commonly related to errors in administration, (wrong vial, and wrong dose).

Recent estimates report that fatal anaphylaxis occurs in about 4% of cases. There is increased risk of death when the body's homeostatic mechanisms are interrupted as when patients are being treated with beta-blockers, angiotensin converting enzyme (ACE) inhibitors, or when there is underlying adrenal insufficiency. Epidemiologic studies have also suggested increased risk of death in patients with asthma.

Diagnosis of anaphylaxis:
The diagnosis of anaphylaxis is made on the basis of clinical setting and clinical presentation. Cutaneous and respiratory findings occur in at least 60% of subjects. Urticaria and angioedema are the most common manifestations and the absence of either should prompt a physician to consider another diagnosis.

The diagnosis can be confirmed in doubtful cases by elevated mast cell enzyme called **tryptase** that remains elevated for up to six hours following anaphylaxis.

Prevention:
Anaphylaxis may be prevented by avoidance of exposure to relevant antigens. Insect avoidance instructions should be given to all patients allergic to Hymenoptera venom. **Venom immunotherapy** reduces the incidence of recurrent anaphylaxis by 95%. When penicillin allergy is suspected and no other antibiotic will suffice, penicillin skin testing and, if necessary, **desensitization** should be performed. If a patient has a history of radiocontrast media sensitivity, a pretreatment regimen of **prednisone together with H1 and H2 antihistamines,** and the use of low osmolality, non-ionic dye reduce recurrent anaphylactoid episodes. Beta blockers and ACE inhibitors should be avoided in patients at risk for anaphylaxis such as those receiving immunotherapy injections, skin tests for allergic disease, or those known to be allergic to Hymenoptera venoms.

Treatment of Anaphylaxis:

A, B, C (Airway, Breathing and Circulation)

Application of a tourniquet proximal to the site of allergen deposition, if possible, retards the systemic circulation of allergen as well as locally released mediators.

Epinephrine is the mainstay pharmacological treatment.
Intravenous fluids, colloids or crystalloids with or without the Vasopressors
May be needed to combat hypotension

Intravenous **diphenhydramine** (H1 blocker antihistamine) will prevent, or possibly reverse, the histamine-induced component of anaphylactic hypotension. Cimetidine H2 blocker may also be used.

Intravenous **glucagon** may reverse the hypotension of patients who have been treated with beta-adrenergic blockers and are unresponsive to epinephrine.

Glucocorticosteroid: Glucocorticosteroid help in by preventing sustained bronchospasm. They also prevent *tissue based* late phase reactions by interfering with the recruitment and activation of eosinophils and neutrophils.

Patients who have experienced anaphylaxis should be referred to an allergy-immunology specialist for diagnosis and counseling. Patients with a history of anaphylaxis to foods, hymenoptera venom, exercise, or unknown causes should be given a **preloaded epinephrine syringe (Prepen) for emergency use**. Demonstration of proper technique with a placebo trainer is recommended since many patients receive improper or no instructions.

6

Infectious Diseases

6.1 Fever in young child without a focus of Infection?

Introduction:

Fever is a common problem in children. Up to 75% of children presenting to emergency room have temperature below 39 c but some 13 % children have fever >39 c. 30% of children below three years with fever have no focus of infection.

Viral infections are common causes for fever in young children, unfortunately there is no simple test available to differentiate between bacterial from viral illness. Secondly some febrile children without focus of infection may have an underlying bacteremia that could prove serious if not treated adequately. It is therefore always a dilemma to decide when to use antibiotics in a febrile young child.

In this chapter we aim to see in what situations a febrile child is more likely to have bacterial infection to justify antibiotic treatment.

Diagnostic criteria for febrile bacteremia:

Fever > 39 c of < 1-week duration
Well looking child
3 - 36 Months of age
No focus of infection on history and physical examination.
With a positive bacterial culture

Incidence:

Various studies have reported the risk of bacteremia in febrile child ranging from 2.3 to 11.6 % (average, 4%). There has been a recent decrease due to HIB immunization

What are the likely organisms?

Strept Pneumoniae: accounts for 85% cases
H. Influenzae (Hib)
Nisseria Meningitidis
Salmonella species

Why Children below 3 years are more susceptible to bacteremia:

Maturational immunodeficiency with low opsonic IgG production to polysaccharide antigen of capsulated Bacteria is the main reason of S. Pneumoniae bacteremia.

Predictive value of temperature and WBC counts:

Temperature of >40c Doubles the risk for presence of bacteremia
WBC: <15000 = 1% Chance of bacteremia
        >15000 = 16% (Especially if associated with polymorphs with Bands & left shift)

Likely outcome of bacteremia:

Spontaneous resolution in 80% of Pneumo coccal infection but only in 5% cases of H. Influenzae bacteremia. Most of persistent bacteremia tends to Localize to an organ causing Pneumonia, Meningitis, Cellulites, Osteomyelitis/ Arthritis.

Management strategy:

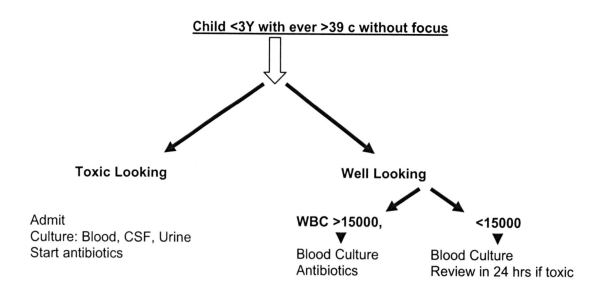

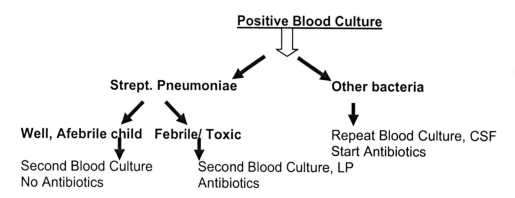

Fever in patients with Sickle cell disease:

These children have high incidence of bacteremia & complications due to:
>Functional Asplenia
>Defect in alternate complement pathways

Bacteriology:
>Pneumococcus, H Influenzae, Salmonella, E Coli

Management:
>Prompt Blood culture, (CSF, Urine, stool, Bone if indicated)
>If sick, Fever >40 c, CBC <5000 or >30000: Admit and start antibiotics
>If not sick: Give one dose of Ceftriaxone and observe for 24 hrs.

Fever > 38 c in an infant <3 Months of age:

Etiology:
Viruses 70%
Unproven infections 15%
Bacteria in only 15% cases:
       Group B Streptococci
       Pneumococcus, Meningococcus, H Influenzae
       Salmonella, E. coli
       Listeria
       Staphylococcal

Management strategy:

A. **Well looking baby:**
    No focus of infection
    WBC 5000-15000, Bands <1500
    Normal Urine-analysis
    Septic work-up and observation

B. **Toxic looking baby**
    WBC <5000 or >15000, Bands >1500
    Perform a septic screen
    Start on Antibiotics: Cefotaxime or Ceftriaxone plus Ampicilline

6.2 Child with Skin Rash

Characteristics of skin rash in common viral exanthemas: Many viral and some bacterial infections present with fever and rash. Some specific characteristics can help in identification.

Primary Lesions

Primary skin lesions provide the most vital clues for making a correct diagnosis. They are the most representative lesions of the disease process without any alteration by the patient due to scratching, rubbing, secondary infection or therapy.

Macules:
> Are flat, non-palpable areas of color change of skin.
> Macules may be erythematous, hypo/or hyper pigmented.
> Examples include café-au-lait spots, vitiligo, Mongolian blue spot and port wine stain etc.

Papules
> They are circumscribed raised skin lesions of less than 0.5 cm in diameter.
> Examples include molluscum contagiosum, warts and miliaria rubra (prickly heat).

Nodules
> Nodules are elevated skin lesions larger that 0.5 cm in diameter.
> They may be located in the epidermis, dermis or subcutaneous tissue.
> Examples include epidermoid cysts fibromas and neurofibromas.

Plaques
> Are well-circumscribed, broad-based lesions often formed by coalescence of a number of papules. The diameter or size of the lesions is greater than its height or elevation.
> A typical example is psoriasis.

Wheals/Urticaria
> They are transient, raised edematous skin lesions with irregular edges.
> The lesions are erythematous with a central pallor.
> Intense itching is usually present.
> They can be seen in dermographism (Darier's sign), urticaria and insect bites.

Vesicles
> The elevated, **fluid-containing** skin lesions of <1.0 cm diameter are called vesicles.
> Examples include chicken pox, herpes simplex or zoster and contact dermatitis.

Bullae
> When vesicles are **larger than 1.0 cm** diameter, they are called bullae.
> They may be intraepidermal or sub epidermal.
> Examples include epidermolysis bullosa and staphylococcal scalded skin syndrome.

Cysts

The circumscribed tumors containing semisolid or fluid contents are called cysts. Typical example is epidermal cysts that occur after puberty on the face and upper back.

Pustules

The elevated well circumscribed skin lesions containing **purulent** material or pus. Unlike the transparent dew drop appearance of vesicles, the pustules may be turbid or opaque. Examples include folliculitis or pyoderma.

Comediennes

These are characteristic skin lesion of **acne** distributed on the face and upper back. Open comedones or **black heads** are 2-5 mm flesh colored papules with black centers.
The closed comedones or **white heads** are 1-3 mm papules with a pin point opening.

Purpura

The leakage of **blood in the skin** is called purpura.
Unlike erythematous macules, purpura cannot be blanched by pressure.

Petechiae

They are small, pinpoint areas of hemorrhages while **ecchymoses** are large areas of extravasations of blood in the skin. Ecchymotic skin patches may be flat or raised above the surface when there is associated vasculitis.
Example: Henoch-Schonlein Purpura and Collagen vascular disorders.

Secondary Lesions

They are produced due to changes affected by scratching, touching, secondary infection and due to local and systemic effects of medications

Crusts

They are formed by drying of blood, serum and any exudates overlying the diseased skin. They are often present in impetigo, in which they appear honey-colored and in infants with weeping eczematous lesions.

Excoriations

They develop as a result of scratching and rubbing. Common examples include contact dermatitis, atopic dermatitis and insect bites.

Ulcers

They occur due to deeper loss of the skin involving both epidermis and a variable depth of dermis or subcutaneous tissue due to infection, vascular insufficiency or burns.

Fissures

Linear clefts deep through the epidermal layer in thickened or chronically inflamed skin.

Lichenification

The exaggeration of skin markings due to chronic rubbing due to allergic or infective skin lesions is called Lichenification.

Atrophy

Atrophy of skin refers to loss or thinning of the epidermis or dermis. Epidermal atrophy is characterized by wrinkling of skin with telangiectases. In dermal or subcutaneous atrophy, the skin is depressed.

Eczematous Skin Lesions

It refers to inflammatory skin lesions which have indistinct margins with erythema and vesiculation in the acute phase. Scaling, crusting and Lichenification may be seen as the disorder progresses.

Hyperkeratosis

It is a thickening of the stratum corneum. The presence of thick rough scales over skin lesions is a good clinical marker of hyperkeratosis.

6.3 Common Childhood Exanthematous fever

Epstein - Barr virus (EBV) infections: Infectious mononucleosis (glandular fever):

EBV infects pharyngeal epithelial cells and then B lymphocytes. These disseminate and proliferate until checked by activated T Cells.

Transmission: saliva, aerosol, kissing disease

Incubation: 30-50 days

Clinical Presentation:

Fever, sore throat, lymphadenopathy, palatal petechiae

Splenomegaly (50%), Hepatomegaly (30%), Hepatitis (80%), Jaundice (5%), Thrombocytopenia Hemolytic anemia

Maculopapular rash (5-15%), 90% if given Ampicillin

Complications

Meningitis, Encephalitis, Guillain-Barré Syndrome, Myocarditis, Splenic rupture, Airway obstruction from Pharyngo tonsillar swelling

Chronic fatigue-like syndrome

Disseminated disease with B cell proliferation in those with T cell immunodeficiencies

Diagnosis

Atypical lymphocytosis on peripheral blood film of CBC

Positive Paul-Bunnell (often negative in young children) or Monospot test, Serology, Heterophile antibodies, PCR

Treatment: Supportive, Steroids for severe airway obstruction

Cytomegalovirus (CMV)

Transmission: close contact, blood, organ transplant

Clinical Presentation:

In normal hosts – often asymptomatic or glandular fever like picture

In Immunocompromised patients – severe disease may occur with Pneumonitis, retinitis, encephalitis, hepatitis and GI disturbance

CMV is the most common **congenital infection**

Diagnosis

Immunofluorescence, intranuclear inclusions, culture, detection of early antigen fluorescence foci (DEAFF) test, Serology and PCR test

Treatment: Symptomatic, IV Gancyclovir and/or IV Foscarnet if immunosuppressed

Herpes Simplex Virus (HSV) Infection

Two types are recognized: HSV-1 (Skin and mucous membranes) and HSV-2 (usually genital)

Primary infections – 85% sub clinical

Recurrent infections – reactivation of latent infection

Incubation: 2-12 days

Transmission: direct contact, very rarely congenital

Clinical Presentation:

Acute herpetic gingivostomatitis – primary infection – acute painful mouth ulcers and fever, most common between 1 and 3 years of age, self-limiting, lasts 4-9 days (may be asymptomatic)

Recurrent stomatitis **"cold sores"** – Vesicular lesions of nasolabial folds
Keratoconjunctivitis and corneal ulcers
Meningoencephalitis
Eczema herpeticum – widespread infection of eczematous skin
Genital lesions – usually in sexually active adolescents, NB: child abuse
Neonatal HSV – acquired from vaginal secretions at delivery – high morbidity and mortality due to meningo-encephalitis

Diagnosis
Electron microscopy of vesicular fluid (very fast), PCR, culture, serology

Treatment
Acyclovir – IV if severe disease, in Immunocompromised host, neonate or in eczema herpeticum patients
Oral, Topical, Eye Drops

Varicella Zoster Virus:

This produces **Chicken Pox** as a primary infection and **Shingles (Herpes Zoster)** as reactivation of dormant virus in dorsal root or cranial ganglia.
Chicken pox can be acquired from contact with chicken pox or shingles patients but shingles can not be acquired from direct contact.

Chicken Pox

Incubation: 11-24 days
Transmission: Direct contact, droplet, airborne; infectious from 24 h before rash until all spots have crusted over (approx. 7-8 days)
Clinical Presentation:
Prodrome of fever and malaise for 24 h; rash appears in crops, first papular then vesicular and itchy, usually start on trunk; crops appear for 3-4 days and each crusts at 24-48 h.

Complications
•Secondary bacterial infection often with group A Streptococcus
•Thrombocytopenia with hemorrhage into skin
•Pneumonia
•Purpura fulminans
•Post-infectious encephalitis, Cerebellitis causing acute ATAXIA
•Immunocompromised – severe disseminated hemorrhagic disease

Diagnosis: Clinical, viral culture
Treatment:
Supportive; Intravenous Acyclovir for immunosuppressed or severely unwell patient (Acyclovir may be given to reduce the severity of the illness with the appearance of the first vesicle. Delayed treatment is of no value)

Prophylaxis:
Zoster immunoglobulin (VZIG) to high riskpatients e.g.: immunodeficiency, or if mother develops chicken pox 5 days before or 2 days after delivery the infant should also be treated with IV Acyclovir.

Herpes zoster

Clinical presentation
Prodrome of pain and tenderness in the affected dermatome with fever and malaise; within a few days rash similar to Varicella appears in distribution of the dermatomes

If infection of the fifth cranial nerve occurs, it may affect the cornea (ophthalmic branch), If eighth nerve involved, paralysis of facial nerve and vesicles in external ear occur (Ramsay-Hunt syndrome)

Complications: dissemination in immunocompromised host.

Treatment: supportive, IV Acyclovir, if severe and Immunocompromised (Routine VZV vaccine available)

Parvovirus B19 (Erythema Infectiosum, Fifth disease)

Affects red cell precursors and reticulocytes in the bone marrow.

Incubation: 1 week

Transmission: respiratory secretions

Clinical presentation:

Very erythematous cheeks (slapped cheeks appearance), then erythematous macular popular rash on trunk and extremities, which fades with central clearing giving the characteristic lacy or reticular appearance, Rash lasts for 2-30 days

Complications:

Aplastic crisis in chronic hemolytic diseases

Aplastic anemia

Arthritis

Congenital infection with anemia and hydrops fetalis.

Diagnosis: Clinical, serology.

Treatment: Supportive.

Roseola Infantum (Exanthem Subitum)

Transmission: Respiratory secretions

Clinical presentation:

Sudden onset of high fever with absence of any localizing signs.

May have **febrile convulsions**.

On day 3-4, child becomes afebrile abruptly and a macular/popular rash appears which usually lasts for less than 24 hours.

Treatment: Antipyretics.

Measles

Incubation: 7-14 days.

Transmission: Respiratory droplets, infectious from 7 days after exposure, i.e. 1 day before rash to 5 days after onset of rash.

Clinical features:

Prodromal stage of 3-5 days with fever, cough, conjunctivitis, **Koplik's spots** (pathognomic white spots on inflamed red base, opposite to lower molars)

Eruptive stage: starts with abrupt rise in temperature to 39-49 ^{0}C associated with macular rash, starting behind ears and along hairline, becomes maculopapular and spreads sequentially to face , upper arms, chest, abdomen, back and legs; lasts approximately 4 days.

Complications:

- Otitis media, laryngitis, bronchitis.
- Interstitial Pneumonitis, secondary bacterial bronchopneumonia, Myocarditis, Encephalomyelitis: mainly post-infectious, demyelinating
- Subacute sclerosing panencephalitis occurs many years later

Diagnoses: Clinical, viral culture, immunofluorescence, serology.

Treatment: Symptomatic, human pooled immunoglobulin less than 5 days of exposure to high risk patients only

Prophylaxis: Immunization- MMR vaccine

Mumps

Incubation: 14-21 days

Transmission: By respiratory droplets; patient is infectious 24 hrs before to 3 days post parotid swelling

Clinical features:

Mild prodrome of fever, anorexia, headache, painful bilateral/unilateral parotid gland swelling. Sometimes may affect sub mandibular glands.

Complications:

- Meningoencephalitis
- Orchitis/epididymitis-15-35 % in adolescents/adults occurs within 8 days of parotitis, abrupt onset of fever, tender, swollen testes. Approximately 30-40% of affected testes atrophy may cause subfertility.
- Pancreatitis, nephritis, Myocarditis, arthritis, deafness, thyroiditis.

Diagnosis: High serum Lipase or amylase levels, clinical, serology

Treatment: Supportive

Prophylaxis: Vaccination-MMR

Rubella (German measles)

Incubation: 14-21 days

Transmission: Respiratory droplets or transplacental

Clinical features:

- Mild coryza, palatal petechiae
- Tender, retroauricular, posterior cervical and sub occipital adenopathy, 24 hrs before rash appears, lasting for one week
- Rash begins on face, spreading quickly to trunk.

Complications:

Arthritis, Encephalitis, Thrombocytopenic purpura

Congenital rubella syndrome (low birth weight, cataract, microphthalmia, retinopathy, lymphadenopathy, splenomegaly, deafness, hepatitis, thrombocytopenia, hemolytic anemia, Microcephaly; severe psychomotor retardation, Diagnosis is by antibody tests for rubella that are positive as soon as the rash appears in the mother; rubella specific IgM antibody in the neonate; rubella virus can also be cultured from nasopharynx or urine of affected baby that could be seen even up to one year of age)

Diagnosis: Clinical, serology

Treatment: Supportive

Prophylaxis: vaccination – MMR

Adenovirus

Transmission: Respiratory droplets, contact, fomites; very contagious, strict infection control policy

Incubation; 2-14 days

Clinical presentation:

- Upper respiratory infection
- Conjunctivitis/Pharyngitis
- Gastroenteritis

Complications: Severe pneumonia, disseminated disease in the Immunocompromised.

Diagnosis: viral culture, serology, PCR.

Treatment: supportive.

Enteroviruses

These include **Polioviruses, Coxsackie and Echoviruses**

Transmission: Fecal/oral and respiratory droplets usually during summer and autumn

Clinical presentation:

- Non specific febrile illness, malaise and myalgia, lasting for 3-4 days.
- Respiratory illness: Pharyngitis, tonsillitis and nasopharyngitis for 3-6 days.
- Gastro intestinal manifestations- diarrhea, vomiting and abdominal pain.
- Skin manifestations;- **Hand foot and mouth involvement (Coxsackie virus A16, enterovirus 71)**; intraoral ulcerative lesions, vesicular lesions on hands and feet, 3-7 mm in size, clearing by one week
- Pericarditis / Myocarditis (Coxsackie B virus)
- Neurological manifestations; Aseptic meningitis (Coxsackie virus B50, encephalitis (echovirus 9), cerebellar ataxia, Guillain- Barré syndrome.

Diagnosis: Viral culture, PCR.

Treatment: Supportive

Prophylaxis: OPV vaccine against polio virus.

Molluscum Contagiosum:

Incubation: 2-8 weeks

Transmission: Direct contact with infected persons.

Clinical presentation: Discrete, pearly papules 1-5 mm on face, neck, axillae and thighs

Diagnosis: Clinical, Microscopy

Treatment: Self limiting, but may last for months or years; in immunodeficiency or widespread disease, cauterization/liquid nitrogen application may be necessary.

6.4 Principles of Anti infective Therapy

The choice of Anti infective therapy is based on following principles:
- Identify the infecting organism and its sensitivity
- Take history of previous adverse reactions to antimicrobial agents
- Check renal and hepatic function
- The choice of antibiotic would also depend on the site of the infection
- Obtain all necessary cultures before prescribing
- Choose narrow spectrum and bactericidal antibiotics if possible
- Use the cheapest, safest and most effective antibiotic
- Prescribe and complete the course of treatment
- In Pediatrics, the dosage should always be based on the weight of the child
- The duration of the treatment would depend on many factors (age, site and type of infection, the organism involved and the immune status of the child)
- Antibiotics should not be prescribed routinely to all patients of fever, especially when the cause of fever is not clear. ***"ANTIBIOTICS ARE NOT ANTIPYRETICS"***

1. SYSTEMIC OR FOCAL SEPSIS

INFECTION	ORGANISM	TREATMENT	ALTERNATIVE
1a. Septicemia 1-3 months age	Group B Strept, H Influenzae Gram-ve Bacteria, Listeria	Ceftriaxone 100mg/kg/d:OD:IV +Ampicillin 200mg/kg/d: q6h:IV	Ampicillin 200mg/kg/d: q6h:IV +Gentamycin 7.5mg/kg/d: q8h:IV
>3 months age	S Pneumoniae, H Influenzae, Gram-ve Bacteria, Salmonella Spp. (e.g.: in SCD), N Meningitis	Ceftriaxone 100mg/kg/d:OD:IV + Gentamycin 7.5mg/kg/d: q8h:IV	Cefotaxime 50mg/kg/dose: q12h:IV + Amikacin 7.5mg/kg/dose: q12h:IV
	Pseudomonas	Peperacillin 50mg/kg/d: q8h:IV + Gentamycin 7.5 mg/kg/d: q8h:IV	Ceftazidime 150mg/kg/d: q8h:IV + Gentamycin 7.5mg/kg/d: q8h:IV
MRSA Septicemia	Methicillin-Resistant S Aureus	Vancomycin* 15mg/kg/dose: q8h: IV (Infuse over 1 hr)	Teicoplanin* 10mg/kg/d: q12h:IV x3 doses; then 10mg/kg/OD:IV
Bacterial Endocarditis	Strep Viridans	Benzyl penicillin 50mg/kg/dose: q4h:IV + Gentamycin 7.5mg/kg/d: q8h:IV	Ceftriaxone 100mg/kg/d: OD:IV
Neutropenia With Infection	Gram-ve, E Coli, Gram +ve, Staphylococci Coag-ve Staph	Ceftriaxone 100mg/kg/d:OD:IV +Gentamycin 7.5mg/kg/d: q8h:IV	Cefotaxime 50mg/kg/d: q6h:IV +Gentamycin 7.5mg/kg/d: q8h:IV
	Pseudomonas	Tazocin 90mg/kg/dose: q6h:IV	Ceftazidime 150mg/kg/d: q8h:IV + Gentamycin 7.5mg/kg/d: q8h:IV
	S Aureus	Cloxacilin 200mg/kg/d: q6h:IV + Gentamycin 7.5mg/kg/d: q8h:IV	

2. RESPIRATORY TRACT INFECTION

INFECTION	ORGANISM	TREATMENT	ALTERNATIVE
Dental Infections	Oral Anaerobes, Microaerophilic and Aerobic	Penicillin V 50mg/kg/d: q6h: PO + Metronidazole 7.5mg/kg: q8h:IV	Co-Amoxiclav 10mg/kg/d: q8h: PO
Otitis Media	S Pneumoniae, H Influenzae, Moraxella	Co-Amoxiclav 30-50mg/kg/d: q8h: PO	Cefprozil 30mg/kg/d: q12h: PO
Pertussis	Bordetella Pertussis	Erythromycin 40mg/kg/d: q6h:IV	
Sinusitis Acute Sinusitis Chronic	As for Otitis Media	Co-Amoxiclav 30-50mg/kg/d: q8h: PO	Cefuroxime 100mg/kg/d: q8h:IV
Tonsillitis	Group A β-Hemolytic Strept.	Penicillin V 50-100mg/kg/d: q8h: PO	Erythromycin 50mg/kg/d: q6h: PO
Lower Respiratory Tract Infection			
Bronchitis	Viral Various Bacteria	Symptomatic: No Antibiotic As for sinusitis	
Pneumonia 1-3 months age	H Influenzae, S Pneumoniae	Cefuroxime 60-100mg/kg/d: q8h:IV To Follow: 5-15mg/kg/d: q12h: PO	
>3 months age	H Influenzae, S Pneumoniae	As above	As above
Bronchopneumonia (severe cases in child <2 years)			
	S Aureus S, Gram-ve Bacteria	Cloxacilin 200mg/kg/d: q6h:IV +Cefotaxime 50mg/kg/d: q6h:IV	
Atypical Pneumonia	M Pneumoniae, Chlamydia	Erythromycin 50mg/kg/d: q6h: PO (3 Day Course)	Moxifloxacin 10mg/kg/d: OD: PO
Respiratory Syncytial Virus: Nil; Aerosol Ribavirin Controversial			
	Coxiella Burnetii	Ciprofloxacin[¤] 10mg/kg/d: q12h: PO **or** 8mg/kg/d: q8h:IV	
Tuberculosis	M Tuberculosis, M Bovis	Rifampicin 10mg/kg/d:OD: PO +Isoniazid 5mg/kg/d:OD: PO +Pyrazinamide 25mg/kg/d: PO +Pyridoxine 5mg OD: PO	
Standard Therapy: 3 Drugs for 2m; Rifampicin and Isoniazid for 4m			

Cystic Fibrosis:
Intermittent Therapy:
Colonization of the respiratory tract with various organisms including Pseudomonas and Staphylococcus Aureus is invariable. Two-Four weeks courses of Amoxycillin, Co-Trimoxazole, Ciprofloxacin or Moxifloxacin PO may reduce exacerbations in selected patients, however, antibiotic resistance develops. Aerosolized Antimicrobials e.g.: Tobramycin are an option.

Acute Exacerbations:

ORGANISM	TREATMENT	ALTERNATIVE
Polymicrobial, H Influenzae, S Aureus, Pseudomonas	Tazocin 50mg/kg/d: q6h:IV +Gentamycin 3mg/kg/d: q8h:IV	Cefipime[¤] 50mg/kg/d: q12h:IV +Tobramycin 6-10mg/kg/d:OD:IV

*NB: Because multi-resistant organisms may be present, rigorous infection control policy is essential to prevent cross infection.

3. Gastro enteral infections

INFECTION	ORGANISM	TREATMENT	ALTERNATIVE
Gastroenteritis	*Non-Typhi Salmonella	None Usually	Co-Trimoxazole
	*Shigella	None Usually	Co-Trimoxazole
	Campylobacter	None Usually	Erythromycin
*Children <6 months of age/immunocompromised with Systemic infection, systemic antibiotics indicated		Ceftriaxone 60mg/kg/d:OD:IV	

4. CNS Infections:

INFECTION	ORGANISM	TREATMENT	ALTERNATIVE
Abscess: Brain	Polymicrobial, Anaerobes S Aureus	Ceftriaxone 100mg/kg/d:OD:IV +Metronidazole 7.5mg/kg/d: q8h:IV +Cloxacilin 200mg/kg/d: q4h:IV	Benzyl penicillin 100mg/kg/d: q4h:IV +Metronidazole 7.5mg/kg/d: q8h:IV +Cloxacilin 200mg/kg/d: q4h:IV
Meningitis	H Influenzae, S Pneumoniae N Meningitidis, Listeria +Neonatal Pathogens	Ampicillin 200-400mg/kg/d:q6h:IV +Ceftriaxone 100mg/kg/d:OD:IV	Chloramphenicol; 100mg/kg/d: q6h:IV 2d, then 50mg/kg/d: q6h:IV/PO
If Gram+ve Diplococci in CSF, add Vancomycin 15mg/kg/d: q8hIV over 1h for possible resistant S Pneumoniae			
	Resistant H Influenzae	+Rifampicin 5mg/kg/d:OD:IV	
Indication For Dexamethasone: H Influenzae Meningitis in child >6 weeks. Start 1h before antibiotics: 0.15mg/kg/d: q6h:IV for 48h.			
Tuberculosis	M Tuberculosis, M Bovis	Rifampicin 10mg/kg/d:OD: PO +Isoniazid 5mg/kg/d:OD: PO +Pyrazinamide 25mg/kg/d: PO +Pyridoxine 5mg OD: PO	
Standard Treatment: All 3 for 2m, Rifampicin +Isoniazid for 7m.+/- Corticosteroids: Indications as in adult section on TB Meningitis			
Toxoplasmosis Abscess	T Gondii	Sulphadiazine 100-200mg/kg/d:OD: PO +Pyrimethamine 200mg PO loading dose: follow-up with 50mg OD x 38d +Folinic Acid 5mg/d:OD: PO	

5. Genito-Urinary infections and Sexually transmitted diseases:

INFECTION	ORGANISM	TREATMENT	ALTERNATIVE
5a. Genito-Urinary Infection Lower UTI	Coliforms, Enterococci	Nalidixic Acid 50mg/kg/d:OD: PO	Co-Amoxiclav 30-60mg/kg/d: q8h: PO
Acute Pyelonephritis	Coliforms, Enterococci, Proteus	Cefotaxime 25mg/kg/d: <4w q12h:IV >4w q8h:IV	Gentamycin 2.5mg/kg/d: q8h:IV

6. Skin and soft tissue infections:

CONDITION	ORGANISM	TREATMENT	ALTERNATIVE
Abscess	S Aureus	Cloxacilin 200mg/kg/d: q6h:IV	Co-Trimoxazole 1.5-3mg/kg/d: q12h:IV
Animal Bite	(+Tetanus Toxoid&Rabies Vaccine) Pasturella Multocida, C Morsitans	Co-Amoxiclav 30-60mg/kg/d: q8h: PO	Cefaclor 20-40mg/kg/d: q8h: PO
If risk of rabies active and passive rabies immunization			
Burns, Infected also Wassim	Streptococci Pseudomonas	Erythromycin 30mg/kg/d: q6h:IV Ceftazidime 150mg/kg/d: q8h: v IV	Benzylpenicillin 400mg/kg/d: q6h:IV
Cellulitis	Streptococci S Aureus	Erythromycin 30mg/kg/d: q6h:IV Cloxacillin 200mg/kg/d: q6h:IV	Benzylpenicillin 400mg/kg/d: q6h:IV Clindamycin 3-6mg/kg/d: q8h: PO **or** IV over 30 mins.
Impetigo	S Aureus, Streptococci	Cloxacillin 200mg/kg/d: q6h: PO/IV **or** Azithromycin 10mg/kg/d:OD: PO	Co-Trimoxazole 1.5-3mg/kg/d: q12h: PO/IV
Necrotising Fascitis	Group A, C, G Strep Polymicrobial Neonate >4 Weeks	Benzylpenicillin 400mg/kg/d: q6h: IV +Metronidazole 15mg/kg Stat:IV; then 7.5mg/kg/d: q12h:IV Q8h	Erythromycin 30mg/kg/d: q6h:IV
Tetanus	C Tetani	Benzylpenicillin 400mg/kg/d: q6h: IV +Tetanus human immunoglobulin 3,000 units IV single dose +tetanus toxoid 1st dose or booster	Erythromycin 30mg/kg/d: q6h:IV
Wound Infection	S Aureus, Streptococci, Coliforms	Cloxacillin 200mg/kg/d: q6h:IV +Gentamycin 7.5mg/kg/d: q8h:IV	Erythormycin 30mg/kg/d: q6h:IV

7. The immunodeficient child

CONDITION	ORGANISM	TREATMENT	ALTERNATIVE
Neutrophilic dysfunction		Treat as patients with neutropenia	
B-Cell Deficiency a) Prophylaxis b) Fever c) Fever>48 hrs d) Chest X-Ray Suggests Pneumocystis	Pneumocystis Gram+ve/-ve	Cotrimoxazole 0.5-0.75m² 480mg:PO 0.76-10m² 960mg:PO (Given Monday, Wednesday, Friday) Cefotaxime 150-200mg/kg/d:IV +Gentamycin 2.5mg/kg/d: q8h:IV +Vancomycinℜ 45mg/kg/d:IV (slow over 1h) Co-Trimoxazole 60mg/kg/d: q12h:IV	Ceftazidime 150mg/kg/d: IV +Amikacin 7.5mg/kg/d: q12h:IV
T-Cell Deficiency a) Prophylaxis	Pneumocystis Jiroveci Other Fungi	Cotrimoxazole 0.5-0.75m² 480mg:PO 0.76-1.0m² 960mg:PO (Given Monday, Wednesday, Friday) Amphotericin B (Infuse 4-6h)	

b) Fever **c)** Fever >48hrs	Gram+ve/-ve Vancomycin[×] 15mg/kg/d: q8h:IV +Amphotericin B 0.5-1.0mg/kg/d OD:IV (4-6h infusion)	Cefotaxime 200mg/kg/d:IV +Gentamycin 2.5mg/kg/d: q8h:IV	Ceftazidime 150mg/kg/d: IV +Amikacin 7.5mg/kg/d: q12h:IV
d) Chest X-Ray Suggests Pneumocystis	Co-Trimoxazole 60mg/ kg/d: q12h:IV		

8. Bones and Joint Infections:

CONDITION	ORGANISM	TREATMENT	ALTERNATIVE
Septic Arthritis Acute Osteomyelitis	S Aureus, H Influenzae, Streptococci	Cloxacillin 200mg/kg/d: 4-6h:IV +Ceftriaxone 100mg/kg/d:OD:IV Treat as for septic arthritis	
Ch Osteomyelitis	Gram-ve Rods, S Aureus, TB MRSA	Await Cultures Vancomycin 15mg/kg/d:q8h:IV over 1h **Or** Rifampicin 10-15mg/kg: PO **or** IV over 3h	

Restricted antibiotics: Thease antibiotics are restricted for specific indications or can only be prescribed by infectious disease specialist.

Tazocin: Dose-90 mg/kg/dose q 6-8 hrs infusion, (especially effective against pseudomonas), Indications-Febrile neutropenia (given with an amino glycoside for synergistic action), severe respiratory infections in immunocompromised children

Meropenem: Dose –10-20 mg/kg/dose every 8hrs, in meningitis 40 mg /kg/every 8 hrs, max-6g/day, indications Hospital acquired infections, Septicemia, febrile neutropenia, meningitis

Imipenem: Dose 15- 20-mg/kg every 6 hrs, (Avoid meningitis due to poor penetration and risk of seizures), Indications- Aerobic and Anaerobic Gram positive and Gram-negative infections.

Cefipime, Ceftazidime, Vancomycin and Teicoplanin: (see above) are also restricted antibiotics and require consent from the ID team.

6.5 Human Immunodeficiency Virus (HIV) Infection

Human Immunodeficiency Virus (HIV) is a retrovirus i.e. it contains the enzyme reverse transcriptase, which allows its viral RNA to be incorporated into host-cell DNA
Two main types are known: **HIV-1** (Widespread) and **HIV-2** (West Africa)
The virus mainly infects CD4 T helper cells. The deficiency of T helper cells leads to acquired immunodeficiency due to B-Cell dysregulation.

Transmission
- •Vertical: From the mother, this is the commonest mode of transmission in children
  - ▪Intrauterine
  - ▪Intrapartum (most common)
  - ▪Postnatally via breast milk
- •Through blood or blood products
  - ▪ In Hemophilia patients
  - ▪ By using contaminated needles
- •Via Mucus Membranes
  - ▪ Sexual intercourse, NB: Sexual Abuse

Diagnosis
1. Viral detection – Viral culture/ DNA PCR/RNA PCR
2. Antibodies – Elisa / Western blot
3. Antigen studies – P24 antigen

The diagnostic tools available are ELISA, Western Blot, DNA & RNA PCR, viral count, P-24 antigen and viral cultures. Good number of vertically transmitted cases can be diagnosed in the first two weeks and almost all by 4-6 months age. The diagnosis of HIV in babies is difficult due to the presence of passively acquired antibodies from the affected mother. An alternative diagnostic test in infants is by detecting the virus or its antigen by PCR or Viral culture on 2 separate specimens taken at different times
Viral load is also used as a parameter to judge the response to treatment as well as a guideline to modify the therapeutic regimen

Management of babies of HIV-positive Mothers:
- Start Zidovudine (AZT, Azidothymidine) orally within 12h of birth
- PCR is 50% positive by 1 week and 90% by 2 weeks
- Check urine for CMV, screen for hepatitis virus
- Look for signs of drug withdrawal
- At 6 weeks: Repeat HIV PCR, stop AZT, start cotrimoxazole Prophylaxis
- At 3-4 months: Repeat HIV PCR
- If all 3 PCRs are negative then there is >95% certainty that baby is not infected, at this point one can stop Cotrimoxazole and just follow-up the baby until HIV Antibody (vertically acquired from mother) are negative.

Follow-Up of HIV Positive Babies/Children:
- To see the baby/child every 3-6 months
- Provide good psychological and social support
- Immunization Information
- Look for the signs of persistent or unusual infections and growth
- 20% of vertically infected children developed AIDS in infancy, approximately

5% of HIV infected children develop AIDS every year
- Most common AIDS-defining illness was presence of a PCP infection
- Hepatitis B, C Viruses, CMV, Toxoplasma status if indicated
- FBC, T cell Subsets/CD4 Count, HIV Viral Load
- Decisions regarding -Pneumocystis Carinii Prophylaxis (PCP) and Highly Active Antiretroviral Treatment (HAART)

Common complications of HIV in children:

1. **Recurrent Bacterial Infections**
   Due to poor CD4 (T-Helper Cell) function, there is B-Cell dysregulation despite often high immunoglobulin levels
   Recurrent serious bacterial infections, such as Pneumonia, Meningitis, Septicemia and Osteomyelitis, may occur. Most common organisms are S Pneumonia, H. Influenzae, Coliforms and Salmonella

2. **Failure to Thrive**
   This is frequently multifactorial:
   Reduced nutrient and fluid intake – psychosocial, oral and esophageal thrush
   Increased nutrient and fluid requirement with chronic disease
   Increased fluid loss with diarrhea – look for gut pathogens, microsporidiosis, cryptosporidiosis, Giardia, atypical mycobacterium and viruses

3. **Lymphocytic Interstitial Pneumonitis (LIP)**
   LIP is caused by diffuse infiltration of pulmonary interstitium with CD8 (cytotoxic) lymphocytes and plasma cells.
   May cause progressive cough hypoxemia and clubbing. Superimposed bacterial infections and bronchiectasis may occur. It is often diagnosed by chest x-ray picture

4. **HIV Encephalopathy**
   This may present with neuro-regression, behavioral difficulties, acquired microcephaly, spastic diplegia, ataxia, and pseudobulbar palsy.

5. **Thrombocytopenia**

6. **Opportunistic Infections**
   i) Protozoa
   Pneumocystis Carinii Pneumonia (PCP) +/- CMV Pneumonitis:
   Most common at 3-6 months of age; presents with persistent non-productive cough, hypoxemia, dyspnea and minimal chest signs
   Chest x-ray typically shows bilateral perihilar "butterfly" shadowing
   Diagnosis is by bronchoalveolar lavage
   Treatment: Supportive, may need to be treated in pediatric intensive care unit, high dose Co-Trimoxazole (Septrin) is given for 21 days. Use steroids in severe disease. Gancyclovir IV if concurrent CMV disease is present. Once stable, commence HAART. Prophylactic low dose Septrin following treatment.

Cerebral Toxoplasmosis:
Rare in childhood HIV infection compared to adults

Cryptosporidiosis:
Cryptosporidium parvum causes severe secretory diarrhea and abdominal pain
Diagnosis by stool microscopy +/-small bowel biopsy
Treatment: Supportive, Paromomycin

ii) Fungal Infections
Candida Albicans
Mostly involving oropharyngeal, esophageal, vulvovaginal or rarely may cause disseminated infection. Treatment: Fluconazole or IV Amphotericin B

Cryptococcus Neoformans: Meningitis (insidious onset), pneumonia
Diagnosis by CSF examination (Indian ink satin, antigen, culture), serum culture and antigen, Treatment: Fluconazole

iii) Viral Infections
CMV: Retinitis, colitis, pneumonitis, hepatitis, pancreatitis
Diagnosis by serum PCR, immunofluorescence and characteristic retinal changes if present; differentiate disease from carriage
Treatment: IV Acyclovir, HAART may help

Herpes Simplex Virus (HSV)
Types 1 and 2 – extensive oral ulceration
Treatment: IV Acyclovir, oral Prophylaxis if recurrent and severe

Measles, Varicella Zoster Virus (VZV), RSV, Adenovirus – all may cause severe disease in HIV infected children, especially pneumonitis

iv) TB and Atypical TB:
Increased risk of TB and Atypical TB, especially disseminated M Avium Complex

7. Tumors
Kaposi's sarcoma: Very rare in children. It is a tumor of vascular endothelial cells, associated with human Herpes Virus-8 (HHV-8) involving skin, gut, lung and lymphatics.
Treatment: HAART, Local Radiotherapy, Chemotherapy if disseminated
Non-Hodgkin's Lymphoma

HIV Treatment

1. Protective Immunizations
2. Antiretroviral therapy
3. Treatment of Opportunistic infections
4. PCP prophylaxis

Indications for starting antiretroviral therapy

1. All children
    a. They are if symptomatic
    b. If there is a drop in CD4 count or rapid increase in the viral load

Highly active Antiretroviral Therapy (HARRT): Time to start treatment in children varies in each country. In Oman, one may start HARRT once child has any of above-mentioned AIDS-defining illness or many B-category symptoms, rapidly increasing viral load or decreasing CD4 counts. Usually 3 drugs are necessary to reduce resistance

Many regimes being evaluated involving protease inhibitors, nucleoside reverse transcriptase inhibitors and non- nucleoside reverse transcriptase inhibitors. *Liaise with tertiary center specialists for further guidance.*

Monitor for efficacy (viral load and CD4 count) and side effects

PCP Prophylaxis: PCP prophylaxis is recommended depending the age of the child, Cd4 count and whether child had PCP pneumonia or not

1. Cotrimoxazole
2. Dapsone
3. Atovaquine
4. Pentamidine

CMV Prophylaxis (Acyclovir): Life-long if ever had CMV retinitis

Breast-feeding:

Although rare but there are reports about transmission of HIV via breast milk, In developing countries breast milk has several other benefits to the child therefore breastfeeding is stopped only if safe alternative is available.

Role of various interventions in preventing HIV transmission:

Stopping breast-feeding reduces transmission to 15%

Use of antiretroviral treatment to mother and baby – reduces rate to 5%

Elective LSCS – reduces transmission to 1%, If Vaginal Delivery is chosen one must avoid invasive fetal procedures, e.g.: fetal blood sampling

MAJOR SIDE EFFECTS OF ANTIRETROVIRAL DRUGS USED IN CHILDREN	
DRUGS	**SIDE EFFECT**
A: Nucleoside Reverse Transcriptase Inhibitors	
1. AZT - Zidovudine	Nausea, bone marrow suppression, Myopathy
2. DDI - Didanosine	Peripheral neuropathy, pancreatitis
3. D4T - Stavudine	Peripheral neuropathy, pancreatitis, raised LFTs
4. 3TC - Lamivudine	Rare – peripheral neuropathy, pancreatitis
5. Abacavir	Life threatening hypersensitivity reactions – usually present as rash and fever
B: Non-Nucleoside Reverse Transcriptase Inhibitors	
1. Efavirenz	Rash, +/-Stevens-Johnson Syndrome
2. Nevirapine	Rash, Hepatitis
C: Protease Inhibitors	
1. Ritonavir	GI side effects common in first 4 weeks, paraesthesia
2. Indinavir	GI disturbances, rashes
3. Nelfinavir	Diarrhea
NB: Protease Inhibitors and D4T are associated with Lipodystrophy	

6.6 Viral Hepatitis
(Please also see chapter 7.5)

Viral hepatitis may be caused by number of viruses. There are six hepatotropic viruses named A to G. In addition many other viruses (CMV, EBV, HIV, Adeno, Entero and Parvo virus B19) can also involve liver as part of multi-system disease

Hepatitis A:
Diagnosis is by detection of the hepatitis virus IgM.

Transmission:

Feco-oral, There is no carrier state and fulminant hepatic failure is very rare (less than 0.1%). The liver function however may be abnormal for up to 1 year.

Prevention:

By either passive or active immunization. Passive immunization is with Immunoglobulins which protects for 3-6 months. Active immunization is with a live attenuated virus. Booster immunization is required after 12-18 months.

Clinical symptoms:

Initially non specific and include anorexia, nausea, fatigue and fever associated with epigastric pain and tender Hepatomegaly. The icteric phase then develops with jaundice, pale stools and dark urine pruritus, persistent jaundice and raised transaminases for a prolonged period are common. The prothrombin time should be monitored. A raised prothrombin time indicates the possibility of severe hepatic necrosis or decompensation of underlying liver disease.

Hepatitis B
Diagnosis:

By detection of the hepatitis B surface antigen (HBsAg).HBeAg positive patients carry a larger virus load and are more infectious. Acute and ongoing chronic infection is associated with anti-HB core IgM. Anti-HBe and anti-HBs antibodies appear as an effective, as an effective immune response develops. All HBs Ag positive children are infective

Transmission:

Parenteral

Perinatal transmission rate is dependent upon the maternal serology. If mother is HBsAg positive and HBeAg negative, the risk is 12-25%. If mother is HBsAg positive and HBeAg positive, the risk is 90%.

It is also known that younger patients have less risk of symptomatic liver disease but they do have greater risk for prolonged viral carriage.

90% OF INFANTS INFECTED IN THE FIRST YEAR OF LIFE BECOME CHRONIC CARRIERS.

Clinical Presentation:

Often asymptomatic, but an acute hepatitis picture can develop with acute liver failure in less than 1 % of patients. The risk of fulminant hepatitis is increased by co-infection with hepatitis D.

Chronicity results in an increased risk of cirrhosis and hepatocellular carcinoma chronically infected children have a 25% life time risk of cirrhosis and hepatocellular carcinoma. Males are more likely to be chronic carriers than females.

Prevention: By both active and passive immunization.

Treatment: Interferon-alpha is the recognized treatment of chronic infection

Vertical transmission of Hepatitis B:

Vertical transmission is thought to account in about 40% of hepatitis B cases worldwide.

The hallmark of ongoing infection is the presence of HBsAg. The presence of anti body to HBsAg alone suggest successful immunization; it's presence along with anti-HBcAg suggests resolved infection.

Hepatitis B immunoglobulin given at birth alone reduces the risk of vertical transmission. Hepatitis B vaccine at birth, 1 and 6 months of age along with hepatitis B immunoglobulin can protect up-to 93% of neonates.

Hepatitis C

Transmission is either perinatal or parenteral. The vertical transmission rate is about 10 % higher in HIV positive mothers.

Diagnosis: By serology with the detection of the anti-HCV antibody.

Clinical features: Infection is usually asymptomatic or may present as acute hepatitis. Fulminant hepatitis is uncommon. HCV RNA detection establishes the presence of viremia confirming infection and infectivity. Chronic infection is common, leading to cirrhosis and hepatocellular carcinoma over 10-15 years.

Treatment is with Interferon-alpha. No vaccine is currently available.

Hepatitis D

Transmission – Parenteral, The virus can replicate and causes the disease only in the presence of hepatitis B virus.

Diagnosis is by detection of anti hepatitis D antibodies and HBsAg in the serum.

It can remain asymptomatic or present as acute hepatitis or fulminant hepatitis.

Successful eradication requires high dose interferon.

Hepatitis E

Epidemics occur in developing countries.

Transmission is Feco-oral.

The clinical course of hepatitis E infection is similar to Hepatitis A. Complete recovery from acute infection occurs and chronic infection has not been reported. Acute fulminant hepatic failure can occur, especially with pregnancy.

Diagnosis is by serology.

No vaccine or prophylaxis is available.

Characteristics of various Hepatotropic viruses:

Characteristics	HAV	HBV	HCV	HDV	HEV	HGV
TYPE	RNA	**DNA**	RNA	RNA	RNA	RNA
INCUBATION	1 month	3 months	2 months	3 months	1 month	?
TRANSMISSION	FECAL	**Parenteral**	**Parenteral**	**Parenteral**	FECAL	**Parenteral**
CHRONICITY	Acute	Chronic	Chronic	Chronic	Acute	Chronic
SEVERITY		**Fatal**		**Fatal**		

7

Digestive System and Hepatology

7.1 Acute Gastroenteritis and Dehydration

Definitions:

Acute diarrhea:
Frequent loose watery stools starting acutely and lasting for less than 2 weeks.

Chronic diarrhea
Diarrhea lasting >2 weeks with failure to thrive.
Mostly secondary to some underlying cause e.g.: Cystic fibrosis, Celiac disease etc.

Persistent diarrhea
Diarrhea that begins acutely but persists for >2 weeks.
Also referred to as post enteritis syndrome

Dysentery
Diarrhea with visible blood and mucous in the stools

Facts about diarrhea
GE is one of the leading causes of morbidity & mortality in children all over the world, causing one billion episodes of illness & 3-5 million deaths annually

Etiology

Predisposing factors

Host factors:
- Lack of breast feeding
- Malnutrition
- Poor hygiene
- Young age
- Immune deficiency disorders
- Maternal illiteracy and poor hygiene

Environmental factors:
- Unhygienic environment
- Day care centers

Causative Agents

Viruses
Rotavirus, Adenovirus, Enterovirus, Norwalk virus

Bacteria
Escherichia coli, Vibrio Cholera, Yersinia Enterocolitica
Salmonella, Shigella, Campylobacter Jejuni

Protozoa
Entamoeba Histolytica, Giardia Lamblia,

Fungal:
Cryptosporidium

Pathogenesis of Diarrhea

1. Secretary Diarrhea
Abnormal secretion of water and electrolytes from the damaged villi into the small bowel e.g. Ecoli, Vibrio cholera, Rotavirus etc.

225

2. Osmotic Diarrhea

Diarrhea due to ingestion of poorly absorbed, osmotically active substance like lactulose, lactose or sorbitol causing osmotic indrawing of water in the lumen.

3. Entero invasive Diarrhea

An infective organism causes invasion of the intestinal mucosa damaging the villi hence decreasing the absorptive surface area as well as loss of the enzymes causing diarrhea. eg. Entero-invasive E. Coli, salmonella and Shigella.

Clinical Signs and degree of dehydration

	Mild = 3-5%	Moderate = 6-9%	Severe = 10-15%
Mucous membrane	Normal/ slightly dry	Dry	Very dry
Eyes/Fontanel	Normal	Sunken	Deeply sunken
Skin turgor	Normal	Prolonged skin fold	Very prolonged
Tears	Present	Reduced	Absent
Extremities	Well perfused	-/+ Delayed cap. refill	Delayed capillary refill >2 sec
Mental status	Alert	Irritable, -/+ lethargic	Lethargic/obtunded
Pulse volume/rate	Normal	Rapid	Rapid, feeble,
BP	Normal	Decreased	Markedly reduced (shock)
Urine output	Normal	Decreased	Absent for > 8 hr
Respiration	Normal	-/+ deep	Rapid /deep

Types of Dehydration: Based on the amount of salt lost in relation to water, the dehydration may be classified into 3 forms

1. Isotonic dehydration: When the net loss of water and sodium is in the same proportion as the extracellular fluid, the serum sodium is normal (130-150 mmol/l) as well as the serum osmolality (275-295 m Osmol/l)

2. Hypertonic dehydration: When the net loss of water in stool is more then sodium or when concentrated formula (ORS or Milk) is fed to the child. Serum sodium concentration is elevated (>150 mmol/l), Serum osmolality is elevated (>295 mOsmol/l).
Since the loss of fluid is more from the cells then the circulation, the signs of dehydration are masked and skin becomes doughy and warm. Seizures may occur due to hypernatremia or on rapid correction of dehydration and sodium levels.

3. Hypotonic dehydration: When the net sodium loss in stools is more then water or if children are given plain water or hypotonic fluid to drink to correct dehydration, it leads to hyponatremia (serum sodium <130 mmol/l) and hypo-osmolality (serum osmolality <275 mOsmol/l). These children are lethargic, irritable and have more marked signs of circulatory failure. Seizures may also develop.

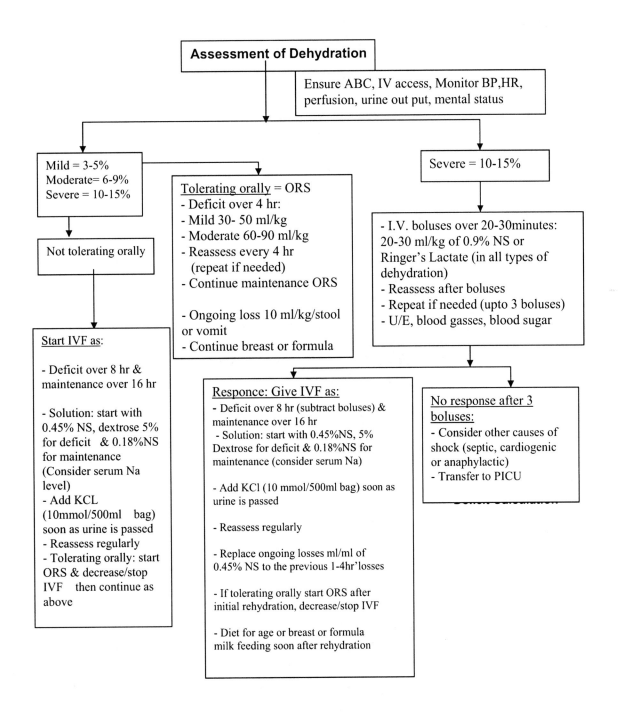

Assessment of Dehydration

Ensure ABC, IV access, Monitor BP,HR, perfusion, urine out put, mental status

Mild = 3-5%
Moderate= 6-9%
Severe = 10-15%

Tolerating orally = ORS
- Deficit over 4 hr:
- Mild 30- 50 ml/kg
- Moderate 60-90 ml/kg
- Reassess every 4 hr
  (repeat if needed)
- Continue maintenance ORS

- Ongoing loss 10 ml/kg/stool or vomit
- Continue breast or formula

Severe = 10-15%

- I.V. boluses over 20-30minutes: 20-30 ml/kg of 0.9% NS or Ringer's Lactate (in all types of dehydration)
- Reassess after boluses
- Repeat if needed (upto 3 boluses)
- U/E, blood gasses, blood sugar

Not tolerating orally

Start IVF as:

- Deficit over 8 hr & maintenance over 16 hr

- Solution: start with 0.45% NS, dextrose 5% for deficit & 0.18%NS for maintenance (Consider serum Na level)
- Add KCL (10mmol/500ml bag) soon as urine is passed
- Reassess regularly
- Tolerating orally: start ORS & decrease/stop IVF then continue as above

Responce: Give IVF as:
- Deficit over 8 hr (subtract boluses) & maintenance over 16 hr
- Solution: start with 0.45%NS, 5% Dextrose for deficit & 0.18%NS for maintenance (consider serum Na)

- Add KCl (10 mmol/500ml bag) soon as urine is passed

- Reassess regularly

- Replace ongoing losses ml/ml of 0.45% NS to the previous 1-4hr'losses

- If tolerating orally start ORS after initial rehydration, decrease/stop IVF

- Diet for age or breast or formula milk feeding soon after rehydration

No response after 3 boluses:
- Consider other causes of shock (septic, cardiogenic or anaphylactic)
- Transfer to PICU

Treatment of Gastroenteritis:

Management Objectives:
- Restoration of adequate hydration
- Replacement of ongoing losses
- Correction of electrolytes/acid base balance
- Maintenance of adequate nutrition
- Treatment of complications
- In selective cases treatment of specific pathogens & prevention of their spread

Fluid Volume required for deficit correction:

Mild dehydration = 30-50 ml/kg
Moderate dehydration = 60-90 ml/kg
Severe dehydration = 100-150 ml/kg

Fluid Volume required for Maintenance:
First 10 kg = 100 ml per kg
Second 10 kg = 50 ml per kg
>20 kg = 20 ml per kg

Oral Rehydration Solution
- Effective in mild & moderate dehydration regardless of type of dehydration
- Can prevent dehydration if given early
- Cheap, easy to administer, can be given by mother at home
- Can be given by spoon, cup, or NGT
- Deficit:
  - Mild = 30-50 ml/kg over 4 hr,
  - Moderate = 60-90 ml/kg over 4 hr
  - Ongoing losses 10 ml/kg /stool or emesis

Composition of various ORS formula:

Glucose Mmol/l	Cl- Mmol/l	K+ Mmol/l	Na+ Mmol/l	Solutions
111	80	20	90	WHO
140	65	20	75	Rehydralyte
14	35	20	45	Pedialyte

Composition of various IV fluids:

Dextrose	Lactate	Cl- Mmol/l	K+ Mmol/l	Na+ Mmol/l	Solutions
0	0	154	0	154	NS (0.9% NaCl)
5%	0	77	0	77	1/2 NS (0.45% NaCl)
4.3%	0	36	0	36	1/5 NS (0.18% NaCl)
	28	109	4	130	Ringer Lactate

Management of specific electrolyte imbalance

Isonatremic dehydration (Na = 130-150 mmol/L)
- Total correction over 24 hrs
- Deficit over 8 hr & maintenance over 16 hr
- Solution used: 0.18% saline with 4% dextrose (Pediatric saline) or 0.45% saline with 5% dextrose

Hyponatremic dehydration (Na <130 mmol/L)
- Total body sodium deficit = (135 - actual serum Na) x 0.6 x body wt
- Sodium maintenance = 2-3 mmol/kg/day
- Correction over 24 hr as isonatremic dehydration
- Solution: according to total sodium deficit (usually 0.45% or 0.9% NS)
- Serum sodium not to be increased >12 mmol/l per 24 hr (risk of central pontine myelinolysis)
- Symptomatic hyponatremia (seizures): give 3% saline 4 ml/kg slowly over 15 min

Hypernatremic dehydration (Na >150 mmol/L)
- Do not allow dropping serum sodium level rapidly (risk of cerebral edema)
- Duration of fluid correction is based upon initial serum sodium level:

* 145-157 mEq/l → 24 hr
* 158-170 mEq/l → 48 hr
* 171-183 mEq/l → 72 hr
* 184-196 mEq/l → 84 hr

- Accepted rate of sodium drop should be 0.5 mmol/hr or not more than 12 mmol/l per 24 hr
- Solution: Start with 0.45% NS
- In severe dehydration first restore intravascular volume by 20 ml/kg of NS over 20-30 min then follow as above
- Symptomatic hypernatremia (seizures) during correction of hypernatremia (Rapid decreased of serum Na level): Give 3% saline 4 ml/kg iv slowly over 15 min, till seizures stop
- Monitor serum sodium, hypocalcaemia, hypoglycaemia and assess the patient regularly

- If serum Na decreases too rapidly → increase Na concentration of IVF or
                                      → decrease the rate of IVF

- If serum Na decreases too slowly → decrease Na concentration of IVF or
                                     → increase the rate of IVF

- Serum Na >/= 200 mmol/l needs peritoneal dialysis & PICU management

Metabolic acidosis in dehydration:
Usually does not require any treatment as it corrects by itself on rehydration
- Correct only if severe pH < 7.1
- 1-2 mmol/kg of sodium bicarbonate solution 8.4% (1-2 ml/kg) over 60 min. infusion
- Bicarbonate deficit = (desired HCO3-actual HCO3) x 0.3 x body wt

Hypokaliemia:
- Potassium should always be added after child has passed urine
- Give KCl as a continuous infusion in the IVF (10 mmol KCl/ 500ml IVF
- Maximum 20 mmol KCl/ 500ml IVF if serum K+ < 3 mmol/l
- Do not give KCl as a bolus
- ECG monitoring required in severe hypokaliemia K+ < 2 mmol/l
- Daily maintenance 2-3 mmol/kg/day

Complications of Diarrhea
- Dehydration
- Metabolic acidosis
- Electrolyte disturbances
- GIT (secondary CHO malabsorption, protein intolerance, persistent diarrhea, intussusception)
- Systemic (septicemia, UTI, bacteremia, arthritis, HUS, renal failure, encephalitis, cerebral venous sinus thrombosis, seizures)
- Malnutrition

Key messages about childhood diarrhea
- Acute watery diarrhea is self limiting
- Diarrhea is a mechanism to get rid of organisms
- Rehydration is best achieved by ORS
- Nutrition should be instituted with ORS, Feeding with age appropriate diets as soon as patients have been rehydrated
- Avoid antidiarrheal and antibiotic drugs
- Teach parents how to prepare & use ORS; recognize the warning symptoms & signs and when to consult a doctor

7.2 Chronic Diarrhea and Malabsorption in children

Definitions:
    Chronic diarrhea: "Diarrhea lasting longer than 2 weeks"
    Intractable diarrhea: "Diarrhea that failed to respond for more than Four weeks"

Etiology of Chronic Diarrhea
    A) Intramural factors

        1) Pancreatic disorders:
          - Cystic fibrosis
          - Shwachman-Diamond syndrome
          - Isolated pancreatic enzyme deficiencies
          - Chronic pancreatitis

        2) Bile acid & hepatic disorders:
          - Chronic cholestasis
          - Terminal ileum resection (Short bowel syndrome)
          - Bacterial overgrowth
          - Primary bile acid malabsorption

        3) Intestinal disorder:
          - Carbohydrate malabsorption
          - Congenital & acquired sucrase, lactase deficiencies
          - Congenital & acquired monosaccharide malabsorption
          - Excessive fruit juice intake
          - Excessive intake of sorbitol, Magnesium hydroxide and lactulose

    B) Mucosal factors

        1) Altered integrity:
          - Infection (bacterial, viral, fungal & parasitic)
          - Cow's milk & soy protein intolerance
          - Inflammatory bowel disease (ulcerative colitis & Crohn disease)

        2) Altered surface area:
          - Celiac disease
          - Microvillus inclusion disease
          - Short bowel syndrome

        3) Altered immune function:
          - Autoimmune enteropathy
          - Eosinophilic gastroenteropathy
          - AIDS
          - Combined immunodeficiency
          - IgA & IgG deficiencies

4) Altered function:
- Defects in CL/HCO3, Na/H & bile acids
- Zinc deficiency, acrodermatitis enteropathica
- Selective folate & B12 deficiencies
- Abetalipoproteinemia & chylomicron retention

5) Altered secretory function:
- Enterotoxin-producing bacteria
- Tumors secreting vasoactive peptides

6) Altered digestive function
- Enterokinase deficiency
- Glucoamylase deficiency

7) Altered anatomic structures:
- Partial small bowel obstruction
- Malrotation

Common causes of chronic diarrhea according to age group:
Infancy
- Cow's milk/soy protein intolerance
- Secondary disaccharidase deficiencies (e.g. lactose intolerance)
Childhood
- Chronic non-specific diarrhea (Toddler's diarrhea)
- Secondary disaccharidase deficiencies
- Giardiasis
- Celiac disease
- Cystic disease
Adolescence
- Irritable bowel syndrome
- Inflammatory bowel disease
- Giardiasis
- Lactose intolerance

Osmotic V/S Secretory Diarrhea:

Secretory diarrhea	Osmotic diarrhea	
>200 ml/24 hr	<200 ml/24 hr	Volume of stool
Diarrhea continues	Diarrhea stops	Response to fasting
>70 mEq/L	<70 mEq/L	Stool Na
Negative	Positive	Reducing substances
>6	<5	Stool pH

Causes of osmotic diarrhea:
a) Malabsorption of water-soluble nutrients
Glucose-Galactose malabsorption (congenital & acquired)
Disaccharidase def. (lactase & sucrase-isomaltase)
b) Excessive intake of carbohydrate fluids
c) Excessive intake of non-absorbable solutes
Sorbitol, lactulose & magnesium hydroxide

Causes of secretory diarrhea:
a) Activation of cyclic AMP:
Bacterial toxins: Enterotoxin of cholera, E.coli (heat labile), Shigella, salmonella, campylobacter jejuni
Hormones: vasoactive intestinal peptides, gastrin, secretin
Anion surfactants: bile acids, ricinoleic acid

b) Activation of cyclic GMP:
Bacterial toxins: E.coli (heat stable) Enterotoxin, Yesinia enterocolitica   toxin

c) Calcium dependent:
Bacterial toxins: clostridium difficile enterotoxin
Neurotransmitters: acetylcholine, serotonin
Paracrine agent: bradykinin

Evaluation of patient with chronic diarrhea
  Phase I
- Clinical history including number & quality of stools, amount of fluid intake/day
- Physical exam including nutritional assessment
- Stool pH, reducing sub, smear for pus cells, fat, ova & parasites and culture
- Stool for clostridium difficile toxin
- Blood studies (CBC, ESR, electrolytes, renal function test, LFT)
  Phase 2
- Sweat chloride test
- Immune profile
- Serology for celiac disease (antiglidin antibodies)
- 72 hr stool collection for fat determination
- Stool electrolytes, osmolality
  Phase 3
- Endoscopic studies: Upper or Lower bowel with Biopsy
- Barium studies
  Phase 4
- Lipoprotein electrophoresis, Hormonal studies: vasoactive intestinal polypeptides, gastrin, secretin, 5-hdroxy indole acetic assays

Scheme of Management of Chronic diarrhea

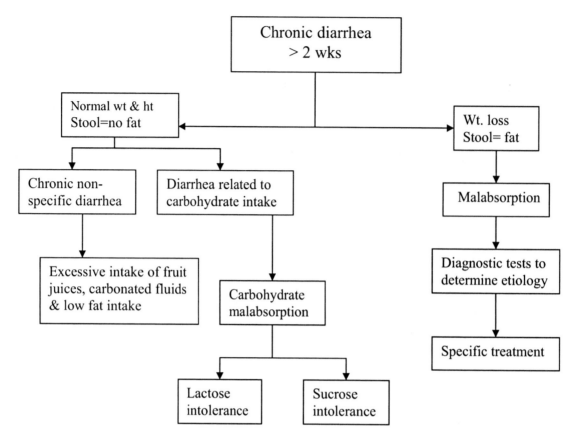

Treatment:
a) Supportive therapy for dehydration, electrolytes & acid base imbalance
b) Treatment of the cause: Parasites, bacteria, celiac disease
c) Replacement of the nutritional deficiencies
d) Non-specific measures: Probiotics, Cholestyramine, Antimotility agents etc.

7.3 Constipation in Children

Common problem in children, 3-5% visits in pediatric OPD, 35% visit to pediatrics gastroenterology clinic are for this problem

Definition: Difficulty in initiation or completion of act of defecation with infrequent or painful passage of dry & hard stools

Functional constipation: Voluntary holding or decreased colonic motility secondary to painful defecation.

Organic Causes:
Dehydration, Polyuria and reduced fluid intake

Abnormalities of colon & ano- rectum
- Anal stenosis, Anal or colonic stricture (post NEC)
- Post-surgical repair of imperforate anus
- Ectopic anus

Spinal cord lesions
- Spina bifida, Meningomyelocele
- Sacral agenesis, Diastematomyelia
- Spinal cord tumors

Neuropathic lesions of GIT
- Hirschsprung disease

Systemic disorders
- Hypothyroidism
- Diabetes mellitus
- Hypercalcemia
- Cerebral palsy / Neuro-muscular diseases

Drugs
- Analgesics esp. Opiate derivatives, Anticholinergics, Iron, Cholestyramine, Antacids,
- Heavy metal toxicity – Bismuth, Lead

Differentiation between Functional Constipation & Hirschsprung diseases:

Hirschsprung disease	Functional	
At birth	2-3 years	Onset
Present	Rare	Abdo. Distention
Poor	Normal	Nutrition growth
Rare	Intermittent or constant	Soiling & retentive behavior
Ampulla my be empty	Ampulla full	Rectal exam.
Ganglion cell absent	Ganglion cell present	Rectal biopsy
Non-relaxation of internal anal sphincter after rectal distention	Normal recto-anal reflex	Rectal manometry
Narrow distal segment with proximal mega colon	Distended rectum	Barium enema

History:

- Age of onset & duration
- Frequency & consistency of stool
- Pain or bleeding on passing stool
- Abdominal pain, nausea, vomiting
- Waxing & waning symptoms
- Stool withholding or fecal soiling
- Toilet training
- Change in appetite & weight loss
- Peri-anal fissures, abscess or fistula
- Current & past treatment
- Family history
- Past medical history: gestational age, time of passing meconium, Surgery
- Delayed growth & development, psychosocial disruption of child or family, School performance, interaction with peers, temperament, toileting at school

Physical Examination:

- General appearance
- Vital signs
- Growth parameters
- Abdomen: distention fecal masses
- Anal inspection: position, stool present around anus/on clothes, Perianal erythema, skin tags, anal fissures
- Rectal exam: anal tone, fecal mass and other masses, consistency of stool, gush of stool on finger withdrawal
- Blood in stool
- Back & spine exam: dimple, tuft of hair
- Neurological exam: tone, power, deep tendon reflexes, and cremasteric reflex

Investigations:

- Plain abdominal X-Ray
- Barium enema
- Ano-rectal manometry
- Rectal biopsy

Management:

- Treat the organic cause if present
- Increased fluid intake and fiber content of diet
- In functional constipation evacuation & disimpaction to be done by oral or rectal medications including **Phosphate enema** (use evening enema for at least 2-3 consecutive days) followed by a maintenance treatment for a minimal of 3-5 months with osmotic laxatives such as **Lactulose** (1-3 ml/kg once or twice per day), subsequently the dose can be adapted to the clinical response.

- **Mineral oil** (lubricant laxative) can also be used as maintenance therapy in

same dose as above
- **Senna or Bisacodyl** (stimulant laxatives) for a short period of 2-3 weeks may be useful in selective patients who are more difficult to manage.

- The treatment period for constipation should be prolonged until the bowel frequency returns to normal (Ideally one bowel movement per day or at least 4 or more times per week)

7.4 Gastro esophageal reflux disease (GERD)

Reflux of gastric contents across the lower esophageal sphincter (LES) into the esophagus.
GER is common during infancy and most often manifest as feed regurgitation. The incidence thereafter decreases to 5% at 10-12 months.

GER- Disease (GERD) is the symptomatic GER.

Regurgitation (spitting): Passive return of gastric content into the mouth/pharynx or out of the mouth without active muscle contraction.

Vomiting: active retrograde transport of gastric content through the mouth caused by periodic contraction of the diaphragm, abdominal & respiratory muscles.

Common causes of vomiting at various ages:

Adolescent	Child	Infant
Gastroenteritis	Gastroenteritis	Gastroenteritis
GERD	Systemic infection	GER
Systemic infection	Gastritis	Overfeeding
Toxic ingestion	Toxic ingestion	Anatomic obstruction
Gastritis	Pertussis syndrome	Systemic infection
Sinusitis	Medication	Pertussis syndrome
IBD	GERD	Otitis media
Migraine	Sinusitis	Congenital adrenal hyperplasia
Medication	Otitis media	Inborn errors of metabolism
Appendicitis		

Rare causes: Inborn error of metabolism, adrenogenital syndrome, brain tumor, increased intracranial pressure, hepatitis, Reye syndrome, peptic ulcer disease, pancreatitis, cyclic vomiting, and renal tubular acidosis.

Pathophysiology of GERD:
        Impaired clearance mechanism (saliva, distal esophageal motility)
        Impaired intrinsic lower esophageal sphincter
        Impaired extrinsic sphincter of diaphragmatic crural fibers
        Delayed gastric emptying

Factors decreasing Lower Esophageal Sphincter pressure thereby increasing reflux:
- Alpha-adrenergic antagonists
- Beta-adrenergic agonists
- Cholinergic antagonists
- Fat, chocolate, ethanol, peppermint

- Calcium channel blockers
- Theophylline, dopamine
- Barbiturates, diazepam, morphine
- Prostaglandin, estrogen, Glucagon

Infants at risk for GERD:
- Premature infants
- Hiatus hernia
- After repair of esophageal atresia
- Cerebral palsy and children with Neuro-disabilities
- Certain disease e.g. cystic fibrosis

Secondary GER:
- GIT (obstruction, peptic ulcer disease, infection)
- Renal (Hydronephrosis, UTI)
- Metabolic (Inherited diseases, electrolyte imbalance)
- Central (meningitis, increased ICP)
- Pulmonary diseases (acute/chronic)
- Food allergy
- Infection (septicemia, hepatitis)

Clinical manifestations of GER:
- Vomiting or regurgitation
- Esophagitis in infants leading to crying, arching, gagging and refusal   to feed Hematemesis
- Failure to thrive
- Aspiration: coughing, chocking, pneumonia, asthma (GER is an important cause of wheezing)
- Apnea in babies
- ENT: posterior laryngitis, strider, dysphonia, hoarseness, otitis media
- Chest pain, Epigastric pain, heartburn in older children

Complications of reflux esophagitis:
- Hematemesis, melena
- Iron deficiency anemia, Failure to thrive
- Dysphasia due to benign stricture

Diagnosis of GERD:
1) History and physical examination
2) 24 hr esophageal pH monitoring pH <4 or >4% of time is diagnostic
3) Upper GI series: barium study for structural lesions
4) Endoscopy for assessment of Esophagitis / biopsy
5) Scintigram (milk scan) for aspiration of milk in lungs

Management of GER (D): (See the flow diagram)
a) Uncomplicated GER:
- Positioning of infant after each feed
  < 3 months of age: nursing on right lateral position 30 degree from the horizontal position
  > 3 months: semi sitting up position preferably on a baby chair

- Dietary manipulation (small amount with increase frequencies)
- Food thickening with cereals or Anti-reflux milk formula (NAN-AR milk formula)
- No drugs

b) GERD (esophagitis):
- Proton pump inhibitors (omeprazole) or
- H2- receptor antagonist (ranitidine)
- Prokinetic drug e.g. Domperidon

c) Surgery: Fundoplication, Indications:
a) Poor response to medical treatment with failure to thrive
b) Risk of aspiration pneumonia
c) Esophageal stricture
d) Hiatus hernia

Key messages:
- Do not wait for spontaneous improvement
- Consider primary v/s secondary GER
- Try hypoallergenic formula for 2 weeks
- Perform Endoscopy before long-term acid suppressive therapy
- Exclude malrotation of mid gut if reflux is bile stained

Scheme of Management of GER in Children:

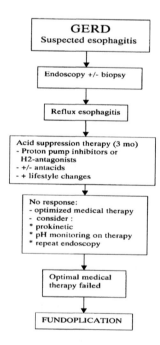

References:
- North American Society For Pediatric Gastroenterology & Nutrition
- J Pediatr Gastroenterology Nutr, Vol. 32, Suppl. 2, 2001

7.5 Acute and Chronic Hepatitis in Children
(Also see Chapter 6.6)

A) Acute Hepatitis

Defined as acute inflammation and necrosis of the liver secondary to infective, toxic, autoimmune or metabolic causes. The most common type is acute viral hepatitis.

Causes:

1. Infection

1) Viruses: Hepatitis A, B, C, D, E; Epstein-Barr virus, Cytomegalovirus, Enteroviruses; Measles, Varicella-Zoster virus, Yellow fever, Herpes viruses, Adenovirus; Dengue; Ebola virus

2) Bacteria (Sepsis, Brucella, Typhoid fever, TB and Leptospirosis)

3) Parasites (Toxoplasmosis)

2. Drugs and Toxins

Isoniazid, Androgens, Paracetamol, Salicylate, Hydralazine, Halothane, Erythromycin esteolate, Iron, Oral contraceptive, Valporate, Phenytoin, Carbamazepine, Methotrexate, 6-mercaptopurine

3. Metabolic & other causes: Reye syndrome

Investigations in a suspected case of Acute Hepatitis:

a) Tests of biochemical activity:
1. Test suggesting Hepatocyte injury: ALT, AST and LDH
2. Tests suggesting Cholestasis:
   Alkaline phosphatase (ALP),
   Bilirubin (total, conjugated and unconjugated)
   Gamma-glutamyl transferase peptidase (GGT)
   5'Nucleotidase (5'NT)
   Urinary urobilinogen
   Serum and urine bile acids

b) Tests of synthetic function
- Albumin, globulin
- Prothrombin time (PT)
- Ammonia (NH_3)
- Plasma amino acids, Tandem MS

c) Other investigations:
- Hepatitis screen
- TORCH titers
- Monospot test for EBV
- Serum immunoglobulins
- Serum ceruloplasmin & copper

- Tissue Auto antibodies
- Serum & urine amino acids

B) Chronic Hepatitis

Persistent clinical features of hepatitis for more than 3 months
Caused by a wide range of diseases, including infection leading to slowly progressive inflammatory damage, fibrosis and eventually cirrhosis of the liver.

Etiology:
a) Chronic Viral Hepatitis:
- Hepatitis B, C and D

b) Autoimmune Hepatitis:
- Anti-liver antigen microsomal antibody positive
- Anti actin antibody positive
- Anti soluble liver antigen antibody positive
- Systemic lupus Erythematosus

c) Drug-Induced Hepatitis

d) Metabolic Disorders Associated with Chronic Liver Disease:
- Wilson disease
- Alpha-1-Antitrypsin deficiency
- Cystic fibrosis
- Tyrosinemia
- Glycogen storage disease type IV
- Galactosemia
- Niemann-Pick disease type 2

e) Bile acid biosynthesis abnormalities

Clinical features suggesting chronicity:
1. History of conjugated hyperbilirubinemia
2. Family history of chronic liver disease (inherited or autoimmune)
3. Relapse of apparent acute hepatitis
4. Persistent clinical features of acute hepatitis for more than 3 months
5. Previous history of hepatitis B, C, or D

Clinical signs of chronic Liver disease:
- Small liver or enlarged left lobe of the liver
- Hard or nodular liver surface
- Firm splenomegaly
- Edema & ascites
- Growth failure & muscle wasting
- Facial telangiectasia, spider angiomata, clubbing or palmer erythema
- GI bleeding
- Extra hepatic manifestations of autoimmune chronic hepatitis,
- Presence of Kayser-Fleischer rings in the eyes

Complications of Chronic Hepatitis:
- Portal hypertension
- GIT bleeding
- Coagulopathy

- Ascites
- Growth failure
- Hepato-renal syndrome
- Hepatic Encephalopathy and End stage hepatic failure

7.6 Hepato-splenomegaly

Enlargement of the liver and/or spleen occurs in many disorders and present as an important clue to the underlying diagnosis. The size, shape, consistency, surface, tenderness, and presence of other associated signs help in differentiating various causes. Thorough examination of abdomen is therefore very crucial. One must remember that a just palpable liver and spleen may be seen in normal infants and small children. 1-2 cm palpable liver is quite commonly seen in children. Palpable spleen is found in most premature and 30% of term babies. Spleen tip may be palpable in 10% of infants by 1 year and 1% of normal children up to 10 years of age.

A. Hepatomegaly

Deciding for the presence of hepatomegaly is not always an easy task; on the other hand a palpable liver may be due to due to a push from the over inflated lungs or diaphragmatic pathology, therefore the actual size of liver as measured by **liver span** is more reliable. Liver span is determined in the right midclavicular line with the patient lying supine and breathing normally. Percussion first establishes the dullness of the upper border, while percussion or palpation may determine the lower border. Remember that forceful palpation may under-estimate the size by pushing the liver up.

Normal range of liver span in infants and children (by palpation method):

Age	Acceptable span (cm)
Pre-term infants	4-5
Healthy term infants	5-6.5
1-5 years	6-7
5-10 years	7-9
10-16 years	8-10

A narrow or a wide costal angel, pectus excavatum, abnormal body posture, accessory liver lobe, Reidel's lobe (a normal elongation of the right lobe), and presence of choledochal cyst can affect the accurate estimation of the liver span.

Examination of liver involves Inspection, Palpation, Percussion and Auscultation. One should carefully look for presence of associated diagnostic clues like jaundice, anemia, clubbing, signs of heart failure, portal hypertension etc. to help in the differential diagnosis.

The hepatomegaly should be described by mentioning following points:
Size below costal margin (in cm. not finger breadth)
Liver span
Shape
Consistency or texture (Soft, firm or hard)
Surface (Smooth or Nodular)
Edges (Rounded or sharp)
Presence of tenderness
Presence of any bruit on auscultation

Important diagnostic clues in the interpretation of Hepatomegaly:

- Firm liver with sharp edges due to cirrhosis or liver fibrosis is always easy to palpate then a soft enlarged liver due to glycogen storage disease.
- Tender liver indicate either infection or congestive heart failure
- Nodular liver indicate cirrhosis
- Presence of Jaundice indicate hepatocellular disease or an obstructive pathology in the hepatobilliary system
- Enlarged spleen and ascites indicate portal hypertension
- A palpable liver may become non-palpable in advanced cases of cirrhosis due to shrinking in size
- A massively enlarged liver is usually due to storage disorders
- Presence of a bruit over liver indicate hemangioma

Important causes of Hepatomegaly by age:

A. Newborn:

Congestive cardiac failure
Hemolytic diseases of newborn
Neonatal Hepatitis
Billiary atresia
Intrauterine Infections (TORCH)
Septicemia
Galactosemia

B. Infancy and Childhood:

1. Infections:
Bacterial: TB, Brucella, Typhoid
Viral: Infective hepatitis, Infectious mononucleosis, CMV, HIV
Protozoal: Malaria, Toxoplasmosis, Amoeba, Kala Azar
Parasites: Hydatid cysts
Fungal: Histoplasmosis

2. Hematological causes:
Hemolytic anemia (Sickle cell, Thalassemia)
Leukemia
Thrombocytopenia

3. Vascular:
Congestive cardiac failure
Constrictive pericarditis

4. Storage / Metabolic:
Glycogen storage disease
Galactosemia
Wilson disease
Lipid storage diseases
Mucopolysaccharidoses

5. Malignancy:
Leukemia
Lymphoma
Hepatoblastoma

   6. Miscellaneous causes:
   Cystic fibrosis
   Congenital hepatic fibrosis
   Malnutrition
   Fatty infiltration
   Cysts and Hemangioma
   TPN therapy

Investigations of a patient with hepatomegaly:

1. CBC :
   - Hemolysis: Anemia, reticulocytosis (Hemoglobinopathies, Autoimmune hepatitis, Wilson disease),
   - Neutropenia (GSD type I, Leukemia, Neuroblastoma),
   - Vacuolated lymphocytes (Storage diseases),

2. Liver functions (LFT's):
   - Total and direct bilirubin differentiates hepatocellular from obstructive causes
   - Liver enzymes (AST and ALT): Elevated in case of liver injury
   - Gamma glutamyl transferase (GGT) and alkaline phosphatase (ALP) are elevated in cases of intra or extra hepatic obstructive conditions,
   - Total serum proteins and albumin: affected in chronic liver disorders (half life of albumin is 21 days),
   - Prothrombin time (PT): is a measure of hepatic synthetic function, it's elevation is a poor prognostic sign

3. Biochemical profile:
   - Serum glucose: decreased in fulminant acute hepatic failure, Rey's syndrome, Galactosemia, Glycogen storage disease
   - Serum ammonia: increased in acute hepatic failure
   - lactic and pyruvic acid, ketone bodies, uric acid, acylcarnitine, amino acids are altered in cases of inborn errors of metabolism
   - α-fetoproteins: Increased in case of Hepatoblastoma or Tyrosinemia
   - Hypophosphatemia: seen in GSD type I, Hereditary fructose intolerance
   - Hypertriglyceridemia seen in Glycogen storage disease
   - Proximal renal tubular dysfunctions (Fanconi syndrome) seen in Tyrosinemia, Hereditary fructose intolerance, GSD type I or Galactosemia

3. Urinalysis:
   - Bilirubinuria is seen in conjugated while urobilinogen in unconjugated hyper-bilirubinemia
   - Ketone bodies, reducing substances, organic acids and amino acids are seen in suspected inborn error of metabolism,
   - Drug screen is required for suspected toxicity

4. Ultrasonography:
   A screening sonogram of the liver and abdomen is the most readily available diagnostic imaging study. It not only evaluates the size of liver but can also indicate underlying pathology

5. Liver biopsy:
Is useful in difficult to diagnose cases as well as to assess disease progression.

B. Splenomegaly

Examination for spleen should be done with child lying supine or in right lateral position, examiner standing on the patient's right side. Examination is performed by the right hand beginning at the right iliac fossa, proceeding obliquely upwards to the left upper quadrant while gently pushing forward the patients left lower rib cage with the left hand thus pushing spleen forward for easy palpation.

Splenic enlargement can be differentiated from other abdominal masses especially the renal by taking notice of following features:
- Spleen enlarges obliquely
- Spleen has a notch
- Upper border of spleen can not be reached
- Renal masses are better felt bimanually and have overlying colonic resonant band on percussion

Causes of splenomegaly:
1. **Infections:**
   See hepatomegaly
   Infective endocarditis
2. **Hematological:**
   See hepatomegaly (Note that spleen is usually not palpable in advance cases of sickle cell disease due to repeated infarctions)
   Severe Iron deficiency anemia
   Hypersplenism
3. **Storage diseases:** See Hepatomegaly
4. **Malignancies:** See hepatomegaly
5. **Miscellaneous:**
   Splenic cysts, Hemangioma, Abscess
   Rheumatoid arthritis, SLE
   Portal Hypertension

Investigations in a case of Splenomegaly:
1. CBC (looking for differential count and blood smear for parasites, blast cells of leukemia and atypical lymphocytosis of viral infections),
2. ESR (high in malignancies and autoimmune disorders),
3. Liver function tests
4. Cultures for suspected endocarditis and other bacterial or fungal infections,
5. Antibodies or PCR for viral hepatitis, EBV, CMV, toxoplasmosis (or TORCH screen), HIV testing
6. ANA, anti dsDNA, rheumatoid factor and ANCA in suspected connective tissue diseases and vasculitis
7. A bone marrow aspiration and biopsy should be done in any child with splenomegaly and pancytopenia (to differentiate bone marrow dysfunction from Hypersplenism)
8. Ultrasonography and nuclear scan: To look for size and underlying pathology

C. Hepato-Splenomegaly

As many features like hematopoiesis and reticuloendothelial functions are common to both liver and spleen, it is therefore no surprise to see the two organs affected together presenting as case of Hepato-splenomegaly.

Causes of Hepato-splenomegaly:
1. **Infections**
2. **Hematological disease**
3. **Storage disease**
4. **Malignancies**
5. **Miscellaneous disorders:**
   Portal hypertension
   Collagen diseases: Rheumatoid and SLE
   Congenital hepatic fibrosis

D. Portal hypertension

Is defined as increase in portal venous pressure by more than 5 mm Hg above the inferior vena caval pressure

The etiological factors can be divided into:
   a) **Pre-hepatic causes**: such as portal vein thrombosis secondary to neonatal omphalitis, umbilical vein catheterization, exchange transfusion and polycythemia.
   b) **Intra-hepatic causes**: such as cirrhosis from any cause, veno-occlusive disease, congenital hepatic fibrosis, and bilharziasis
   c) **Supra-hepatic causes**: Hepatic vein thrombosis (Budd-Chiari syndrome), congestive cardiac failure and constrictive pericarditis.

- Clinically, pre and supra-hepatic causes present with tender smooth hepatomegaly.
- Cirrhosis is a dynamic process that includes hepatocellular injury, fibrosis as a response to injury, and nodule formation from regenerating hepatocytes. It is the end-stage of many chronic liver diseases. Clinically, cirrhosis presents with a firm non-tender, nodular liver, together with *signs of portal hypertension which include a firm splenomegaly, esophageal varices, ascites and hypersplenism.*

Respiratory System

8.1 Common upper airway infections
(Please also refer to Chapter 14.2)

1. Common cold (URTI)

The common cold is an acute, highly infectious viral disease of the nasopharynx and paranasal sinuses. It is characterized by nasal stuffiness, sneezing, coryza, throat irritation and little or no fever. It can occur many times per year and is caused by over 100 different viruses

Rhinoviruses, which cause about 50% of colds, and corona viruses, which cause 10 to 20%, are the most important pathogens. RSV, PIV, influenza virus, adenovirus, and some entero viruses also cause colds.

Pathogenesis
The Inhalation or self-inoculation of viruses onto nasal mucosa or conjunctiva leads to epithelial cell infection, which causes increased nasal secretions, submucosal edema and shedding of ciliated epithelium. Increased numbers of neutrophil locally produce the mucopurulent discharge

The greatest viral concentration is from the nasal discharges, and the maximum viral shedding is from day 2-7, but some may continue shading up to 2 weeks

Clinical manifestations
Adults and older children with rhinovirus colds typically have prominent upper respiratory tract symptoms (i.e. sneezing, nasal discharge, nasal obstruction, sore or scratchy throat, and cough) and often have headache but little fever or few systemic complaints other than malaise. Physical findings are nonspecific like nasal discharge and mucosal erythema

Infants are usually irritable, and febrile with temperatures around 38-39 ˚C. The nasal obstruction can interfere with feeding and sleep. They may also develop vomiting and diarrhea (Parenteral diarrhea)

Differential diagnosis:
Allergic rhinitis, pertussis, bacterial nasopharyngitis, and, rarely nasal diphtheria or bacterial nasal infection should be excluded. If there is persistence nasal symptom adenoiditis or sinusitis must also be ruled out

Common cold usually have excellent out come. Some patients may have complications like otitis media, tonsillitis, sinusitis and lower respiratory tract infections

Management:
Disease usually resolves quickly with no specific treatment. Many well-designed studies failed to show any benefits of the common cold preparation over placebo

Treatment is directed toward specific symptoms like Paracetamol for fever; Saline nasal drops and gentle suction are effective for nasal obstruction causing difficulty in feeding or sleep. Adequate hydration. Avoiding tobacco smoke exposure. There is no role for antibiotics

2. Pharyngitis

It is an infective inflammatory illness of the mucous membrane of the throat and/or tonsils leading to tonsillitis, tonsillopharyngitis or nasopharyngitis

Pharyngitis is commonly caused by viruses like Adenovirus 1-7, Influenza A&B, Parainfluenza 1-4, Entero viruses and EB Virus. Uncommon viruses include: RSV, Rhinovirus, Rotaviruses, HSV, CMV, Measles and Poliovirus

Exudative Pharyngitis is seen with specific organisms, like Adenovirus, Herpes simplex, EBV or bacteria like Streptococcus pyogenes, Diphtheria or fungi like Candida

Clinical manifestations
Sudden onset of fever, sore throat, anorexia, headache and malaise
Physical examination may show enlarged, tender cervical nodes, pharyngeal erythema (exudate, follicles, ulcers), and petechiae. It is a self limited, illness lasting 4-10 days.
Only 0.3-3.0% of untreated S. infection may lead to rheumatic fever
Other complications of bacterial Pharyngitis includes: Retropharyngeal abscess, and rarely septicemia or toxic shock syndrome.

Diagnosis:
Throat swab culture to diagnose Streptococcal pyogenes infection. A rapid antigen detection test is also available that can give result within 10 minutes, thus can help physician to decide which patient require antibiotic treatment, although the sensitivity of this test varies from 31-95% but has high specificity

Management
Symptomatic relief with warm fluids, saline gargles and analgesics. In older child use of soothing lozenges may be of help. There is no place for decongestants or antihistamines. Antibiotics are used only to treat proven S. pyogenes infection. Penicillin is still effective up to 9 days after the onset of acute infection to prevent rheumatic fever. Dose of Penicillin V is 250 mg bid and if the child is older then 12 y 500 mg bid for 10 days (Erythromycin is used in allergic patients)

3. Viral Croup

Viral croup or **acute laryngotracheobronchitis** is the most common cause of upper airway obstruction in children from 6 months to 6 years of age. The peak age is second year. Croup affects about 15% of children. Below 6 months of age croup is unknown and other diagnosis like subglottic stenosis, hemangioma or laryngotracheomalacia should be suspected.
Croup is a clinical syndrome of barking cough, inspiratory stridor, hoarse voice and respiratory distress of varying etiology mostly of viral like Parainfluenza 1-3, Influenza A &B, and RSV. Other less common causes are Adeno, Rhino, Entero, HSV and Reo viruses

Pathophysiology
The viral infection causes Inflammation and edema of the larynx, trachea, and bronchi and increased production of mucus. The subglottic trachea is the narrowest part of

a child's upper airway, it gets even more critically narrowed with the edema and it is placed outside the pleural cavity, the negative pressure generated on inspiration tends to narrow the airway further increasing the airway resistance and obstruction. Patient will have severe airway compromise with inspiratory strider, difficulty of breathing and hypoxia. Swelling of the vocal cord, on the other hand, results in hoarseness of voice. The barking cough is the result of inflammation in the larynx and trachea.

Clinical manifestation:

Disease starts with rhinorrhea, sore throat and mild fever followed by barking cough, hoarseness and inspiratory strider. It may cause severe upper airway obstruction mostly at night.

On physical examination patients may be hypoxic, anxious, restless and cyanosed. Child will have tachycardia, tachypnea, nasal flaring, and inspiratory stridor.

Chest examination will show in drawing and paradoxical chest & abdominal movements also may have depressed consciousness

Differential Diagnosis

Spasmodic croup
Epiglotitis
Bacterial tracheitis
Foreign body
Vocal cord paralysis
Angioneurotic edema
Laryngospasm (hypocalcemic tetany)

Diagnosis

The diagnosis of viral croup is mainly a clinical one based on the history and physical findings. Diagnostic tests are not usually necessary.

Radiographs of the neck should be considered when aspirated foreign body is suspected or when the diagnosis is in doubt or when the response to standard treatment is unsatisfactory.

A "pencil tip" or "steeple sign" of subglottic edema on the AP view and an over distended hypo pharynx on the lateral view are classical findings.

Management

More than 80% of children have mild symptoms. In approximately 60% to 95% of children, the symptoms resolve spontaneously within 2 to 5 days

Home treatment with warm mist from hot bathroom shower can help to minimize the discomfort.

Hospital treatment depends on the severity of the illness and may include any or all of the following modalities: general supportive measures, corticosteroids, Nebulized epinephrine, supplemental oxygen, and endotracheal Intubation.

Corticosteroids: Is the mainstay of therapy, they suppress local inflammation, cause shrinkage of lymphoid swelling and reduce capillary permeability.

1. **Systemic Dexamethasone**: is a potent corticosteroid with an anti-inflammatory effect ten times that of prednisone It can be given orally or intramuscularly Oral form is preferred because it is inexpensive, easy to administer, readily available, and relatively well tolerated .The dose is 0.6 mg/kg/dose The maximal effect is reached

at 6 hours and half-life is 36-54 hours

2. **Inhaled Budesonid** is a synthetic glucocorticoid with relatively strong topical anti-inflammatory effects and low systemic activity. Nebulized Budesonide have been found equally effective to dexamethasone but nebulization can be distressing. The dosage is 2 mg as single dose.

Intramuscular Dexamethasone or Nebulized Budesonide is reserved for children unable or unwilling to take the oral dexamethasone.

Croup improves in 1-2 days and there is no need to repeat the dose

Nebulized Epinephrine: Racemic epinephrine is a 1:1 mixture of the dextrorotatory (D) and levorotatory (L) isomers of epinephrine, of which the L form is the active component. It acts by stimulation of the α-adrenergic receptors in the airway with resultant mucosal vasoconstriction and decreased subglottic edema and by stimulation of the β-adrenergic receptors with resultant relaxation of the bronchial smooth muscle.

Nebulized epinephrine should be reserved for children with moderate to severe croup and should be used with caution in children who have tachycardia or ventricular outlet obstruction. Recommended dose of L-epinephrine is 5 ml of a 1:1,000 solution diluted in 2 to 5 mL of saline solution. The onset of action is within 10 to 30 minutes and the duration of action is approximately 2 hours, at which time patients return to their baseline severity (rebound phenomenon). Adverse effects of Nebulized epinephrine include tachycardia and circumoral pallor.

Progression

Although the simultaneous use of corticosteroid helps to reduce the rebound phenomenon and obviates the need for hospitalization, patients still should be observed for a minimum of 2 hours following treatment

Hospitalization should be considered in children who have stridor at rest with chest-wall indrawing, toxic look, poor oral intake and infant below 6 months age.

Endotracheal Intubation with or without assisted ventilation is rarely required except for those who have impending respiratory failure despite Corticosteroids and epinephrine

8.2 Bronchiolitis

Definition

Bronchiolitis is an inflammation of the terminal bronchioles, resulting from a viral infection mainly Respiratory syncytial virus. It is usually a self-limited disease and typically has no long-term complications.

Bronchiolitis is a clinical syndrome characterized by acute respiratory symptoms in a child < 2 years of age. Typically, the initial symptoms of upper respiratory tract infection, such as fever and coryza, progressing within 4 to 6 days to include lower respiratory tract leading to cough wheezing and respiratory distress

Epidemiology

Bronchiolitis occurs mostly in children younger than 12 months of age. Infants younger than 6 months are at highest risk of clinically significant disease.

Bronchiolitis is a seasonal disease commonly occurring from **December to May** months. There is a male predominance (1.5:1). Environmental and genetic factors contribute to the severity of disease. Daycare attendance, exposure to passive smoke, and household crowding are associated with increased risk factors. Some studies have suggested that there might be a genetic predisposition found in families with family history of asthma or other wheezing disorders.

Etiology

Sixty to ninety percent of children with Bronchiolitis have Respiratory syncytial virus (**RSV**) as the primary pathogen. Other viruses, including parainfluenza, adenovirus, rhinovirus, and influenza, cause the remainder of cases; *Mycoplasma pneumonia* can cause a similar disease. Coinfection of RSV with other organisms is also found in up to 5% to 10% of cases of RSV lower respiratory tract infections

Pathogenesis:

The clinical symptoms of obstructive lower respiratory tract infection are a consequence of the partial occlusion of the distal airways. Histological examination of the lungs of affected children often reveals necrosis of the respiratory epithelium, monocytic infiltration with edema of the peribronchial tissues, and obstruction of the distal airways with mucus and fibrin plugs. Infants are predisposed to develop wheezing and other symptoms of airway obstruction because of the small caliber of their distal airways and the absence of active immunity to RSV and other respiratory viruses.

Clinical manifestations:

An infant with Bronchiolitis typically presents with illness during the winter months, although sporadic cases appear throughout the year. More than half of affected children are between 2 and 7 months of age. Parents often report that a child attends daycare or has a household contact with cold-like symptoms. Early in the illness, infants usually experience copious rhinorrhea. Typically, infants develop a tight wheezy cough associated with poor feeding 4 to 6 days after the initial onset of symptoms. Overall, infants with RSV-associated Bronchiolitis are often febrile at the time of presentation; Fever is much higher in patients with adenovirus- or influenza-associated Bronchiolitis.

1. **Mild infection** the symptoms include rhinorrhea, mild cough, irritability, and low-grade fever for 1-3 days.
2. **Moderate infection** and infections in infants and young children often present with more pronounced cough, wheezing, moderate fever and poor feeding.
3. **Severe infection**: As the condition progresses the infant work harder to breathe, nasal flaring, grunting, tachypnea, and retractions develop. If the infant does not receive supportive therapy he will become listless, hypoxic with diminished breath sounds, may experience **Apneic spells**, and can rapidly progress to cyanosis and respiratory failure

Examination:

May reveal Hyper-inflated resonant chest with audible wheezing, fine rales, rhonchi, poor air movement and prolonged expiratory phase. There may be associated conjunctivitis, rhinitis, and otitis media. Many infants have a distended abdomen caused by hyperinflation of the lungs.

Diagnosis

The diagnosis of Bronchiolitis is made by history and physical examination. Diagnostic criteria include exposure to persons with URI symptoms, a prodromal phase of URI symptoms followed by wheezing occurring during the winter months.

Differential diagnoses

Include asthma, pneumonia, cystic fibrosis, heart failure, foreign body aspiration and pertussis.

In infants and children with moderate or severe respiratory symptoms, a chest x-ray is often ordered to rule out other respiratory conditions. **Radiographic examination** typically reveals hyperinflation, patchy Atelectasis, and peribronchial wall thickening and can usually differentiate between pneumonia and Bronchiolitis.

Definitive diagnosis of RSV as the causative agent for Bronchiolitis is accomplished by enzyme-linked immunosorbent assay **(ELISA)** that detects viral antigen. A **nasopharyngeal aspirate** specimen is obtained by deep nasal suction in an enclosed container. The test has a sensitivity of 80%-90%. However, routine laboratory screenings such as RSV assays, complete blood counts (CBCs), and chest x-rays provide little additional information beyond a thorough history and physical examination.

Management

Controversy surrounds the treatment of Bronchiolitis. Management of Bronchiolitis in infants and young children is predominantly by supportive measures.

Treatment includes: Maintenance of adequate fluid and sufficient caloric intake to meet the increased basal metabolic needs associated with a respiratory illness

Rest, use of nasal saline drops to promote ease of breathing,

Use of antipyretics/mild analgesics to control fever and minimize irritability.

Most infants and young children with Bronchiolitis can be treated at home.

Pulse oxymeter readings should be taken on all infants

Close follow up and careful instructions should be given to the parents to document:

(a) Signs of increasing respiratory distress
(b) Signs of dehydration
(c) Guidelines for oral intake

(d) Fever management and antipyretic use, and

(e) How to access health care services if symptoms worsen.

Hospitalization

Is required for younger infants with toxicity, apnea, tachypnea >70, marked retractions, oxygen saturation <93%, lethargy, history of poor fluid intake or if the infant belongs to high risk group like underlying cardio-pulmonary disease.

The degree of medical intervention is usually determined by the child's level of oxygenation as indicated by pulse oximetry. Use of humidified oxygen by hood, Isolette, or nasal prongs in concentrations sufficient to alleviate dyspnea and hypoxia. Clinicians must carefully monitor signs of impending respiratory failure, such as the inability to maintain adequate oxygen saturations or rising arterial carbon dioxide levels. Ventilatory assistance (i.e., Intubation) should be considered for infants with recurrent apnea or severe oxygen desaturation. Adequate hydration is important, however, oral fluid intake may be contraindicated because of tachypnea, weakness, and/or fatigue with a risk of aspiration. Parenteral fluids are usually provided in the hospitalized infant until the acute stage of the disease has passed.

Bronchodilators:

1. Salbutamol had been shown to have short-term positive effects on respiratory status but did not alter hospitalization rates. Flores and Horwitz (1997) found no improvement in oxygenation or reduction in hospitalization rates with its use. In a wheezing infant a trial may be given with pre and post assessment to see the response. Discontinue if no or minimal response is obtained.

2. Racemic Epinephrine has both a-adrenergic and b-adrenergic activity. Menon, Sutcliffe, and Klassen (1995) found it to be better than Salbutamol. They found that only 30% of the 21 infants treated with racemic epinephrine required hospitalization as compared to 75% of the 21 infants treated with Salbutamol. Some other authors found no difference in the effectiveness of therapy for infants hospitalized with Bronchiolitis.

Corticosteroids:

Research has shown that Corticosteroids, systemic or inhaled, do not seem to exhibit any beneficial respiratory effects and are not recommended

Antiviral drugs:

Many studies have not found Ribavirin (anti RSV) therapy to reduce either mortality rates or duration of mechanical ventilation. Thus, Ribavirin appears to have limited clinical efficacy in previously healthy infants with severe RSV infection

Prevention:

The most important aspect of prevention is by parental education, especially when the infant is at high risk. The most important method for reducing the transmission of RSV, as well as other infectious diseases, is frequent and consistent hand washing. (AAP 1998). Additional preventative measures include eliminating cigarette smoke and exposure to crowds (e.g., day care).

There are two medical methods for preventing RSV infection in high-risk patients:

1. Monthly intravenous RSV-IGIV to be given during the high season or

2. Monthly intramuscular palivizumab (Synagis) which is a humanized RSV neutralizing monoclonal antibody, it received FDA approval for the prevention of lower respiratory tract infection in infants at high risk for developing severe RSV disease.

8.3 Bronchiectasis

Definition

The term Bronchiectasis is derived from the Greek word *bronchion,* meaning windpipe, and *ectasis,* meaning stretched. The term implies **permanent irreversible alteration in the anatomy of the airway**, it is usually a consequence of a lower respiratory tract infection with accompanying persistent obstruction or underlying congenital disease that predispose to lung infections like cystic fibrosis or those rare disorders that affect the bronchial supporting structures

Pathophysiology

Bronchiectasis, a permanent irreversible destruction of airways and is generally the result of obstruction and inflammation of the airway that may result from:

- o Congenital muco-ciliary abnormalities (e.g., cystic fibrosis, ciliary dyskinesia),
- o Anatomic obstruction (e.g., foreign body, external compression) causing Intrinsic airway destruction
- o Destruction caused by infections (e.g., adenovirus, measles, TB, HIV, immunodeficiency Dis.)
- o Allergic disease and asthma.

Frequency

In developed countries, the frequency is low (an approximate incidence of 1.1-0.2/10,000.children) the frequency is much higher in the developing world, where measles, pneumonia, tuberculosis, and HIV infection are all on the rise and inadequately treated

History

The diagnosis should be considered in children with a daily productive cough of longer than 6 weeks' duration. The cough is not always productive. It often occurs first thing in the morning and improves throughout the day. Cough is almost universal symptom, and it is frequently described as productive in older children or loose in toddlers and infants. Because small children rarely expectorate, the clinician may observe the child with a loose-sounding cough who often swallows sputum after coughing.

Hemoptysis is a rare complication, but it should strongly suggest bronchiectasis. The diagnosis of asthma or reflux-associated lung disease does not preclude bronchiectasis. In fact, bronchiectasis may be a complication of these diseases.

Physical Examination

Observation of a productive cough by the clinician, coupled with localized crackles or coarse rhonchi, suggests bronchiectasis, especially over the left lower lobe, lingula, and right middle lobe areas of the chest.
Digital clubbing is reported in 37-51% of patients with bronchiectasis. In some patients, the clubbing gets cleared after the affected section of the lung is surgically removed. Or can improve in those treated medically
Repeated exacerbation of respiratory infections with poor health and failure to thrive and poor exercise tolerance is seen in chronic cases.

Lab Studies: Laboratory evaluation should eliminate many of the possible etiologies of bronchiectasis. Evaluation includes the following tests:

- Sweat chloride
- Evaluation for acute bronchopulmonary aspergillosis (ABPA) - Immunoglobulin E (IgE), eosinophil count, and serum precipitants for Aspergillus; sputum culture for fungus; and an Aspergillus skin test
- Complete blood cell count
- Serum IgG, IgM, IgA, IgG subclasses
- HIV test
- Sputum culture or deep oropharyngeal swab in younger children
- Antinuclear antibody and rheumatoid factor
- **Radiography:** P/A and lateral chest radiography is an important initial step; however, normal findings on radiography do not rule out bronchiectasis.
- **Computed tomography:** Today, the diagnosis is made by thin section high-resolution computed tomography (HRCT) based upon the presence of an internal bronchial diameter greater than the adjacent pulmonary artery, lack of tapering of the bronchial lumina, and visualization of the bronchi within 1 cm of the pleura.
- **Gastro esophageal reflux:** Evaluate patients suspected of having bronchiectasis for gastro esophageal reflux (GER), especially infants and young children.
- **Fiber optic bronchoscopy** is used to assess the caliber and appearance of the airways and to provide broncho-alveolar lavage for evidence of chronic aspiration (lipid-laden macrophages) or infection (quantitative cultures and white blood cell counts).
- **Histological Findings:** Examination of the bronchoalveolar fluid reveals inflammatory cells in the presence of chronic inflammation or infection. Hemosiderin-laden macrophages generally suggest the presence of alveolar blood for more than 7 days.
- **Lipid-laden macrophages** suggest chronic aspiration but may also be observed in other forms of severe airway disease.

Medical Care:

Chest physiotherapy, postural drainage, and antibiotics, are the mainstay of treatment. **Inhaled corticosteroids** may be helpful to modulate the host response and curb inflammatory damage. **Bronchodilators** are indicated when evidence of bronchial hyper reactivity exists because they help to improve ciliary beat frequency and facilitate mucus clearance. However, some patients with bronchiectasis have a paradoxical bronchoconstriction with beta agonist therapy. Therefore, assessing bronchodilator response before beginning such therapy is essential. Exercise generally promotes increased muco-ciliary clearance, which may enhance airway clearance.

Surgical Care:

Pulmonary segmental resection may be beneficial when damage is severe, well localized and uncontrollable on medical therapy. Surgery be delayed, unless symptomatically necessary, until the patient is aged 6-12 years because of the possibility of clinical improvement.

8.4 Asthma and wheezing in children

Types of wheezing in young children:

1. **Transient early wheezing**: Starting in the first year of life, generally not associated with a family history of asthma or allergic sensitization. Mostly resolves around 3 years age.
   Risk factors for this phenotype are:
   - Reduced pulmonary function in infancy
   - Prematurity,
   - Male gender,
   - Exposure to siblings and other children at day care centers,
   - Prenatal maternal smoking and postnatal exposure to tobacco smoke

2. **Nonatopic wheezing (or 'VIRAL induced wheeze')** the attacks are triggered by recurrent viral infections. Factors such as a specific or enhanced immune response, or histological or functional alterations of the airways may play a role

3. **Persistent 'ATOPIC' wheezing**: Episodic wheezing with symptom-free intervals, symptoms worse at night, family history of asthma, elevated serum IgE and peripheral blood eosinophilia. They do respond to bronchodilators and corticosteroids treatment. These children are very likely to develop asthma in later childhood, mostly after the first birthday.

Definition of Asthma

Asthma is a chronic inflammatory disorder of the airways characterized by obstruction to airflow that may be reversed completely or partially with or without specific therapy.

In susceptible individuals, airway inflammation may cause recurrent or persistent bronchospasm, which causes symptoms including wheezing, breathlessness, chest tightness and cough particularly at night or after exercise.

Pathophysiology:

Multifactorial disorder in which there is an interaction between environmental and genetic factors that results in airway inflammation, limiting airflow and leads to functional and structural changes in the airways in the form of bronchospasm, mucosal edema, and mucus plug formation.

Airway obstruction causes increased resistance to airflow and decreased expiratory flow rates. These changes lead to a decreased ability to expel air and may result in hyperinflation, which alters pulmonary mechanics and increases the work of breathing. Uneven distribution of air and alterations in circulation due to hyperinflation leads to ventilation-perfusion mismatch and hypoxia. CO_2 accumulation is not a problem until a late stage of disease, therefore high CO_2 in any asthmatic child is an ominous sign.

Chronic inflammation of the airways is associated with increased bronchial hyper-responsiveness (BHR), which leads to bronchospasm and typical symptoms of wheezing, shortness of breath, and coughing after exposure to allergens, environmental irritants, viruses, cold air, or exercise

Airway inflammation in asthma may represent a loss of normal balance between two "opposing" populations of Th lymphocytes. Two types of Th lymphocytes have been characterized: Th1 and Th2. Th1 cells produce IL-2 and IFN-a, which are critical in cellular defense mechanisms in response to infection. Th2, in contrast, generates a family of cytokines (IL-4, -5, -6, -9, and -13) that can mediate allergic inflammation.

Frequency:

Worldwide, 130 million people suffer from asthma. The prevalence is 8-10 times higher in developed than the developing countries. In developed countries, the prevalence is higher in low-income groups in urban areas and inner cities.

The international study on Asthma and allergy (ISAAC) has shown that the prevalence of asthma among school age children is 10%. The Omani part of the study however have shown that asthma prevalence in **Omani children** age 13-14 years old is as high as 20% in comparison to 10 % in the 6-7 years old.

Sex: Before puberty, the prevalence is 3 times higher in boys. During adolescence, the prevalence is equal. Adult-onset asthma is more common in women than in men.

Age: In most children, asthma develops before they are aged 5 years, and, in more than half, before 3 years. Among infants, 20% have wheezing with only upper respiratory tract infections (URTIs) and 60% no longer have wheezing when they are aged 6 years.

Mortality/Morbidity:

Globally, morbidity and mortality associated with asthma have increased over the last 2 decades. This increase is attributed to increasing urbanization. Despite advancements in our understanding of asthma and the development of new therapeutic strategies, the morbidity and mortality due to asthma has definitely increased between 1980 and 1995.

Clinical diagnosis

To establish the diagnosis of asthma, the clinician must establish the following:
  (a) Episodic symptoms of airflow obstruction are present,
  (b) Airflow obstruction or symptoms are at least partially reversible,
  (c) Alternative diagnoses are excluded

Other important points in the history
  • Precipitating factors
  • Present treatment and response
  • Previous hospital admission
  • Typical exacerbations
  • Home and school environment
  • Impact of asthma on lifestyle (e.g. exercise)
  • History of atopy (eczema, allergic rhinitis)
  • Prolonged URTI symptoms
  • Family history

Physical examination

Physical findings vary with the absence or presence of an acute episode and its severity,

The absence of physical findings at the time of examination does not exclude asthma

Look for sign of chronic illness such as:

- Harrison sulci
- Hyperinflated chest
- Signs of atopy or allergic rhinitis, such as conjunctival congestion, hypertrophied nasal turbinate and pale violaceous nasal mucosa/polyps
- Eczema or dry skin
- Clubbing of the fingers is not a feature of straightforward asthma and indicates a need for more extensive evaluation and work-up to exclude other conditions, such as cystic fibrosis
- Lung examination may reveal prolongation of the expiratory phase, expiratory wheezing, coarse crackles, or unequal breath sounds

Look for signs of acute exacerbation:

- Tachypnea,
- Tachycardia,
- Reduced air entry
- Wheeze,
- Use of accessory muscles
- Cyanosis,
- Drowsiness,

Lab Studies:

Pulmonary function test (PFT) results are not reliable in patients younger than 5 years. In young children (3-6 y) and older children who can't perform the conventional spirometry maneuver, newer techniques, such as measurement of airway resistance using impulse oscillometry is being tried. Measurement of airway resistance before and after a dose of inhaled bronchodilator may help to diagnose responsiveness and reversibility of obstruction

Spirometry: In a typical case, an obstructive defect is present in the form of normal forced vital capacity (FVC), reduced FEV1, and reduced forced expiratory flow over 25-75% of the FVC (FEF 25-75). Documentation of reversibility of airway obstruction after bronchodilator therapy is central to the definition of asthma. In an outpatient or office setting, measurement of the **peak flow rate** can provide useful information. However, a normal peak flow rate does not necessarily mean normal airway.

Plethysmography: Patients with chronic persistent asthma may have hyperinflation, as evidenced by an increased total lung capacity (TLC) at Plethysmography. Increased residual volume (RV) and functional residual capacity (FRC) with normal TLC suggests air trapping. Airway resistance is increased when significant obstruction is present.

Bronchial provocation tests: Bronchial provocation tests may be performed to diagnose BHR. These tests are performed in specialized laboratories by specially trained personnel to document airway hyper responsiveness to substances (e.g., methacholine, histamine). Increasing doses of provocation agents are given, and FEV1 is measured. The endpoint is a 20% decrease in FEV1 (PD20).

Exercise challenge: the diagnosis of asthma can be confirmed with this test in a patient with a history of exercise-induced symptoms (e.g., cough, wheeze, chest tightness or pain), In a patient of appropriate age (usually >6 y), the procedure involves baseline spirometry followed by exercise on a treadmill or bicycle to a heart rate greater than 60% of the predicted maximum, with monitoring of the electrocardiogram and oxy-hemoglobin saturation

Blood testing: Eosinophil and IgE levels may help when allergic factors are suspected

Chest radiograph: Is not required at each visit in an uncomplicated case of recurrent obstruction and wheeze. A base line X-ray may be done on initial workup if the asthma or when child does not respond to therapy as expected. In addition to typical findings of hyperinflation and increased bronchial markings, a chest radiograph may reveal evidence of parenchymal disease, Atelectasis, pneumonia, congenital anomaly, or a foreign body. In a patient with an acute asthmatic episode that responds poorly to therapy, a chest radiograph helps in the diagnosis of complications such as pneumothorax or pneumomediastinum.

Allergy testing: can be used to identify allergic factors that may significantly contribute to the asthma. Once identified, environmental factors (e.g., dust mites, cockroaches, moulds, animal dander) and outdoor factors (e.g., pollen, grass, trees, molds) may be controlled or avoided to reduce asthmatic symptoms. Allergens for skin testing are selected on the basis of suspected or known allergens identified from detailed environmental history.

Classification of severity of chronic asthma: According to the Global Initiative for Asthma (GINA):

STEP 1: Mild intermittent disease. Patients have symptoms fewer than 2 times a week, and pulmonary function is normal between exacerbations. Exacerbations are brief, lasting from a few hours to a few days. Night time symptoms occur less than twice a month. The variation in peak expiratory flow (PEF) is less than 20%.

STEP 2: Mild persistent asthma. Patients have symptoms more than 2 times a week but less than once a day. Exacerbations may affect activity. Night time symptoms occur more than twice a month. Pulmonary function test results (in age-appropriate patients) demonstrate that the forced expiratory volume in 1 second (FEV1) or PEF is less than 80% of the predicted value, and the variation in PEF is 20-30%.

STEP 3: Moderate persistent asthma. Patients have daily symptoms and use inhaled short-acting beta2-agonists every day. Acute exacerbations may occur more than 2 times a week and last for days. The exacerbations affect activity. Nocturnal symptoms occur more than once a week. FEV1 and PEF values are 60-80% of the predicted values, and PEF varies by more than 30%.

STEP 4: Severe persistent asthma. Patients have continuous or frequent symptoms, limited physical activity, and frequent nocturnal symptoms. FEV1 and PEF values are less than 60% of the predicted values, and PEF varies by more than 30%.

Important to Note that:

- The presence of one severe feature is sufficient to diagnose severe persistent asthma.

- The characteristics in this classification system are general and may overlap because asthma is highly variable.
- The classification in a patient may change over time.
- Patients with asthma of any level of severity may have mild, moderate, or severe exacerbations.
- Some patients with intermittent asthma have severe and life-threatening exacerbations separated by episodes with almost normal lung function and minimal symptoms; however, they are likely to have other evidence of increased BHR (exercise or challenge testing) due to ongoing inflammation

Management of chronic Asthma

Goals of asthma therapy are:
1. To prevent chronic and troublesome symptoms,
2. Maintain normal or near-normal pulmonary function,
3. Maintain normal physical activity levels (including exercise),
4. Prevent recurrent exacerbations of asthma,
5. Minimize the need for emergency department visits or hospitalizations,
6. Provide optimal pharmacotherapy with minimal or no adverse effects
7. Meet the family's expectations for asthma care.

Medical care includes treatment of acute asthmatic episodes and control of chronic symptoms, including nocturnal and exercise-induced asthmatic symptoms.

Pharmacologic management includes:

- Use of control agents such as inhaled Corticosteroids, long-acting bronchodilators, Theophyl line and leukotriene modifiers

- Use of relief medications such as short-acting bronchodilators and systemic corticosteroids,

Non pharmacologic management includes measures to improve patient compliance and adherence. For all but the most severely affected patients, the ultimate goal is to prevent symptoms, minimize morbidity from acute episodes, and prevent functional and psychological morbidity to provide a healthy (or near healthy) lifestyle appropriate to the age of child.

Step-wise approach
Based on the asthma severity classification system emphasizes the initiation of high-level therapy to establish prompt control and then decreasing therapy.
- Treatment should be reviewed every 1-6 months; a gradual stepwise reduction in treatment may be possible.
- If control is not maintained despite adequate medication and adherence and the exclusion of contributing environmental factors, increased therapy should be considered.
- Long- and short-term therapy is based on the severity of asthma, as follows:
- **STEP 1 Mild intermittent asthma**

  o **Quick relief**: Short-acting bronchodilators in the form of inhaled beta2-agonists should be used as needed for symptom control.

- o The use of short-acting inhaled beta2-agonists more than 2 times a week may indicate the need to initiate long-term control therapy.

- **STEP 2 Mild persistent asthma**

  - o **Long-term control**: Anti-inflammatory treatment in the form of low-dose inhaled corticosteroids or nonsteroidal agents (e.g., cromolyn, nedocromil) is preferred. Some evidence suggests that leukotriene antagonists may be useful as first-line therapy in children.

  - o **Quick relief**: Short-acting bronchodilators in the form of inhaled beta2-agonists should be used as needed for symptom control. Use of short-acting inhaled beta2-agonists on a daily basis or increasing use indicates the need for additional long-term therapy.

- **STEP 3 Moderate persistent asthma**

  - o **Long-term control**: Daily anti-inflammatory treatment in the form of inhaled corticosteroids (medium dose) is preferred. Otherwise, low- or medium-dose inhaled corticosteroids combined with a long-acting bronchodilator or leukotriene antagonist can be used, especially for the control of nocturnal or exercise-induced asthmatic symptoms.

  - o **Quick relief**: Short-acting bronchodilators in the form of inhaled beta2-agonists should be used as needed for symptom control. The use of short-acting inhaled beta2-agonists on a daily basis or increasing use indicates the need for additional long-term therapy.

- **STEP4 Severe persistent asthma**

  - o **Long-term control**: Daily anti-inflammatory treatment in the form of inhaled corticosteroids (high dose) is preferred. Other medications, such as a long-acting bronchodilator, leukotriene antagonist or Theophyl line, can be added.

  - o **Quick relief**: Short-acting bronchodilators in the form of inhaled beta2-agonists should be used as needed for symptom control. The use of short-acting inhaled beta2-agonists on a daily basis or increasing use indicates the need for additional long-term therapy.

Management of Acute asthma

1. **Assessment of Severity** of the episode from history (cough, wheezing, breathlessness, triggering factors) and physical examination(respiratory rate, color, respiratory effort, and conscious level) and classifying according to this table

	Mild acute asthma	Moderate acute asthma	Sever acute asthma
Altered conscious level	No	No	Yes

Physical exhaustion	No	No	Yes
Speech	Sentences	Phrases	Words
Pulsus paradoxus	No	May be present	Present
Central cyanosis	No	No	Yes
Wheeze	Yes	Yes	Silent chest
Use of accessory muscle	Absent	Moderate	Marked
Sternal retraction	Absent	Moderate	Marked
Initial PEF	> 60%	40-60%	Less then 40%
SaO2	>93%	91-93%	Less then 90%
Admission	Unlikely	May be needed	Needed /ICU

2. **Criteria for admission**:

- Failure to respond to standard home treatment

- Failure to response to nebulized treatment in mild to moderate cases

- Relapse within 4 hours of nebulized beta2 agonist

- Severe acute asthma

3. **Treatment goals** for acute asthma are:

- Correction of significant hypoxemia with supplemental oxygen: In severe cases, alveolar hypoventilation requires mechanically assisted ventilation.

- Rapid reversal of airflow obstruction by using repeated or continuous administration of an inhaled beta2-agonist:

- Early administration of systemic corticosteroids (e.g., oral prednisone or intravenous hydrocortisone) in children with asthma that fails to respond promptly and completely to inhaled beta2-agonists.

- Achieving these goals requires close monitoring by means of serial clinical assessment of the severity of airflow obstruction and its response to treatment.

- Improvement in airflow after 30 minutes of treatment is significantly correlated with a broad range of indices of the severity of asthmatic exacerbations,

Complications:

- Pneumothorax status asthmaticus with respiratory failure

- Fixed (nonreversible) airway obstruction

- Death

Prognosis:

- Of infants who wheeze with URTIs, 60% are asymptomatic by age 6 years; however, children who have asthma (recurrent symptoms continuing at age 6 y) have airway reactivity later in childhood.

- Some findings suggest a poor prognosis if asthma develops in children younger than 3 years, unless it occurs solely in association with viral infections.

- Individuals who have asthma during childhood have significantly lower FEV1 and airway reactivity and more persistent broncho-spastic symptoms than those with infection-associated wheezing.

- Children with mild asthma who are asymptomatic between attacks are likely to improve and be symptom-free later in life.

- Children with asthma appear to have less severe symptoms as they enter adolescence, but half of these children continue to have asthma.

- Asthma has a tendency to remit during puberty, with a somewhat earlier remission in girls. However, compared with men, women have more BHR.

Patient Education:

- Patient and parent education should include instructions on how to use medications and devices (e.g., spacers, nebulizer, MDIs). The patient's MDI technique should be assessed on every visit.

- Discuss the management plan, which includes instructions about the use of medications, precautions with drug and/or device usage, monitoring symptoms and their severity (peak flow meter reading), and identifying potential adverse effects and necessary actions.

- Write and discuss in detail a rescue plan for an acute episode. This plan should include instructions for identifying signs of an acute attack, using rescue medications, monitoring, and contacting the asthma care team.

- Parents should understand that asthma is a chronic disorder with acute exacerbations; hence, continuity of management with active participation by the patient and/or parents and interaction with asthma care medical personnel is important.

- Emphasize the importance of compliance with and adherence to treatment.

- Incorporate the concept of expecting full control of symptoms, including nocturnal and exercise-induced symptoms, in the management plans and goals (for all but the most severely affected patients).

- Avoid unnecessary restrictions in the lifestyle of the child or family. Expect the child to participate in recreational activities and sports and to attend school as usual.

8.5 Evaluation of a Child with Wheezing

Definition

Wheezes are continuous musical sound, more commonly expiratory and usually associated with harsh breath sounds (short inspiratory and prolonged expiratory phase). They can be of single pitch (monophonic) or multiple pitches (polyphonic). Sometimes it is difficult to distinguish wheeze from upper airway sound such as stridor or snoring. A monophonic wheeze that is both inspiratory and expiratory suggests obstruction of a large central airway, whereas a polyphonic and expiratory wheeze reflects peripheral airway obstruction

Differential diagnosis

Although asthma is the most common disorder associated with wheezing, "NOT EVERY CHILD WITH WHEEZE HAS ASTHMA" nor does every child with asthma wheeze.

The differential diagnosis varies with the age of the child

1. Early infancy: **Congenital anomalies** for example tracheo bronchomalacia and vascular ring
2. Late infancy: **Bronchiolitis** in a less the 12 months old infant, with acute onset symptoms
3. Infant borne prematurely and had a period of mechanical ventilation: **Bronchopulmonary dysplasia**
4. Chronic infection with suppurative lung disease in a toddler: **Cystic fibrosis**
5. Chronic aspiration secondary to **gastro esophageal reflux** or a neurologic abnormality with dysfunctional swallowing may present wheeze at any age
6. **Foreign body aspiration**, pulmonary or esophageal, classically presents as a monophonic, unilateral wheeze and usually in more then 6 months old infant
7. **Congestive heart failure** may lead to wheezing secondary to lymphatic engorgement and compression of the airways in the peribroncho-vasculer sheath
8. **Vocal cord** malfunction in an older child

Evaluation

The evaluation of a child with wheezing starts with a careful history to look for the above mentioned differential diagnosis according to the age of the child, then followed by a thorough physical examination. If the child has signs and symptoms of increase work of breathing or distress, it is important to start some medical intervention to stabilize before etiologic evaluation can be done

Depending on the age of the child and the suspected cause following tests can be done

1. Radiological tests: chest radiography, CT scan, MRI, esophagogram, swallowing study
2. Pulmonary function tests with bronchoprovocation or bronchodilator response
3. Microbiologic studies especially looking for respiratory syncytial virus in infants
4. Empiric trail of bronchodilators
5. Bronchoscopy evaluation may also be needed in some patients

8.6 Asthma Drugs, Doses and Devices

Device		Preventer	Reliever	Age
MDI + Spacer with facemask (Infant Aero chamber - orange)		Beclomethasone MDI 50µg/ 250µg puff 50-500µg every 12H	Salbutamol MDI 100µg /puff 100-200µg up to x 4 daily prn	**Birth To 6 mo**
MDI + Spacer with facemask		Beclomethasone MDI 50µg/ 250µg puff 100-500µg 12H	Salbutamol MDI 100µg /puff 100-200 µg up to x 4 daily prn (Max 1200µg/day)	**6 mo To 6 years**
(Child Aero chamber – yellow)		Sod cromoglycate MDI 5mg/puff 10mg 6-12H		
Direct Powder Inhalation (DPI) device	Turbohaler	Budesonide turbuhaler 100/200/400µg puff 100-400µg bd	Salbutamol MDI 100µg puff 100-200µg qds prn (Occasional use only)	**6 years**
		Symbicort: Budesonide 80 / Formoterol 4.5µg per puff 2 puff bd, reduce to 1 puff bd		
	Diskus	Salmeterol 50µg puff 1 puff bd (add on therapy)	None	**To**
	Aerolizer	Formoterol 12µg puff 12-24µg bd (add on therapy)	None	
MDI + Spacer with mouthpiece	MDI + Volumetric or Blue Aero chamber	Beclomethasone MDI 50/250 µg puff, 100-500µg bd	Salbutamol MDI 100µg/puff 100-200µg up to x 4 daily prn (Max 1200µg/day)	**10Years**
		Sod cromoglycate MDI 5mg/puff 5-10mg 3-4 times daily		
		Salmeterol MDI 25µg puff 25-50µg bd (add on therapy)		
MDI alone		Beclomethasone MDI 50/250µg puff 100-500µg bd (max 1mg bd)	As Above	**10 years Upward**
		Seroflo MDI Flutic250/Salmet25/ puff 1-2 puffs bd		
		Salmeterol MDI 25µg/puff 25-50µg bd (add on therapy)		
		Sod cromoglycate MDI 5mg/puff 10mg up to qds		

8.7 Pneumonia in children

A. Pneumococcal Pneumonia

90% of cases are due to serotypes 1, 14 and 19.

Pathological stages:
In an untreated case the pathological course undergoes four stages:
1. **Congestion**
   Reactive edema of alveolar walls → ↓ gas exchange → hypoxia and acidosis → Rapid breathing.
2. **Red Hepatization**
   Two days later, alveolar sac becomes full of inflammatory exudates → consolidation → **crepitations** are heard on auscultation + opacity on x-rays.
3. **Gray Hepatization**
   Exudate is transformed into pus, which fills the alveoli → ↓elasticity → breathing movements will lead to **Chest indrawing**. Clinically there is ↓ **breath sounds**. X-Rays also shows **opacity** of affected lobe.
4. **Resolution**
   On the 4th - 7th day, complete resolution may take another 1-3 weeks. The above-mentioned stages are not seen if antibiotics are given early.

Tachypnea and chest indrawing are the two most important signs of LRTI

Clinical picture:
Onset of pneumonia in both infants and children is usually preceded by an URTI.
In older Children: It usually presents as **lobar pneumonia**
In Young Infants: It usually presents as **Bronchopneumonia**

In older children
- Shaking chills, high fever
- Drowsiness + intermittent restlessness
- Dry irritating cough
- Fast breathing: rapid shallow respiration (tachypnea)
- Child prefers to lie on affected side to minimize pleuritic pain

- **General Signs**
- Fever, and signs of respiratory distress

- **Chest Signs**
- During stage Of Congestions
    * Rapid breathing ◄———| **EARLIEST SIGN** |
- During stage Of Consolidation
    *Inspection: ↓Movement, sub costal and intercostals retraction
    *Palpation: Increased tactile vocal fremitus

*Percussion: Impaired note
*Auscultation: ↓Breath sounds, bronchial breathing, ↑vocal resonance ± fine

crepitations
•During stage of Resolution
        *Bronchial breathing replaces crepitations
        *Cough becomes productive

•Other Signs
•Right lower lobar pneumonia may be associated with right lower quadrant abdominal pain simulating appendicitis
•Upper lobar pneumonia may be associated with meningismus (neck stiffness)

In Young Infants:
•**Onset** (Initial URTI followed by)
EARLIEST SIGN
•Sudden rise of temperature
•Fast Breathing: (60/minute or more in infants <2 months) ← | EARLIEST SIGN |
        and (50/minute or more in infants aged 2-12 months)
•Restlessness
•Respiratory distress manifested by:
        *Pneumonia Triad: Grunting + Working ale nasi + Inverted Breathing
        *Chest Indrawing (lower ribs and sternum) during inspiration
        *Dyspnea ± cyanosis in severe cases

•Subsequent course
•Cough may be absent or appears late
•Signs of consolidation: usually not apparent (lesion patchy in distribution)
•Dullness, if present may denote complicating empyema
•Chest Findings:
        *Crepitations: bilateral, usually heard over both lung bases
        *No bronchial breathing except over areas of confluent (extensive) bronchopneumonia
        *Vocal resonance is normal except over areas of confluent bronchopneumonia
•Abdominal distension (due to air swallowing or to paralytic ileus)
•Liver may be palpable (due to pushing down of diaphragm or to congestive heart failure
•Neck stiffness (meningismus): may be found with involvement of the right upper lobe

Remember, the sequence of appearance of signs in pneumonia is as follows
1. Fast Breathing   3. Chest Indrawing
2. Fine Crepitations   4. Opacity in X-Rays

Chest X-Ray
•In Older Children: Picture of lobar pneumonia (consolidation ± pleural reaction)
•In Infants: Bronchopneumonia, less commonly, lobar pneumonia ± pleural reaction
Blood tests
•CRP is ↑

▪Blood Gases: done only in severe cases: $PaO_2\downarrow$, $PaCO_2\downarrow$ at the start, then ↑
▪Leucocytosis (15,000-40,000 WBC/mm^3) with predominant Polymorphs
▪**Cultures:** Identification of the causative organism: This is usually laborious, slow and not clinically useful. The definitive diagnosis requires isolation of the organism from the blood, pleural fluid or lung. Blood cultures are positive in only 20% of children with Pneumococcal pneumonia.

Treatment:

•General Measures: Rest, Oxygen, Fluids and Antipyretics
•Specific Measures: Crystalline Benzyl Penicillin G intravenously for 10 days was considered the first line treatment for a long time. Nowadays, many strains of Pneumococci are resistant to penicillin. In such cases, parenteral Cefuroxime (75-150 mg/kg/day) is used.

B. Staphylococcal Pneumonia

Age: More common in infants, 70% occur in babies <1 year.

Etiology:

Staphylococcus Aureus secretes a variety of toxins and enzymes: hemolysin – leukocidin – staphylokinase and coagulase.

Pathology

•Confluent **Bronchopneumonia:** Unilateral or more prominent on one side
•Extensive areas of hemorrhage necrosis and irregular areas of cavitations (multiple abscesses)
•Pleura covered by thick fibrino-purulent exudates
•Multiple small abscesses → Rupture of sub pleural abscesses leading to Bronchopulmonary Fistula Empyema or Pyopneumothorax

Clinical Picture

•Age: Infant <1 year
•Affected Side: Right side 65%, Bilateral 20%
•History of staphylococcal skin infection (furunculosis) or maternal breast abscess
•URTI for few days→ acute onset of high fever, cough and respiratory distress
•Rapid progression of symptoms (in few hours) → tachypnea, grunting, acting alae nasi, sub costal and
  sternal retractions, lethargy (if left undisturbed) and irritability (if aroused)
•In Severe Cases: Dyspnea, cyanosis and shock-like state
•Early Signs: Those of bronchopneumonia: ↓ breath sounds + scattered crepitations
•Later Signs: Those of Empyema or Pyopneumothorax

Diagnosis

•X-Rays: Picture of bronchopneumonia + small abscesses ± pneumatoceles ± effusion ±   Pyopneumothorax in 25%
•Other Investigations: Like Pneumococcal pneumonia.

Complications

• Empyema or Pyopneumothorax

- Pericarditis, Meningitis, Osteomyelitis
- Metastatic soft tissue abscesses

In all cases of Staphylococcal Pneumonia, one should test for Immunodeficiency and Cystic Fibrosis

Treatment
- General measures: Rest, Oxygen, Fluids and Antipyretics
- Specific Measures: Parenteral Cefotaxime + Vancomycin or Clindamycin
- Treatment of Complications: (see treatment of empyema)

C. Viral Pneumonia

Is most common in infants and young children

Etiology
- Respiratory Syncytial Virus (RSV)
- Influenza Virus
- Parainfluenza Virus
- Adenovirus
- Enterovirus

Clinical Characteristics:
- Temperature is lower and child does not appear to be very sick compared to bacterial pneumonia
- Wheezes may be heard due to associated bronchitis
- Respiratory distress in young infants
Clinical course is usually self-limited
- X-Ray → diffuse perihilar infiltrates + hyperinflation
- Normal or mild leucocytosis with lymphocytes

Treatment:
Supportive
- Oxygen
- Hydration (oral or parenteral fluids)
Antiviral Agents {Oral Amantadine **(for type A Influenza)** or Aerosolized Ribavirin **(for RSV)** may be used in cases with immunodeficiency.

D. Mycoplasma Pneumonia or Primary Atypical Pneumonia

Mostly seen in **school age children**. The disease is suspected when *symptoms are more severe then the chest signs and the x-ray findings*.
- Persistent non-productive (Dry) paroxysmal hacking cough and/or wheezes especially in older children (10-13 years of age)
- X-Ray → interstitial infiltrates
- CBC normal
- Cold hemagglutinins test (positive)

• Treatment is with Erythromycin or Azithromycin.

N.B. Mycoplasma is resistant to Penicillin because it has no cell wall.

E. Aspiration Pneumonia

Etiology: Can be caused by aspiration of
  •Amniotic fluid or meconium (in newborns)
  •Foreign Body
  •Zinc Stearate (baby powder)
  •Food (in cases of neurologically handicapped child or in tracheoesophageal fistula
  •Lipoid Material → Lipoid Pneumonia (Ghee, Oil drops)
  •Hydrocarbons (like kerosene) →Kerosene Pneumonia

Hydrocarbon (Kerosene) Pneumonia

Etiology
  Aspiration of hydrocarbons like (kerosene, furniture polish, gasoline)
  Aspiration may occur during: vomiting, swallowing, gastric lavage (contraindicated)

Pathology
  •Pulmonary surfactant is inactivated → lung collapse
  •Alveolar macrophages are injured
  •Pulmonary edema, inflammation and hemorrhage

Complication
  •Secondary Infection (suspect if fever re-appears)
  •Pneumothorax (subcutaneous emphysema of the chest wall – pneumatoceles)
  •Pleural Effusion

Treatment
  •If ingested amount is small: **Don't** induce vomiting of gastric lavage (risk of aspiration)
  •If ingested amount is large: **Cautious** nasogastric suction. Better insert a cuffed endotracheal tube before suction, to avoid aspiration during suction/gastric lavage.
  •A Cathartic (purgative) is usually given
  •Antibiotics: Used only if there is secondary infection (detected by re-appearance of fever after 3-5 days), treated with Penicillin G and Tobramycin
  •Corticosteroids have **No role** and may be harmful
  •Supportive Measures: Oxygen, Physiotherapy and in severe cases assisted ventilation

Decision Tree for the management of a case of Kerosene Pneumonia:

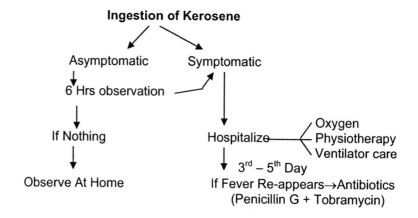

Ingestion of Kerosene

Asymptomatic Symptomatic

6 Hrs observation

If Nothing Hospitalize —— Oxygen / Physiotherapy / Ventilator care

Observe At Home $3^{rd} - 5^{th}$ Day
If Fever Re-appears→Antibiotics
(Penicillin G + Tobramycin)

F. Recurrent Pneumonia and Incomplete resolution

When you see recurrent pneumonia or failure of resolution, think of:
- Gastro-esophageal Reflux Disease (GERD)
- Foreign Body
- ↓ Gag Reflex (Cerebral palsy or neurodegenerative diseases)
- Immunodeficiency diseases
- ↑Pulmonary blood flow (Left to Right shunts)
- Congenital Anomalies (cleft palate, T-E fistula, congenital anomaly, immotile cilia)
- Cystic Fibrosis
- Immunodeficiency diseases

8.8 Common Pleural Diseases

Pleural Effusion

Pleural Effusion is a broad terminology that means an accumulation of fluid (inflammatory, non-inflammatory, blood, etc) in the pleural cavity. Its terminology will differ according to the type of accumulated fluid.

1.   **Inflammatory Fluid (Exudate)**
▪Serofibrinous effusion as in pneumonia, SLE, etc
▪Empyema (purulent effusion) as in pneumonia (staphylococcal, Pneumococcal), rupture of lung abscess etc.

2.   **Non-Inflammatory Effusions**
▪Hydrothorax **(transudate)**: as in Nephrotic syndrome. It is usually bilateral
▪Hemothorax (blood in pleural cavity): as in malignancies, bleeding tendencies & trauma
▪Chylothorax (chyle in the pleural cavity): as in congenital anomaly or operative trauma of the thoracic duct and to the thoracic duct.

Pleurisy

Etiology and clinical types:
    1.   **Dry (plastic) pleurisy**
        ▪Pneumonia
        ▪URTI (Enteroviruses pleurodynia (Bornholm Disease)
        ▪Rheumatic Fever
        ▪Tuberculosis
    2.   **Serofibrosis**
        ▪Pneumonia
        ▪Connective Tissue Disease (SLE, juvenile rheumatoid arthritis)
        ▪Inflammatory conditions of abdomen, mediastinum
    3.   **Purulent (Empyema)**
        ▪Pneumonia (staphylococcal, Pneumococcal, Haemophilus, etc)
        ▪Rupture of lung disease
        ▪Surgical trauma to thoracic cavity (e.g.: rupture of esophagus)

Empyema

Means pus within the pleural cavity

Symptoms
    This usually appears with symptoms of the underlying cause (e.g.: pneumonia)
    Followed by an interval of few days during which the antibiotic therapy is usually inadequate or inappropriate, finally there is development of empyema leading to fever, respiratory distress and patient appears more toxic and sick.

Physical Signs:
    •Signs of the original illness (e.g.: pneumonia)

- •Inspection　　(full intercostals spaces + ↓ movements
- •Palpitation　　↓ tactile VF
- •Percussion　　Stony dull
- •Auscultation　↓air entry, ↓vocal resonance

X-Ray findings

- •Homogeneous density obliterating normal markings of underlying lung
- •Obliterated costo-phrenic angle
- •Shift of mediastinum to other side if the empyema is considerable
- •X-Ray findings of the underlying cause (TB, pneumonia, tumor, etc)

How can you demonstrate small amount of fluid in the pleural cavity

- •X-Ray (wide interlobar fissure)
- •By Ultrasonography

Lab investigations

- •CBC (leucocytosis)
- •ESR (elevated)
- •Thoracocentesis should always be performed when empyema is suspected. Remove as much pus as possible. The sample should also be sent for:
  - ○　Chemical Analysis
  - ○　Gram and Ziel Nielsen stain
  - ○　Bacteriological Culture

Difference Between Exudate And Transudate		
	Transudate	**Exudate**
Appearance	-Clear	-opaque
Specific Gravity	-<1015	->1015
Protein	-<3 gm/dl	->3 gm/dl

Treatment

- •Treatment of the original cause
- •Systemic antibiotic therapy
- •Closed drainage of the effusion by an underwater seal of continuous suction
- •Surgical decortication is done if there are extensive fibrinous changes on the surface of collapsed lungs

Pneumothorax

Means air within the Pleural cavity

Etiology:

Common Causes

- •Staphylococcal Pneumonia
- •Accidental (Thoracocentesis)
- •Spontaneous

Other Causes

- •Trauma (surgery, thoracotomy)
- •Rupture of cyst, emphysematous bleb
- •Cystic Fibrosis

Clinical picture:

Depends on the extent of lung collapse and on the underlying lung disease
- Respiratory Distress
- Shift of the mediastinum to the opposite side
- Tympanitic percussion note

If there is Tension Pneumothorax
- There is limited expansion of the contralateral lung
- Cardiovascular compromise and pulsus paradoxus

If there Is Bronchopleural Fistula
- Amphoric Breathing will be heard
- Grunting sound with respiration
- Fills rapidly after aspiration

Differential Diagnosis:
- Emphysema (localized/generalized) -Cyst/Cavity
- Gaseous distension of stomach
- Diaphragmatic Hernia
- Large bleb

X-Ray can help in reaching the correct diagnosis

TREATMENT
- Treatment of the cause
- Analgesics
- Treatment of Pneumothorax depends upon:

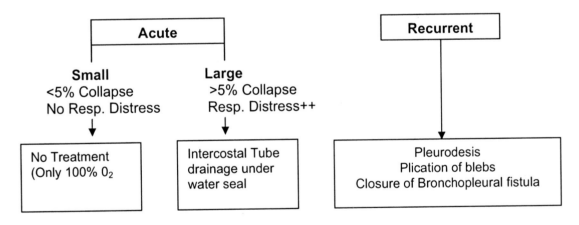

Pleurodesis (formation of adhesion between lung and chest wall) may be achieved by:
- Chemical (local injection of tetracycline or silver nitrate)
- Basilar Pleural Abrasion
- Stripping of the pleura

9

Cardiovascular System

9.1   Common congenital heart diseases (CHD)

Congenital heart disease refers to a group of anatomic abnormalities of the heart that are generally present at birth, although majority of them may not be symptomatic at birth.
The overall **incidence** of CHD has been estimated at 6-8 per 1000 live births.
No definite **etiological factor** can be identified in the vast majority of children with CHD, and the disease is believed to have a multifactorial origin.

- Chromosomal problems (Down Syndrome, Turner syndrome)
- Intrauterine infections (congenital rubella)
- Maternal medications (sodium valproate, Phenytoin) are associated with CHD
- Specific inheritable gene defects (Holt Oram syndrome).

Classification

A   Left to right shunts (mostly acyanotic)
  1   Ventricular septal defect
  2   Patent ductus arteriosus
  3   Atrial septal defect
  4   Atrioventricular septal defect (endocardial cushion defect)

B.   Right to left shunts (mostly cyanotic)
  1.   Tetralogy of Fallot
  2.   Transposition of great arteries
  3.   Truncus arteriosus
  4.   Total anomalous pulmonary venous drainage

C.   Obstructive lesions
  1. Coarctation of the aorta
  2. Aortic stenosis
  3. Pulmonary stenosis

D. Complex heart diseases
  1. Hypoplastic left heart
  2. Hypoplastic right heart

A.   Left to right shunts

These are a group of disorders where there is an abnormal communication between the right and left sides of the heart. As the pressures are greater on the left side, blood flows from the left to the right side of the heart. The excess blood entering into the lungs causes congestion resulting in symptoms like breathlessness, feeding difficulties, irritability, poor weight gain and recurrent chest infections. The shunt and above symptoms are minimal or absent in neonatal period due to high pulmonary resistance but get marked in late infancy due to natural drop in pulmonary resistance. Exception is patent ductus arteriosus in the preterm baby. If left untreated, complications include infective endocarditis, and irreversible pulmonary hypertension with reversal of blood flow **(Eisenmenger syndrome)**.

A1.   Ventricular septal defect (VSD)

VSD is the most common CHD, accounting for almost 25% of the CHD patients. Manifestations depend mainly on the size of the defect and degree of pulmonary hypertension. Smaller defects present with prominent pansystolic murmur best heard over the lower left sternal border, without any other abnormal cardiovascular signs. These babies are asymptomatic, and in many of them the defect closes spontaneously by 3 years age.

Large VSDs are associated with significant left to right shunt and become symptomatic in the late neonatal period (2-4 weeks). Physical examination reveals evidence of failure to thrive, chest deformity and labored breathing. Tachypnea, tachycardia and hepatomegaly denote heart failure. The precordium is deformed, with clinically detectable cardiomegaly. Left parasternal heave reflects right ventricular hypertrophy and palpable second heart sound indicates pulmonary hypertension. Systolic thrills over the lower left sternal border can occasionally occur even with large defects, although more commonly thrills indicate small to moderate defects. Second heart sound is loud on auscultation, and there is a pansystolic murmur over the lower left sternal border. Increased venous return flowing though a normal mitral valve may gives rise to an apical mid-diastolic murmur. Chest X-ray reveals cardiomegaly and pulmonary congestion (Plethoric lung fields). ECG shows biventricular hypertrophy, with left atrial or bi-atrial enlargement. Echocardiography localizes the defect, detect other associated anomalies, and can measure the pulmonary artery pressures.

Large defects in the presence of heart failure require anti-heart failure therapy, and if symptoms persist necessitate surgical closure of the defect with an open-heart operation. Some of the larger defects can become smaller, and even close spontaneously; therefore if symptoms are controlled and pulmonary hypertension does not develop, they may be followed up medically. Best age for surgical closure of large VSD is between the ages 6-12 months. Infective endocarditis prophylaxis is required to cover at risk procedures.

A2. Patent ductus arteriosus (PDA)

Ductus arteriosus has an important role in fetal circulation by enabling the systemic venous return to reach the placenta for oxygenation. After birth, the fall in pulmonary vascular resistance and rise in systemic vascular resistance results in a left to right flow across the ductus, which remains patent for up to 48 hours in majority of neonates. Abnormal persistence of the ductus may either be due to the immaturity of its muscle as in preterm babies, or due to an abnormal musculature. The resultant blood flow from aorta to pulmonary artery tends to increase pulmonary blood flow and lead to symptoms of heart failure.

Small PDA just produces a continuous or systolic upper parasternal murmur, without any symptoms, and is best dealt with non-surgical closure using coils or an umbrella device before school going age.

Large PDA is associated with heart failure. Examination reveals high volume collapsing pulse with a wide pulse pressure, cardiomegaly, loud second heart sound, and a continuous upper parasternal murmur, which is widely conducted. The murmur extends through the whole of systole, peaks at the second sound and flows into early part of diastole, and is marked by multiple 'clicks' (machinery murmur, 'train in tunnel' murmur). Chest X-ray shows cardiomegaly, and pulmonary congestion. ECG reveals LVH with left or bi-atrial enlargement. Echocardiogram confirms the diagnosis and assesses the suitability for device closure.

Preterm neonate with symptomatic PDA may respond to indomethacin or ibuprofen. Surgical closure is now resorted to only for the neonate or infant who is in heart failure and symptomatic preterm who fails to respond to indomethacin, or where the drug is contraindicated. Infective endocarditis prophylaxis is required to cover at risk procedures.

A3. Atrial septal defect (ASD)

Foramen ovale is an interatrial communication that enables the fetal heart to convey the oxygenated umbilical venous blood to the left side of the heart and from there to the brain. After birth, the defect is sealed by its edges, but the flow may still be present for 2-3 weeks. Abnormal persistence of this defect or presence of other defects in the atrial septum is a common form of CHD. The resultant left to right shunt is minimal in infancy, but becomes more as age advances, hence these lesions are asymptomatic in infancy and early childhood. Mostly they come to attention from the associated pulmonary flow murmurs on routine examination. Occasionally, ASD can present with recurrent chest infections or even heart failure. In the presence of a large ASD, cardiac examination reveals normal pulses, left parasternal heave, wide fixed splitting of the second heart sound, and an ejection systolic murmur over the pulmonary area.

Chest X-ray shows cardiomegaly, prominent pulmonary artery segment, and increased pulmonary vascularity. ECG shows RVH and an incomplete right bundle branch pattern (rsR' in right chest leads.) Echocardiography serves to confirm the diagnosis and assess the size of the defect and suitability for device closure. Most ASDs can now be closed by device closure in the preschool age. However, ASDs, which are not suitable for device closure on account of their location or, those which present in infancy with heart failure require surgical closure. Pulmonary hypertension is a late event. Infective endocarditis prophylaxis is not recommended except during the 6 months following closure by device or surgery.

A4. Atrioventricular septal (endocardial cushion) defects (AVSD)

These include defects in the lower part of atrial septum (primum ASD), upper (inflow) ventricular septum along with cleft anterior mitral leaflet and variable mitral regurgitation. Incomplete defects with isolated primum atrial septal defect and/or mitral regurgitation are also common. AVSD is more common in children with **Down syndrome**. AVSD allows flow of blood across both atrial and ventricular septa, and also from the left ventricle into the right atrium. Besides, the associated mitral and tricuspid regurgitation complicate the hemo-dynamics and auscultatory findings. Pulmonary hypertension is early in onset and progression. Cardiac auscultation reveals a loud second heart sound and a prominent pansystolic murmur over the lower left sternal border. The latter is usually due to the tricuspid regurgitation, and not the VSD. Early surgical repair of the defect is recommended before the age of 6 months. Isolated primum ASD may be repaired like secundum ASD before the school going age. Infective endocarditis prophylaxis is required to cover at risk procedures.

B1. Tetralogy of Fallot (TOF)

TOF is the prototype of a right to left shunt. The defect is combination of four associations, hence named tetralogy.
1. Infundibular pulmonary stenosis
2. Large sub aortic VSD.
3. Right ventricular hypertrophy and
4. Over-riding aorta above the VSD.
Symptoms vary widely and depend mainly on the severity of pulmonary stenosis. PS often

increases in severity with age and majority of infants develop cyanosis in the second 6 months of life. Cyanosis and shortness of breath on exertion including feeding and hyper-cyanotic spells are the usual manifestations in infancy. Hypercyanotic spells are characterized by periods of increasing cyanosis with crying, fast breathing and irritability, sometimes leading on to unconsciousness and even anoxic seizures. These are believed to be due to pulmonary infundibular spasm. Older children may present with effort intolerance and squatting (sitting with bent hip and knee joints). Squatting helps by increasing systemic vascular resistance, thereby promoting pulmonary blood flow. *Heart failure does not occur in uncomplicated TOF.*

Physical examination reveals central cyanosis and clubbing of fingers and toes. Pulses are normal and there is no precordial bulge or deformity. Left parasternal heave may not be prominent, and thrills are uncommon. Second heart sound is single (aortic) and there is a long parasternal systolic murmur of infundibular stenosis.

Chest X-ray shows an upturned cardiac apical shadow, with concave pulmonary bay (boot shaped heart), and pulmonary oligemia. ECG confirms RVH. Echocardiography confirms the diagnosis, assesses the severity and identifies any associated anomalies. Cardiac catheterization and angiography is now performed only in selected patients.

Management includes attention to nutrition, prevention and treatment of iron deficiency, infective endocarditis prophylaxis. Hypercyanotic spells may require oxygen inhalation, knee chest position, morphine, correction of metabolic acidosis, intravenous fluids, and sometimes intravenous propranolol or general anesthesia for resistant cases. Spells can be minimized by correction of iron deficiency and use of prophylactic propranolol. Presence of spells indicates the need for surgical intervention – either palliative shunt surgery or total repair if feasible. Total correction of TOF is indicated in all symptomatic infants around 6 months to 1 year. This involves resection of the infundibular muscle and patch closure of the VSD.
Infective endocarditis prophylaxis is required to cover at risk procedures.

C1. Coarctation of the aorta

This refers to a narrowing of the aorta at the junction of the arch with descending aorta, opposite the insertion of the ductus arteriosus. In severe cases, the blood supply to descending aorta comes through the ductus, and when it closes in the first week of life, baby presents in shock. Heart failure in the neonatal period is another mode of presentation. Less severe types may present later with hypertension, cardiac murmur or weak/absent femoral pulses. Co-existing intracranial aneurysms or complications like infective endocarditis could occasionally lead to the diagnosis. Associated cardiac anomalies include VSD and bicuspid aortic valve. Coarctation is more common in children with *Turner syndrome*.
Cardiovascular findings include weak femoral pulses, brachio femoral or radio femoral delay, and fall in systolic blood pressure in the lower limbs compared to upper limbs. Auscultatory findings are variable, and may include loud aortic second sound (with hypertension), aortic ejection click (with bicuspid aortic valve), right parasternal systolic murmur (with bicuspid aortic valve), and short systolic murmurs over the left upper parasternal region below the clavicle or interscapular region (coarctation murmur). It is worth remembering that in the neonate presence of a large PDA may lead to good femoral pulses even with severe coarctation. Surgical repair of any significant coarctation is indicated once the diagnosis is confirmed. Infective endocarditis prophylaxis is required to cover at risk procedures.

C2. Aortic stenosis

The narrowing may be valvular, subvalvular or supravalvular. Bicuspid aortic valve is the most common cause. Williams's syndrome is associated with supravalvular AS. Most children are asymptomatic. Severe AS may be associated with dyspnea or easy fatigability. Critical AS (tight AS) presents in the neonate with heart failure.

Cardiovascular signs include a systolic thrill over the aortic area, conducted to the neck. AS produces an ejection systolic murmur, preceded by a fixed ejection click, sometimes better heard over the cardiac apex. ECG is normal except in severe AS, where is shows LVH with strain pattern. Echocardiography helps to confirm diagnosis, assess severity, and detect any associated anomalies. Majority of children do not require intervention, but moderate to severe types benefit from balloon angioplasty or surgical repair. Infective endocarditis prophylaxis is required to cover at risk procedures.

C3. Pulmonary valve stenosis

Most children are asymptomatic. Severe PS may be associated with dyspnea or easy fatigability. Critical PS (tight PS) presents in the neonate with poor feeding, tachypnea with or without cyanosis. **Noonan syndrome** is associated with dysplastic pulmonary valve and PS.

Cardiovascular examination reveals normal pulses, no cyanosis or clubbing, left parasternal heave, systolic thrill over pulmonary area. Auscultation shows an ejection systolic murmur best audible over the pulmonary area, and preceded by an ejection click that is audible in inspiration. Chest X-ray shows prominent post-stenotic dilatation of the pulmonary artery, with mostly normal pulmonary vasculature (Except in severe PS – pulmonary oligemia). ECG shows RAD and RVH, in moderate to severe cases, and normal in mild cases. Echocardiogram helps to diagnose and assess severity. Treatment is indicated for moderate to severe cases. Most cases are amenable to balloon angioplasty. Surgical repair is necessary in the neonate with critical PS. Infective endocarditis prophylaxis is required to cover at risk procedures.

Prognosis and counseling in CHD

It is important to explain the nature of the disease and natural history to parents, with help of diagrams of models. Despite successful therapy for most diseases being feasible, children require long-term follow up, in view of the late complications including sudden death.

9.2 Rheumatic fever and Rheumatic heart disease

Definition
Acute rheumatic phenomenon is an abnormal immunologic reaction to throat infection by rheumatogenic strains of group A beta-hemolytic streptococci.
The attack rate following streptococcal pharyngitis ranges from 0.3 to 3%.

Predisposing factors include family history of rheumatic fever, low socio-economic status and age 6 to 15 years. The disease involves various tissues as outlined below. The heart bears the major brunt of the attack and may be associated with chronic residual valvular disease.

Acute rheumatic fever

Diagnostic criteria (Revised Jones Criteria):

Major criteria	Minor criteria
Polyarthritis	Fever
Pancarditis	Acute phase reactants (ESR, CRP, WCC)
Chorea	Prolonged PR on ECG
Subcutaneous nodules	Arthralgia (Joint pain)
Erythema marginatum	Previous history of rheumatic fever

Supporting evidence of preceding streptococcal throat infection is an **essential criterion** that could be represented by evidence of recent streptococcal infection, in the form of elevated ASO / DNAase B titre, scarlet fever, or positive throat swab culture for the organism.

The diagnosis requires presence of either **two major criteria or one major and two minor criteria, with evidence of recent streptococcal throat infection.**

Clinical manifestations:

1. Rheumatic arthritis sets in about 3-6 weeks after the streptococcal throat infection, and involves predominantly the larger joints like knee, ankle, elbow or wrist joints. It is associated with fever and joint pain and swelling. The affected joints are tender, with limitation of movement and evidence of fluid accumulation in the joint spaces. Classically the arthritis is flitting, meaning the symptoms move from one joint to another, the earlier affected joint starts resolving when a new joint is affected. Joint involvement is self-limiting, and resolves in 3-4 weeks even if left untreated. Arthralgia without signs of acute inflammation is considered as minor criteria only.

2. Pancarditis: Meaning combined Peri, Myo and Endo Carditis. This also sets in about 3-6 weeks following the infection, but manifestations may have a delayed onset in those with chronic carditis. Severity may vary from mild asymptomatic murmur of mitral regurgitation to florid heart failure. Symptoms include chest pain, palpitation, dyspnea, shortness of breath and dependent edema in the presence of heart failure. Cardiac findings include tachycardia, cardiomegaly, muffled heart sounds, soft mid-diastolic apical murmur (Carey Coombs murmur), pansystolic apical murmur of mitral regurgitation, early diastolic murmur of aortic regurgitation, and pericardial rub (in the presence of Pericarditis). Pericardial effusion may be significant, but cardiac tamponade is rare. Chest X-ray may show cardiomegaly, and shape of the cardiac shadow could raise the suspicion of pericardial effusion. ECG shows prolonged PR interval, and low voltage complexes. Echocardiogram helps to define the cardiac involvement. Mitral regurgitation is the most common lesion, followed by aortic regurgitation.

3. Rheumatic chorea is a delayed manifestation of rheumatic fever, with onset 6 weeks to 6 months after the throat infection. It is characterized by abnormal involuntary movements that involve the face as well as extremities, described as quasi-purposive and non-repetitive. The movements increase with excitement and disappear in sleep. Muscle hypotonia and emotional lability are other associated features of rheumatic chorea. Several physical signs have been described with rheumatic chorea, like the Milkman's sign, jack-in-the-box sign and pronator sign. Being a late manifestation, it may not be possible to fulfill the diagnostic criteria for rheumatic fever – chorea for which there is no other obvious cause like medications or neurologic disease is considered as rheumatic in origin. 25% of children with rheumatic chorea have associated clinical or subclinical carditis, which may be picked up on echocardiogram. Chorea is self-limiting, and resolves in due course (6-18 months), but some children may require medications.

4. Subcutaneous nodules are hard, painless, mobile swellings, which are distributed along the extensor aspect of elbow, knee and other large and small joints, over the scalp or along the spine. They may last for weeks, and have a significant association with Carditis.

5. Erythema marginatum refers to Non pruritic serpiginous or annular erythematous rashes that appear on the trunk or proximal extremities; it is of an evanescent (transient) nature.

Differential diagnosis
- Post streptococcal reactive arthritis – lacks the classical features of rheumatic Polyarthritis, often smaller joints are also involved, respond poorly to Salicylate
- Juvenile chronic arthritis – often younger age of onset, smaller joint involvement, presence of other manifestations like eye involvement
- Hematological conditions like sickle cell disease and leukemia may also to be considered in atypical cases
- Other collagen vascular diseases including SLE etc.

Management
Requires confirmation of the diagnosis, cardiac assessment including echocardiogram, and parental counseling, including advice on prophylaxis.
Specific therapy depends on the manifestations. Arthritis requires Salicylate 60-100 mg/kg/day in 4 divided doses to be continued for 4-6 weeks. Carditis if mild requires no additional medications. Carditis with heart failure (severe Carditis) is usually treated with Prednisolone 2 mg/kg for two weeks and then tapered off in the next 2-4 weeks. Salicylate is added when Prednisolone is tapered, to continue for a total of 6-12 weeks. Rheumatic chorea may require Haloperidol or sodium valproate. Heart failure if present requires diuretics and ACE inhibitors therapy – Digoxin is contraindicated because of risk of inducing dangerous arrhythmias.

Residual streptococcal infection is treated with a single injection of Benzathine penicillin 0.6 to 1.2 million units deep IM. For children allergic to penicillin, erythromycin 40 mg/Kg in 4 divided doses for 10 days is prescribed.

Prevention of recurrence

Benzathine penicillin 0.6 to 1.2 million units deep IM once in 3-4 weeks is effective in prevention of recurrences. Children who are allergic to penicillin can be given erythromycin 250 mg twice a day. Compliance to therapy needs to be monitored in both these situations.

Prevention of infective endocarditis

Additional prophylactic antibiotics are required in patients with established heart disease when they undergo procedures at risk for endocarditis. See chapter 9.4.

Chronic rheumatic valvular heart disease

Mitral regurgitation is the most common rheumatic valve disease in children. Clinical features depend on the severity of the regurgitation and presence of any co-existing mitral stenosis. Mild mitral regurgitation may just present as an asymptomatic cardiac murmur, without any other abnormal findings. Severe MR generally is symptomatic with fatigue, and chest pain. Complicating endocarditis or frank heart failure are other modes of presentation. Cardiac examination reveals cardiomegaly, systolic thrill over the apex. Second heart sound may be closely split, due to shortening of LV ejection, and S3 is often audible. The hallmark of MR is the loud, pansystolic murmur best heard over the apex and conducted to the axilla and back. Increased forward flow across the mitral valve causes a short low-frequency diastolic rumble at the apex, even in the absence of organic mitral stenosis (Carey Coombs murmur).

Chest X-ray may show cardiomegaly and prominent upper lobe veins, and ECG shows LVH with or without left atrial enlargement. Older children may show also atrial fibrillation. Echocardiogram confirms the presence of MR assesses severity and also diagnoses other associated valve lesions including co-existing mitral stenosis.

Medical management includes exclusion of rheumatic activity, treatment of heart failure when present, advice on infective endocarditis prophylaxis. ACE inhibitor therapy is believed to be helpful to reduce symptoms. Surgical repair or replacement of the mitral valve is required in the presence of persistent heart failure, progressive cardiomegaly or pulmonary hypertension.

Aortic regurgitation is the second most common valve lesion in acute rheumatic fever and unlike mitral regurgitation that occurs in the acute stage is less likely to resolve with time. Severe AR leads to exercise intolerance and even frank heart failure. Late features include anginal chest pain and palpitation (frequent ventricular premature beats). The pulses are bounding and radial pulse shows a high volume collapsing nature. The pulse pressure is wide. A high pitched decrescendo diastolic murmur best audible in the 3rd or 4th left intercostals space and accentuated in expiration, is the hallmark of significant AR. The increased forward flow across the aortic valve gives rise to an additional ejection systolic murmur over the aortic area and carotids even in the absence of organic aortic stenosis. Chest X-ray shows cardiomegaly, and dilated ascending aorta and prominent aortic knuckle. Upper lobe pulmonary veins may be engorged. ECG shows LVH. Echocardiogram reveals dilated left ventricle, and aortic regurgitation. Medical management includes exclusion of rheumatic activity, treatment of heart failure when present, advice on infective endocarditis prophylaxis. ACE inhibitor therapy is believed to be helpful to reduce symptoms, and delay progression of LVH. Surgical replacement of the aortic valve is required in the presence of persistent heart failure, and is recommended even in those with no symptoms in the presence of significant cardiomegaly, early LV dysfunction on echocardiogram or exercise related symptoms. Besides replacement, repair of the aortic valve is also been considered in more and more children with significant AR.

Mitral stenosis is late sequelae of rheumatic mitral valve involvement, and usually develops 5-15 years after acute rheumatic fever. However, in certain parts of the world, MS can develop even at an earlier age. Dyspnea with or without exertion, orthopnea, nocturnal dyspnea and palpitations indicate significant MS. Hemoptysis and atrial fibrillation are late manifestations. Cardiac examination reveals a tapping cardiac apex, with left parasternal heave, and loud P2 in the presence of pulmonary hypertension. First heart sound is loud at the apex, and a low frequency apical diastolic rumble, best heard in the left lateral position is the hallmark. Severe MS may be associated with dilatation of the tricuspid valve ring and give rise to pansystolic murmur of tricuspid regurgitation. Chest X-ray shows a straightening of the left cardiac border contributed by the dilated pulmonary artery segment, dilated left atrium and hypertrophied right ventricle. Lung fields show pulmonary venous congestion, and Kerley's B lines denote interstitial edema. ECG reveals right axis deviation, right ventricular hypertrophy and left or biatrial enlargement. Echocardiogram helps to assess severity of the MS, and detect any other valve lesions. Medical management includes diuretics for heart failure, and prevention of rheumatic recurrence and infective endocarditis. Anticoagulation may be indicated in the presence of atrial fibrillation. Balloon angioplasty to dilate the mitral valve can be considered in symptomatic children. Open valve repair or replacement is required in the presence of significant MR, or calcification of the leaflets. Patients who receive prosthetic mitral valve replacement have to be anticoagulated with warfarin and coagulation status monitored periodically.

9.3 Congestive heart failure in children

Definition

Congestive heart failure (CHF) refers to a symptom complex resulting from an inability of the heart to pump enough blood to meet the demand. The consequent symptoms and signs are the result of both poor tissue perfusion and build up of backpressure in the venous circulation.

Aetiology

Usually secondary to an underlying heart disease, problems outside the heart can also result in a similar symptom complex.

Cardiac causes	Extra-cardiac causes
Congenital Heart Diseases	Birth Asphyxia
Left to right shunts – VSD, PDA, ASD	Meconium Aspiration
Right to left shunts – TGA+VSD, TAPVC, Truncus arteriosus	Metabolic Acidosis
Obstructive lesions – Coarctation, AS, PS	Hypoglycemia
Complex heart disease – single ventricle, Hypoplastic left heart	Sepsis
Myocarditis and Cardiomyopathy	Pneumonia
Rheumatic Heart Disease	RDS
Cardiac Arrhythmias	Anemia
Kawasaki disease	Fluid Overload
Infective Endocarditis	Upper Resp. Obstruction
Hypertension	Cystic Fibrosis
Pericarditis	Neuromuscular disorders
Drugs - Anthracyclines	Storage disorders

Clinical recognition

Symptoms: Presenting features differ in infants and older children.
- **Infants** present either acutely with pallor, sweating, poor feeding, irritability, breathlessness, wheezing, decreased urine output, hypotension, or more insidiously with cough, chest recessions or failure to gain weight.
- **Older children** may present with chest pain, chest discomfort, palpitation, shortness of breath, orthopnea, paroxysmal nocturnal dyspnea, abdominal pain or syncope.

Signs:
- **Infants** demonstrate failure to thrive, tachypnea, tachycardia and hepatomegaly. Weak peripheral pulses and cold extremities are common findings. In extreme cases, hypotension is pronounced.
- **Older children** show dependent edema, elevated jugular venous pulses and fine crepitations in the lung bases.

Cardiac examination may give a clue to the underlying cause. Gallop rhythm (S3/S4) may point to heart failure and loud P2 if pulmonary hypertension co-exists. Underlying disease dictates the cardiac murmurs, but absence of murmur does not exclude CHF.

Lab investigations
- Acute management may require other investigations like full blood counts, C-reactive proteins, electrolyte profile, renal functions and liver functions.
- Chest X-ray may show cardiomegaly, and pulmonary edema
- ECG may reveal a cardiac arrhythmia or evidence of underlying heart disease
- Echocardiography and Doppler studies serve to assess cardiac function and diagnose underlying heart disease.

Management
Management involves stabilization of the patient, confirmation of the diagnosis and identification of any treatable causes.
- In the acute stage, diuretics form the mainstay of therapy. These are combined with angiotensin converting enzyme inhibitors (captopril, enalapril).
- Selected patients may benefit from Digoxin.
- Underlying heart disease and any aggravating factors require attention.
- In children with dilated cardiomyopathy, it may be necessary to use additional diuretics, intravenous Frusemide and dobutamine infusion. β-Adrenergic receptor blockers with vasodilator action like carvedilol may improve quality of life.

Complications
Severe failure to thrive, recurrent infections, cardiac arrhythmias, pulmonary hypertension, other complications related to the cause of heart failure and related to medications

Prognosis and counseling
Depends on the underlying cause of heart failure. Where specific cure is possible, prognosis is generally good. Patients with congenital heart disease have better outcome with corrective surgery or non-surgical intervention.

9.4 Infective Endocarditis and its Prophylaxis

Definition
Infective endocarditis is an infection of the endocardial surface of the heart, which could also involve septal defects, mural endocardium or intravascular implanted devices. Endarteritis that involves arteries including the ductus arteriosus, the great vessels, aneurysms or arteriovenous shunts also comes under this definition.

Aetiology:

Predisposing heart diseases	Predisposing procedures
Prosthetic cardiac valves	Dental procedures known to induce bleeding
Previous infective endocarditis	Tonsillectomy and adenoidectomy
Most congenital heart diseases (except ASD)	Bronchoscopy with rigid bronchoscope
Surgically created systemic to pulmonary artery shunts	Laparoscopy / cystoscopy
Acquired valvular heart diseases	Urethral dilatation or catheterization
Mitral valve prolapse with mitral regurgitation	Cardiac surgery
Hypertrophic cardiomyopathy	Incision and drainage of infected tissue
	Presence of indwelling devices including long lines

Infective agents
1. Streptococci – Alfa hemolytic (Strep Viridans – most common), Enterococci
2. Staphylococci – Staph aureus, coagulase negative Staph
3. Gram negative agents – HACEK group
4. Fungi – Candida species

Clinical recognition
Onset is usually insidious with fever, fatigue, loss of appetite and pallor. Acute endocarditis with Staph aureus or post-operative endocarditis with coagulase negative Staph or fungi can have an acute onset with high fever and heart failure. Other symptoms may include chest pain, palpitation, joint pains and hematuria or other thrombo-embolic episodes.
High-grade fever and new or changing cardiac murmur are two hallmarks of endocarditis.
Splenomegaly is common. Skin changes include petechiae on skin and mucosa, splinter hemorrhages, Osler's nodes, and Janeway lesions. Embolic phenomenon to other organs like kidney and brain are present is almost 50% of patients. Clubbing of fingers can develop as fast as 2 weeks. Signs of heart failure may appear, and murmurs of mitral regurgitation or aortic regurgitation may mark involvement of these valves.

Lab investigations
Positive blood cultures form the gold standard for microbiologic diagnosis. Repeated blood samples, at least three, taken at intervals of half to 2 hours apart especially at the peak of febrile episodes are recommended to maximize positive yield. Bacteria may be

recovered from skin lesions if scraped and examined under the microscope. Full blood count shows anemia, polymorph leucocytosis with shift to left. C-Reactive proteins and ESR are elevated. Microscopic hematuria is present in 30% cases.

Chest X-ray may show cardiomegaly, and ECG points to any predisposing heart disease. Echocardiography and Doppler studies may demonstrate vegetations, and/or evidence of mitral/aortic regurgitation. This also serves to assess cardiac function and diagnose underlying heart disease.

Management

Management involves stabilization of the patient, confirmation of the diagnosis and parent counseling. High doses of intravenous antibiotics form the mainstay of therapy. Initial therapy may be started with a combination of penicillin and Gentamycin, and Cloxacillin may replace penicillin if Staph. Infection is suspected. Vancomycin may be required as the initial antibiotic in the presence of indwelling devices. Once culture results are available antibiotics may required to be changed as per the sensitivity. Therapy is to be continued for 4-6 weeks.

With control of infection or when infection fails to come under control despite appropriate antibiotics, surgical intervention may have to be considered on an urgent basis.

Complications

Heart failure, aortic ring abscess, renal failure, cerebrovascular accidents, peripheral gangrene, bowel ischemia and complications of therapy.

Prognosis and counseling

Varies with the underlying disease and causative agent. Prognosis is guarded, as the infection may remain uncontrolled despite antibiotics, and complications may leave long-term sequelae.

Prevention

Appropriate guidelines for antibiotic cover should be followed while performing at risk procedures in patients who are prone to develop endocarditis (see table).

Procedure	Antibiotic prophylaxis
Dental, oral, respiratory or esophageal procedure	Amoxycillin 50 mg/Kg PO 1 hour before or IV 30 minutes before procedure
In patient allergic to penicillin	Clindamycin 10 mg/Kg PO 1 hour before procedure OR Vancomycin 20 mg/Kg infusion over 10 min given 15 minutes before procedure
Genito-urinary or gastrointestinal (except esophageal) procedure	Amoxycillin 50 mg/Kg, PO 1 hour before procedure OR IV 30 minutes before
In high risk patients	Amoxycillin 50 mg/kg iv before procedure, repeat 25 mg/kg 6 hrs later PLUS Gentamycin 2 mg/kg iv before procedure
In patients high risk and allergic to penicillin	Vancomycin 20 mg/kg infusion over 1 hr ending 15 min before procedure PLUS Gentamycin 2 mg/kg iv before procedure

9.5 Cardiomyopathies in children

Definition:
Cardiomyopathies are the cardiac muscle disorders of uncertain aetiology leading to myocardial structural and functional defect.

Classification:
    A.   **Dilated**
    B.   **Hypertrophic**
    C.   **Restrictive cardiomyopathy**

Dilated cardiomyopathy is the most common type seen in Oman.

A. Idiopathic dilated cardiomyopathy:

This refers to congestive cardiac failure secondary to dilatation and poor function of the ventricles (predominantly left side) in the absence of an identifiable underlying disease. IDCM is the most common type of heart muscle disease in children. The diagnosis is reached after excluding secondary causes of myocardial disease as listed in table

Secondary causes	Examples
Infections	Coxsackievirus B, Adenovirus, HIV, echovirus, rubella, varicella, mumps, E B virus
Congenital heart diseases	Anomalous left coronary artery from pulmonary artery
Neuromuscular diseases	Duchenne muscular dystrophy, Friedreich ataxia
Hematological disorders	Thalassemia, sickle cell disease
Metabolic disorders	Glycogen storage diseases, Carnitine deficiency, Fatty acid oxidation defects, Mucopolysaccharidoses
Collagen vascular diseases	Rheumatic fever, SLE, Kawasaki disease
Drugs and medications	Anthracycline, cyclophosphamide, chloroquine, iron overload
Endocrine diseases	Hypo or hyper-thyroidism, hypo-parathyroidism
Nutritional disorders	Kwashiorkor, pellagra, thiamine or selenium deficiency

Clinical recognition:

Symptoms:
- Presenting features are those of unexplained heart failure, often precipitated by LRTI.
- Older children may present with chest pain, chest discomfort, palpitation, orthopnea, abdominal pain or syncope.
- Occasionally infective endocarditis, neurologic deficit, cardiac arrhythmia or cardiomegaly detected on a chest radiograph leads to the diagnosis.
- History of a preceding viral illness is found in about half and a positive family history in about 10-25% patients.

Signs:
- Infants demonstrate failure to thrive, tachypnea, tachycardia and hepatomegaly. Weak peripheral pulses and cold extremities are common findings.
- Older children show edema, elevated JVP and fine crepitations in the lung bases.
- Precordium is generally quiet. Careful palpation of the cardiac apex shows it to be displaced downward and outward indicating significant cardiomegaly. Auscultation reveals gallop rhythm (S3/S4), loud P2 and systolic murmurs of mitral and tricuspid regurgitation.

Lab investigations
- Chest X-ray shows cardiomegaly, and pulmonary edema
- ECG reveals LVH with strain pattern
- Echocardiography and Doppler studies serve to make the diagnosis and exclude congenital heart diseases. Shows dilated LA/LV with varying degrees of mitral regurgitation, tricuspid regurgitation and pulmonary hypertension.
- Acute management may require other investigations like full blood counts, C-reactive proteins, electrolyte profile, renal functions and liver functions.

Differential diagnosis
- Viral myocarditis: usually acute onset, elevated myocardial enzymes and positive viral titres.
- Anomalous left coronary artery from pulmonary artery: Carefully performed echocardiography and cardiac catheter studies and angiography in doubtful cases.
- Other types of congenital heart disease: echocardiogram helps to identify these.
- Systemic Carnitine deficiency: Diagnosed by Tandem MS

Management
Management is essentially similar to that of heart failure (CCF) using a combination of diuretics, angiotensin converting enzyme inhibitors (ACEI) and Digoxin. Use of additional diuretics, intravenous Frusemide, Dobutamine infusion and β-adrenergic receptor blockers help to improve quality of life in resistant patients. Management of end stage CCF is cardiac transplant.

Complications
- Intercurrent infections
- Worsening heart failure despite initial control
- Thrombo-embolic events
- Cardiac arrhythmia and Infective endocarditis

Prognosis and counseling
In general, approximately one third of patients die, one third continue to have chronic heart failure requiring therapy, and one-third experience improvement in their condition. Recent studies have reported 85% survival at 5 years. Causes of death include worsening heart failure, intercurrent infections and ventricular fibrillation.

B. Hypertrophic cardiomyopathy:

The hallmark of the disorder is myocardial hypertrophy of the left ventricle (LV) especially involving the interventricular septum, resulting in obstruction of the LV outflow tract.

Etiology:

The disease is transmitted as **autosomal dominant**, and positive family history of sudden death often initiates investigations that lead to the diagnosis. May be associated with maternal diabetes mellitus. Echocardiogram usually shows hypertrophy of the ventricular septum, and sometimes the hypertrophy is severe enough to cause obstruction to left ventricular outflow tract. Majority of babies do not require any specific therapy, and it resolves by itself.

Clinical presentation

- Recognized as a **cause of sudden death in pre-adolescents and adolescents** due to sudden left ventricular outflow obstruction and cardiac arrhythmias.
- Dyspnea on exertion, syncope, angina, dizziness, palpitations and frank heart failure.
- Physical findings may include cardiomegaly, double cardiac apical impulse, third/ fourth heart sounds and murmurs of mitral and/or aortic regurgitation.

Investigations:

- ECG shows ST-T wave changes and LV hypertrophy +/- Cardiac arrhythmias.
- Echocardiography confirms the LV hypertrophy, measures any obstruction to LV outflow, and excludes other forms of heart disease.

Treatment:

- Options include Bea-blockers and in later stages diuretics. Surgical resection of obstructing muscle bundles and implantable cardioverter defibrillators are used in selected patients.

Hematological System

10.1 Anemia in children

Definition:

Decrease in hemoglobin concentration and RBC mass compared with the values in age-matched controls. Anemia occurs for different reasons:

- Decreased production of red blood cells
- Increased Destruction of red blood cells
- Increased blood loss from the body

1. Iron Deficiency Anemia

Most frequently encountered anemia in children. In developing countries it is the most common nutritional problem, affecting about 50 – 90% of children. In Oman its overall prevalence is coming down with the ongoing socio-economic improvement.

Stages of iron deficiency:

Children have 55 mg/kg of iron in the body. 70% of iron is in the form of Hb, 26% is in stores and about 4% is in myoglobin and other iron containing enzymes. Iron balance in the body is achieved mainly by control of absorption of iron rather than its excretion. Most of the iron is re-cycled in the body. The iron deficiency anemia develops in progressive stages:

1. Pre iron deficiency: At this stage the only abnormalities are decreased iron stores and increased iron absorption from the gastrointestinal tract. It is characterized by reduced serum ferritin, reduced iron concentration in the marrow and liver tissue. Hemoglobin, serum iron, total iron binding capacity (TIBC) are still within normal limits.

2. Latent iron deficiency: In this stage, in addition to already reduced iron stores (decreased serum ferritin), serum iron and transferrin saturation also become low with increased total iron binding capacity. However hemoglobin level is still normal

3. Overt iron deficiency anemia: By now the production of erythroid cells in the marrow is impaired resulting in drop in hemoglobin level and development of progressive microcytic, hypochromic anemia. Thus, Hb, MCV, MCH & MCHC are reduced, in addition to already decreased serum iron and increased TIBC and decreased transferrin saturation. Transferrin saturation below 12-16% is diagnostic of iron deficiency state.

Causes of Iron deficiency:

a) **Inadequate intake-** Reduced dietary intake & poor bio-availability is the most common cause. In Oman toddlers are highly vulnerable for IDA due to poor dietary habits in children relying mostly on packet of crisp and sugar based flavored drinks ("Sun Top")

b) **Decreased absorption** e.g.: malabsorption due to chronic diarrhea, malabsorption syndromes, milk allergy leading to GI Bleed, sprue, partial or total gastrectomy and rarely genetically determined absorptive defect.

c) **Increased requirement**: as seen in premature babies during first few months of rapid growth and later during adolescence

d) **Chronic blood loss** - Often these bleeds are occult and unsuspected e.g. Hookworm infestation, occult GI. bleeding as in cow milk intolerance or allergy, Meckel's diverticulum etc.

Clinical features:

Age: Biphasic, between 6 months - 3 years and 11 – 17 years

Features due to anemia: In mild anemia there may be no signs and symptoms. In severe deficiency fatigue, breathlessness, irritability, anorexia, may be seen. Spleen may be enlarged slightly.

Changes in Epithelial cells: These include koilonychia, platyonychia, angular stomatitis, atrophic glossitis

Growth retardation

Exercise intolerance

Behavioral changes, reduced attention span, irritability, and poor school performance

Altered host response: IDA affects both cell mediated as well as humoral immunity

Pica is a well documented symptom but unexplainable. It is a habitual ingestion of unusual substances, the most common of which is eating mud or clay (Geophagia), laundry starch (amylophagia) and ice (pagophagia). Pica usually is the manifestation of iron deficiency and is relieved when condition is treated.

Investigations:

Red cell count, hemoglobin and hematocrit are all decreased in IDA.
Red cell indices like MCV, MCH, MCHC & are also decreased but
RDW is increased (i.e. most red cell population is of different size, this is in contrast to thalassemia trait in which RDW is low).
The peripheral blood film shows hypochromic, microcytic red cells. Reticulocyte may be normal or decreased.
Thrombocytosis may be seen
Serum Ferritin is less than 10-12 ng/ml, Serum iron is reduced to < 6, TIBC is increased and Transferrin saturation is low.
Bone marrow aspiration is not routinely indicated. Prussian blue staining for iron particles revealing little or no stainable iron is diagnostic.

Management:

Successful treatment depends on Replenishment of reduced body iron & Correction of underlying factors. In 80-85% of patients, it is possible to determine the cause.

Oral Iron therapy: Ferrous salts are absorbed better than ferric salts and **Ferrous Sulphate** is the cheapest preparation. The dose is 4-6 mg/kg/day of elemental iron given for 3 months after Hb returns to normal so as to also replenish the stores. Dose is given in between meals (empty stomach) because cereals and milk retard absorption, it is conveniently given with orange juice as acidic media and vitamin C increase the absorption. A positive response to treatment can be confirmed by developing reticulocytosis within 3 to 5 days of initiation of treatment, reaching a peak at 7-10 days Side effects are probably related to dose and amount of elemental iron. They include gastrointestinal symptoms - heart burn, nausea, abdominal cramps, diarrhea, constipation, blackish discoloration of tongue and teeth (avoided by brushing or rinsing teeth after the dose).

Nutritional Strategies:

A detailed assessment of patients' diet and appropriate counseling, keeping in mind the bioavailability of the food iron is essential. A protein rich balanced diet is advised. The best dietary sources of iron are the foods containing "heme" iron e.g. meat and fish as it is easily absorbed and used by the body (12 - 20% bioavailability). Iron is also found in green vegetables, staple grains, cereals and legumes, but the absorption of this form -- "non-heme" iron -- is highly variable (1 to 7%). Eating a vitamin C-rich food enhances iron absorption, whereas tea, coffee, egg yolk and bran can inhibit absorption of non-heme iron.

Iron containing Foods:

Red Meat, Organ meat, Fish & Seafood, Pulses & Legumes, Soya bean, Green Leafy vegetables e.g. Spinach, Nuts, oil seeds and Dates etc.

Community measures such as Food fortification, health education and **timely introduction of weaning food thus avoiding prolonged milk feeds.** Fortification of milk formula with iron

2. Sickle Cell Disease

Background:

Sickle cell disease is an Autosomal recessive disorder of hemoglobin synthesis. The polymerization of deoxy HbS molecules causes sickling of RBCs and chronic hemolytic anemia and vaso-occlusive phenomenon. Sickle cells produce thrombosis and obstruction in small vessels, leading to ischemia and necrosis of distal tissue

Pathophysiology:

Sickle hemoglobin results from a single amino acid substitution (valine for glutamate) in position 6 of the beta-globin chain of hemoglobin. The polymerization of deoxy HbS molecules causes a chronic hemolytic anemia and vaso-occlusive phenomenon. When patient is homozygous for Hb S (Hb SS) it is called Sickle cell Anemia. Even double heterozygotes, where Hemoglobin S exist with one other abnormal hemoglobin (e.g. B Thal, C, D E etc.), this behave in a similar fashion and grouped under Sickle cell disease syndromes.

Frequency:

In Oman: According to Genetic Blood disorders survey prevalence rates for the sickle-cell trait was estimated to be 6% and of sickle cell homozygous was 0.2%.
Internationally: Sickle disease occurs in about 0.15% of African American newborns. The disease is also prevalent in GCC states, parts of India, Middle East, and Mediterranean region

Diagnosis:

Newborn screening for sickle hemoglobinopathies is mandatory in the tertiary care centers of Oman (SQUH). Screening of high risk newborns (+ve F/H etc.) is done in other centers. Specific diagnosis is confirmed with hemoglobin electrophoresis performed in specialized reference laboratories. Apart from low Hb, reticulocyte count is usually elevated. These values may vary depending on the extent of baseline hemolysis. The peripheral smear will show sickle cells

Clinical features:

The clinical course of sickle cell disease is one of chronic illness precipitated by multiple acute exacerbations that can become life threatening at any time. Generally, child becomes symptomatic from 6 months of age as the level of Hb F drops and the Hb S level rises. The spectrum of clinical disease varies from a severe to a mild course.

1. Vaso-occlusive crisis:

A painful crisis is the most frequent clinical symptom of sickle cell disease. In infants, painful symmetrical swelling of the hands and feet (dactylitis or hand-foot syndrome) caused by infarctions of the small bones may be the initial manifestation of the disease. Most bony vaso-occlusive events occur primarily in the bone marrow cavity, they are multifocal and associated with mild tenderness and localized edema. As the child matures, the painful episodes usually affect the long bones, hips and knees, chest wall and back. Abdominal pain often occurs as excruciating pain with diffuse tenderness, distension, and muscular rigidity of the abdominal wall and may mimic an Acute Abdomen.

2. Splenic Sequestration:

This crisis is a distinct form of acute Hypersplenism, most commonly seen in young children. It may be associated with pain abdomen, sudden onset of pallor and hypotension

3. Acute Chest Syndrome (ACS):

Is more common in older children and presents as chest pain, cough, dyspnea, or tachypnea and sudden desaturation. The etiology may be infectious (e.g., pneumonia), vaso-occlusive, or both. This syndrome often results in hypoxia and, occasionally, death

4. Cerebro Vascular Accidents (CVA):

Occlusion occurs in large or small cerebral vessels. A neurologic event may occur. Patients may develop hemipareses, gait disturbances, paresthesias, aphasia, altered consciousness, or seizures. MRI findings or high flow on transcranial Doppler sonography of silent lesions are associated with a high risk of stroke

5. Hyper hemolysis: It is more common with associated G6PD deficiency.

6. Priapism: Prolonged, acute, and painful erection due to venous occlusion.

7. Aplastic Crisis: is secondary to infection by the parvovirus B19.

8. Other problems:
Susceptibility to infection with encapsulated organisms especially Pneumococcus and salmonella due to failure of opsonisation function of spleen
Growth retardation, avascular necrosis of femoral head is seen in some cases.
Patients with **sickle trait** have erythrocytes that contain only 30-40% HbS. Heterozygosity for the sickle gene has a benign clinical course. Sickling does not occur under physiologic conditions

Factors precipitating Sickling process:

Hypoxia, Dehydration, Hypertonicity of plasma, Acidosis, Infection, Exposure to cold, Fatigue and Psychosocial stress

Management:

1) **Hydration** should be administered to meet maintenance needs, as well as correct preexisting deficits. Administer intravenous (IV) isotonic sodium chloride solution at a rate of 1-1.5 times the maintenance rate if oral hydration cannot be sustained. In older children IVF of more than maintenance should be given with caution.
2) **Aggressive pain management** with Morphine, Pethidine in addition to standard NSAIDs
3) **CVA:** Patients with suspected stroke require immediate exchange transfusion sufficient to decrease the percent of sickle hemoglobin to less than approximately 25-30%. Long-term transfusion therapy is required to prevent recurrent strokes.
4) **Priapism** is treated with analgesia, hydration, and transfusion therapy sufficient to decrease the sickle hemoglobin level to less than 30%. Surgical evacuation may be needed in rare instances
5) **Acute Chest Syndrome** requires immediate exchange transfusion, antibiotics and supportive care.
Top up PRBC transfusion is given to manage **splenic sequestration, Hyperhemolytic crisis & aplastic crisis** followed by serial CBCs.

Further outpatient care:
All SCD children should be managed under a Comprehensive clinical care program (CCCP). **Pneumo coccal Vaccine, Penicillin prophylaxis** for encapsulated organisms, **folic acid** and therapy with **Hydroxyurea** in selected cases is instituted. **Counseling** of parents and teachers in addition to **pre marital screening** should never be forgotten

3. Thalassemia - Major

Thalassemia is an inherited disorder of hemoglobin synthesis arising from a defect in the globin chain production. In normal adult hemoglobin (Hb A) 2 alpha & 2 beta globin chains exist at a ratio of 1:1. Due to defective production of one type of chain an excess of the other normally produced type accumulates in the red cell as an unstable product, leading to the destruction of the cell. When B chains production is affected it is called B thalassemia and when alpha chains are involved it is termed as Alpha thalassemia. B Thalassemia major (homozygous) is the commonest of Thalassemia syndromes.

Frequency:

In Oman, the prevalence of beta-thalassemia trait is 2 per cent and homozygous beta-thalassemia 0.07 per cent.

Beta thalassemia has a significant presence in Mediterranean countries such as Greece, Italy and Spain, in North Africa, Gulf countries, the Middle East, India and Eastern Europe. It is getting more common in UK & USA due to the increasing immigrant population.

Clinical features:

Symptoms of anemia start in infancy when the gamma chain production is switched off and the beta chains fail to form in adequate numbers. Manifestations of anemia include extreme pallor and enlarged abdomen due to Hepato splenomegaly. The findings vary widely, depending on how well the disease is controlled. Inadequate management results in massive splenomegaly, bone deformities (frontal bossing, prominent facial bones), growth retardation and peculiar facies and 80% of them may die within the first 5 years of life. Patients may also develop diabetes, thyroid disorder, or other endocrine involvement. These stigmata are typically not observed in patients who are optimally treated and any complication they develop is usually due to adverse effects of the treatment (transfusion or chelation).

Diagnosis:

- Blood film- peripheral blood film reveals severe hypochromia and microcytosis, marked anisocytosis, fragmented RBCs, polychromasia, and nucleated RBCs.
- Hemoglobin electrophoresis shows an elevated Hb F level. In beta-0 thalassemia, only Hb A_2 and Hb F are found, no Hb A is detected; while in beta + pts small amount of Hb A is present.
- X-Ray: Bony changes may be severe, resulting in osteopenia and a characteristic radiologic picture of skull x ray (hair on end appearance).

Management:

1. Blood transfusion:

To maintain a pre transfusion Hb level of 9-9.5 g/dl at all times.

Transfused blood should always be leukocyte poor; 10-15 mL/kg, PRBC at the rate of 5 mL/kg/h every 3-5 weeks is usually adequate to maintain the pre-transfusion Hb level needed. A pre-transfusion workup should include RBC phenotype, hepatitis B vaccination and hepatitis profile.

Iron overload: Large amounts of iron with each blood transfusion and excessive iron absorbed from the GI tract are responsible for this condition. Tissue toxicity in iron overload is due to peroxidation of cell membrane and is probably the major cause of organ damage. Serum ferritin level is usually helpful in detecting iron overload because Ferritin correlates well with total body iron burden.

2. Chelation therapy:

The introduction of agents capable of removing excessive iron from the body has dramatically increased life expectancy. **Deferoxamine** (DFO Desferral), a complex hydroxylamine with high affinity for iron is administered as 8-12 hrs subcutaneous infusion in a dose of 30-40 mg/kg/d for 5 d/wk by a mechanical pump. The aim is to achieve a negative iron balance (i.e. excreting more iron than acquired from both intestinal absorption and transfusion). The optimal time to initiate chelation therapy is dictated by the amount of accumulated iron, this usually occurs after 1-2 years of starting the transfusion regimen. **IV Desferral** is given as continuous infusion as an adjuvant to SC Desferral in cases of increased iron overload.

Oral Chelation with Deferiprone was tried but is not practical due to toxicity and less than optimal chelation. It is now being used as an adjuvant to SC chelation in selected cases. A New oral drug **IL 670** has recently been introduced but is still not in regular usedue to its prohibitive cost.

Complications of chelation therapy include local reactions, hearing deficit and other Neurosensory deficits and occasionally slowing of growth.

3) Stem cell transplant may be curative in selected cases
4) Counseling of high-risk families and community awareness for pre marital screening

4. G6PD Deficiency

The Glucose 6 Phosphate Dehydrogenase (G6PD) enzyme deficiency was detected in about 27% of Omani males compared with 11% of females. It is an X-linked recessive.
Diagnosis: By cord blood sampling or when suspected by a screening tests done on peripheral blood

Clinical features:
> Chronic hemolysis causing mild anemia with slightly raised reticulocyte count.
> Neo-natal Hyperbilirubinemia: The most serious clinical complication.
> Acute hemolytic crisis: In the most frequent variants of this disease hemolysis occurs during stress, imposed for example by infection, "oxidative" drugs or after ingestion of fava beans or Henna application leading to acute hemoglobinuria (Cola urine) and acute anemia.

Treatment:
> Top up PRBC transfusion followed by folic acid during the acute phase.
> Education for patient and health professionals' on avoiding the agents known to trigger acute hemolysis.
> Distribution of cards to patients with a list of incriminating agents should be supplied to the patient as warning to prescribing doctors.

10.2 Leukemia in children

Acute Leukemia represents a clonal expansion of blast cells and arrest at a specific stage of normal myeloid or lymphoid hematopoiesis. It is the commonest childhood malignancy accounting for one third of all childhood malignancies.

Clinical classification:
1. Acute Lymphocytic Leukemia (ALL) 75-80%
2. Acute Myeloid Leukemia (AML), also known as Acute Non-Lymphocytic Leukemia (ANLL) 15-20%
3. Acute Undifferentiated Leukemia (AUL) <0.5%
4. Acute Mixed Lineage Leukemia (AMLL) V. rare

Acute Leukemia: constitute 97% of all childhood leukemia

Chronic Leukemia constitute only <5% of childhood leukemia and is of two types:
1. Philadelphia Chromosome Positive (Ph[1] positive)
2. Juvenile Chronic Myelogenous Leukemia (JCML)
   (Note: CLL does not exist in childhood)

Annual Incidence:
25 new cases per million population of <13 years age
Peak incidence between 2 and 5 years of age

Etiology: Unknown. Following risk factors may be associated:

1. Ionizing Radiation
2. Chemicals (e.g.: Benzene, Heavy Metals, Pesticides, Petroleum distillates) in AML
3. Drugs: Alkylating Agents in combination with radiotherapy increases risk of AML (2nd tumor effect)
4. Genetic factors:
   - Identical twins: 20% risk if one twin develops it during the first 5 years of life
   - Incidence of leukemia in siblings is four times greater than general population
   - Down syndrome
   - Chromosomal breakage or defective DNA repair (e.g.: Fanconi's Anemia, Ataxia Telangiectasia)
   - Immunodeficiency Syndromes (e.g.: Wiskott-Aldrich)

Assessment of a Child with Suspected Leukemia (See Algorithm)

Clinical Manifestations:

1. **Central nervous system (CNS):**
   Occurs in < 5% of children with ALL at initial diagnosis. In some cases this may be the presenting feature.

2. **Leukemic Involvement of the Testis:**
    Usually presents with painless enlargement of the testis
    Occurs in up to 1/3 of boys during the course of the disease
    Risk factors for the development of testicular involvement
    - T-Cell ALL type
    - High Leukocytosis at diagnosis (>20,000/mm^3)
    - ↑Tumor burden

3. **Ovarian Involvement:** Ovarian Involvement occurs less commonly.

4. **Priapism:** Occurs rarely.

5. **Renal Involvement**
    Appreciated in many patients by ultrasonography
    Occasionally may present with hematuria, hypertension and renal failure

6. **Gastrointestinal Involvement**
    Occurs frequently in ALL
    The most common manifestation is bleeding
    Usually clinically silent until terminal stages when necrotizing enteropathy might occur. The most common site for this is the caecum, leading to a syndrome known as 'Typhlitis'

7. **Bone and Joint Involvement**
    Bone pain is one of the initial symptoms in 20% of patients. It may result from direct leukemic infiltration of the periosteum, bone infarction or expansion of marrow cavity by leukemic cells.
    Radiologic Changes Seen Most Frequently Include
    - Osteolytic lesions involving medullary cavity and cortex
    - Transverse metaphyseal radiolucent bands
    - Transverse metaphyseal lines of increased density (growth arrest lines)
    - Subperiosteal new bone formation

8. **Other Organs:** May become involved because of leukemic infiltrates or hemorrhage.

Poor Prognostic factors in ALL:
- WBC >50 x 10^9/L
- Age < 2 or >9 years
- Male sex
- Presence of Philadelphia chromosome
- Hypodiploidy in blast cells
- Presence of CNS disease
- Late responders to steroid therapy

Acute Lymphoblastic Leukemia

Classification: (FAB classification)
Based on cell size, shape and nuclear chromatin/nucleoli into L1, L2 and L3 types. It is further classified by the cell membrane antigens from a panel of antibodies (Flow cytometry) into:
- Early Precursor B
- Precursor B
- Mature B cell
- T cells ALL.

Treatment:

A: Treatment phases

    1.   Induction of remission

    2.   Consolidations or intensification

    3.   CNS prophylaxis

    4.   Maintenance (2 drugs for 3 years) plus reinforcement therapy monthly

B: Supportive Care:

    1.   Emotional support for the patient and family throughout

    2.   Control of bleeding and anemia by platelet transfusion and packed red cells

    3.   Combating side effects of chemotherapeutic drugs

    4.   Good nutrition and hygiene

    5.   Prophylactic Co-Trimoxazole to prevent pneumocystis carinii infections

Treatment course usually lasts for 3 years in boys & 2 years in girls

Bone Marrow Transplant is selected for individual cases (High Risk category)

5-year survival rates in standard risk ALL is now about 80%

Mature B cell ALL cases are treated with short-term intensive chemotherapy.

Acute Myelocytic Leukemia

- Is divided into 7 sub-types depending on morphology and immuno-phenotype characteristics
- Chromosomal abnormalities occur at least 80% of cases
- Treatment is more intensive but shorter than ALL
- 5 year survival rates are now $\geq$ 50 %
- BMT is required in relapsed or high-risk sub-types

Side Effects of Chemotherapy are:

- Mucositis
- Hair Loss (Temporary)   } **General**
- Febrile Neutropenia

- Tumor lysis syndrome
- Bleeding due to ↓platelets or deranged coagulation
- Neuropathy (Vincristine)
- Cardiomyopathy (Anthracyclines)   } **Specific Agents**
- Hyperglycemia (L-Asparaginase)

Late Effects of Therapy:

- Majority of children who complete treatment lead a normal life
- Depends on the intensity of treatment regimen
- Most are mainly due to irradiation e.g.
  - Slow growth& short stature
  - Delayed puberty & occasionally loss of fertility
  - Lower IQ
  - Increased risk of secondary neoplasm

Main Causes of Death in leukemia:

- Infections, •Hemorrhage, •Infiltration of Vital Organs •Relapse

Risk for relapse is greatest in the 1ˢᵗ year post therapy and falls progressively

ALGORITHM FOR THE ASSESSMENT OF A CHILD WITH SUSPECTED LEUKEMIA

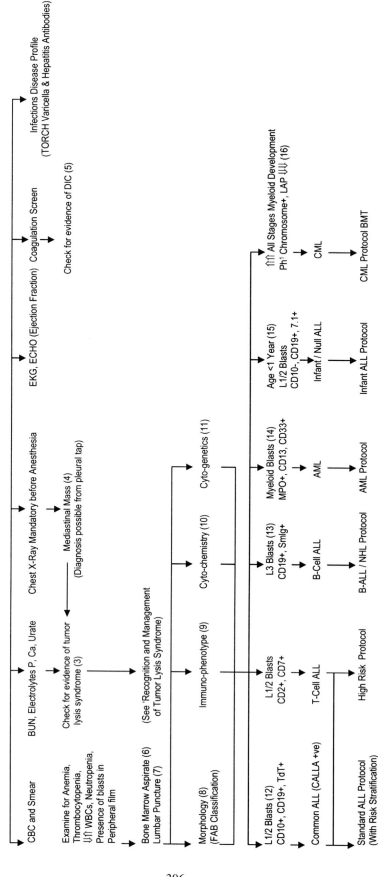

History (1) – Anemia, Bruising, Bleeding, Fever, Infection, Bone Pain, Limping

Examination (2) – Pallor, Lymphadenopathy (especially supraclavicular and other non-cervical and/or large, non-tender glands), Bruising, Petechiae, Hepatosplenomegaly

For the numbers in bracket, please follow the legends to algorithm on next page:

Legend to Algorithm
(Please refer to the numbers shown in the algorithm)

1. Among children with ALL at the time of diagnosis, approximately 60% have fever, 50% have bleeding, 40% pallor and over 20% have bone pain or limp. The symptoms are similar in children with AML although the proportion affected is somewhat less.

2. Bulky non-tender lymph nodes ± splenomegaly in an afebrile child are highly suggestive of a malignant process. Supra-clavicular adenopathy is especially concerning.

3. Recognition and management of tumor lysis syndrome is important.

4. Refer for the differential diagnosis of mediastinal mass. The presence of an anterior mediastinal mass in a child with suspected leukemia is almost always associated with the presence of a T-Cell ALL or non-Hodgkin's Lymphoma. Mediastinal masses can be a medical emergency. General anesthetic and sedation should be avoided as the muscle relaxation on the operating table allows the mass to fall posteriorly and compress the trachea deep within the mediastinum beyond the reach of a standard endotracheal tube. Often such cases are associated with pleural and/or pericardial effusion; a simple aspirate of the effusion usually yields adequate cells to allow a diagnosis to be reached and often enough to set up cytogenetic cultures. However, it is still important to perform a bone marrow aspirate to establish the degree of infiltration as soon as possible and certainly within 3 days of starting chemotherapy. Less than 20% blasts within the bone marrow would generally be called T-Cell non-Hodgkin's Lymphoma that has slightly better prognosis requiring less aggressive treatment.

5. Most common with acute promyelocytic leukemia (M3). Also found in monocytic leukemias and to a lesser extent in other subtype of leukemia. Partial Thromboplastin Time (PTT) and Prothrombin Time (PT) tests should be performed as a minimum coagulation screen.

6. Even if the diagnosis of leukemia is not obvious at this stage, it is usual to aspirate sufficient marrow to allow all listed investigations to be performed. Occasionally, the marrow can be fibrotic and aspiration alone is insufficient; a trephine bone marrow biopsy then becomes essential. Leukemia is suspected when Bone Marrow contains >5% Blasts

7. If the diagnosis is clearly ALL on the blood film, then it is usual to give the first intra-thecal chemotherapy at this juncture (assuming the coagulation screen is normal or has been corrected according to institutional guidelines). However, a clean tap must be obtained first as the presence of CNS blasts at diagnosis may infer a worse prognosis.

8. The FAB (French, American, British) classification is based on morphology.

9. Most laboratories have large standard panels of antibodies for Flowcytometry that are performed in a designated order (according to morphology); only the characteristic antigens have been shown in the above algorithm. Terminology assigns a CD (cluster

differentiation) number to identify most antigens. Flowcytometry has become a very powerful tool and enables the leukemic subtype to be confirmed within a few hours of the bone marrow aspirate. The most specific markers are noted in bolded text.

10. Cytochemistry has been replaced by Flowcytometry in the majority of laboratories, but can be useful in difficult cases when it is hard to separate ALL from AML.

11. Chromosomal translocations are the most significant prognostic factor in AML. In ALL, translocations are less frequent and often of adverse prognostic significance t (4; 11), t (9; 22). However, standard G-Banding (Karyotype) techniques can determine the number of chromosomes at mitotic metaphor stage (Hyperdiploidy, Pseudodiploidy, Diploidy and Hypoploidy) but as they produce results after 14 days they cannot be used in the initial assessment. It is quicker to perform the interphase advanced molecular cytogenetics (FISH) that compliments conventional molecular tests (PCR) to identify specific translocations.

12. Morphologically (FAB classification), a homogeneous population of cells with a very high nuclear/cytoplasmic ratio and the absence of prominent nucleoli typify L1 morphology. L2 cells have more pale blue cytoplasm and nucleoli. Distinction between the two is not of prognostic significance, but they must be separated from L3 blasts. L3 blasts signify a different disease, which needs different treatment and responds poorly with standard ALL therapy.

13. L3 blasts are striking for their deep blue vacuolated cytoplasm. However, care still needs to be applied, as not all cases are as obvious as those in hematological atlases.

Their immunophenotypes is characterized by the presence of immunoglobulin on the cell surface, signifying a more mature cell of origin than that of common ALL; risk of tumor lysis syndrome is very high.

14. Myeloid blasts are typically larger and have more cytoplasm. Often the presence of myeloperoxidase positive granules or Auer rods confirms their lineage. However, it is not always possible to separate L2 ALL from AML and it is on this occasion where Cytochemistry and extensive immunophenotyping become invaluable.

15. Infant ALL is characterized by the presence of 11q 23 chromosomal translocations and a much worse prognosis than childhood ALL. The '7.1' antibody recognizes a surface antigen, which is only expressed by cells carrying 11q 23 translocation. An accurate same-day diagnosis can thus be achieved. This is important for the child in the second year of life, as there is increasing evidence that those children without 11q23 have better prognosis and do not need the aggressive and dangerous infant chemotherapy.

16. CML is usually easily diagnosed. WBC averages 250,000 and only a few blasts are noted; the platelets are ⇑ or normal. ⇑⇑⇑ Blasts only occur with conversion from chronic to blast phase. Juvenile myelo-monocytic leukemia (juvenile CML) is a rare but distinct entity, occurring at <2 years of age. It is Ph' chromosome negative and associated with elevated fetal hemoglobin.

10.3 Bone Marrow Examination

Bone marrow examination (aspiration and biopsy) is carried out to permit cytological assessment of marrow cells. Before examination, one should review the patient's medical history, physical examination, CBC and blood film reports.

Indications:
Evaluation of hematological disorders
To stage lymphoproliferative disorders
Diagnostic workup of PUO as it may reveal TB, fungal infection, malaria or typhoid,
Diagnosis of storage disease like Gaucher and Niemann pick disease.

Technique for Bone Marrow aspiration: Site: anterior or posterior iliac crest. Under aseptic conditions local anesthetic is in filtered up to periosteum. The bone marrow aspiration needle with a stylet in place is inserted and advanced by rotating clock and counter clock wise till a sudden give in resistance is noted when marrow cavity is entered stylet is then removed. Using 20 cc syringe 1-2 cc of bone marrow is aspirated.
Technique/procedure/ Bone marrow Biopsy; the patient is prepared as above. The needle is held with palm and index finger and the stylet is locked in place, once needle touches the bone stylet is removed. By using firm pressure advance it to bone marrow cavity by rotating it in clock and counter clock wise motion to cut the bone specimen, needle is then slowly pulled out After procedure several layers of Gauze pressure should be applied.

Complications; infection and bleeding, chronic pain, fracture of bone

Contra indications; Hemophilia, other coagulation disorders and local infection, Thrombocytopenia is not a contra indication for BMA and biopsy
Reporting:
Staining of slide, H&E stain for focal infiltrates, granuloma Iron stain
Low power examination: For assessment of cellularity and detection of focal lesions
Low to medium power: For megakaryocytes number, bone structure.
High power examination: For fine details of fungal (histoplasmosis) protozoal infections, leukemias, lymphomas, and megaloblastic anemia.

Cellularity:	For example normo cellular particles, smear cellular
Erythropoiesis:	Active or Inactive
Megakaryocytes:	Plentiful or Few
Granulopoiesis:	All stages of maturation should be seen
Lymphocytes:	Normal or abnormal

Other Cells: Differential on 200-500 cells

Blasts % should be   < 5%
Promyelocytes   %
Myelocytes   %
Basophils   %
Lymphocytes   %
Monocytes   %
Plasma cells   %
Erythroid precursors %
Myeloid to Elytroid ratio

10.4 Oncologic Emergencies

1. Tumor lysis syndrome

Definition: Acute tumor lysis Syndrome is a triad of:
- Hyperuricemia
- Hyperkalemia
- Hyperphosphatemia (with hypocalcemia)

This occurs as a result of the release of a large amount of the above mentioned substances from the breakdown of large number of tumor cells, following the start of treatment, at a rate that exceeds the excretory capacity of kidneys. If unrecognized, it may result in cardiac arrhythmias, renal failure, seizures, coma and even death. The condition is preventable and treatable; the mortality rate has therefore fallen from 85% to 15% in the past four decades due to advances in supportive care.
Most commonly seen in ALL and NHL.

Risk Factors
Patients with large tumor mass/load, decreased urinary flow, renal failure, pre-existing hyperuricemia, dehydration and acidic urine are at high risk of developing **TLS**.

Prevention and/or Treatment
1.	Data to Be Monitored
- Blood: Renal profile, Calcium, Magnesium, Phosphates, Uric Acid, Coagulation Profile
- Urine: Electrolytes, Crystal urea, Creatinine Clearance and GFR
- Fluid intake and output charting
- Body weight
- BP, Cardiac monitor for arrhythmias
2.	Fluid Therapy and Hydration:
- Give Normal saline 10-20 ml/kg bolus if sign of under perfusion or dehydration is present, repeat the bolus if no improvement.
- Continuous hydration 3000 ml/m^2 to maintain urine output of 3 ml/kg/hour in a child less than 9 years and 90 ml/meter square/hour in older child.
3.	Diuresis
- Start only after adequate hydration: use Mannitol 500 mg/kg I/V rapid infusion or Frusamide 1 mg/kg I/V every 4-6 hours.
4.	Anti-hyperuricemic measures
- Alkalinization with sodium bicarbonate to maintain urine pH at 6.5 to 7.5
- Allopurinol 300-500 mg/m2 per day (maximum 800 mg/day)
- Acetazolamide 150 mg/kg Q 6-8 hourly to alkalinize the urine.
- Discontinue alkalinization as soon as uric acid is normal.
- Rasburicase: new drug for hyperuricemia, it is a pure recombinant form of urate oxidase, dose 0.15mg - 0.20 mg/kg I/V QID for 5-7 days.
5.	Anti hyper viscosity measures, when WBC counts >3,000,000
- Avoid non-essential PRBC transfusion
- Do not raise Hb more than 6-8G/dl
- Exchange transfusion
- Cranial radiation to prevent intracranial hemorrhage

2. Electrolyte imbalance

Hyperphosphatemia
- Avoid IV Phosphate administration
- Aluminum Hydroxide Gel 50-150 mg/kg/day Q4-6 hourly
- Ensure urine output >3 ml/kg/hour
- Use dialysis in severe cases

Hypocalcemia
- No therapy if asymptomatic
- Symptomatic: Calcium Gluconate 50-100mg/kg I/V slow infusion under cardiac monitoring

Hyperkalemia
- Do not administer I V potassium
- Hydration, alkalinization
- Administer Rectal enema of Polystyrene sulfonate dose 1 gm/kg/dose 6-8 hourly
- If Serum Potassium rises more than 7 meq/dl use the following:
  - Calcium Gluconate 50-100mg/kg IV with cardiac monitoring
  - Insulin 0.1 unit/kg with glucose 0.5 gm/kg as continuous infusion
  - Hemodialysis

Hypercalcemia: Serum Calcium >12 mg/dl; symptoms may include nausea, vomiting, constipation, polyuria
- Hydration: Correct electrolyte imbalance
- Diuresis with normal saline 2-3-fold maintenance with Frusemide
- Bisphosphonate
- Prednisolone 1-2 mg/kg/day
- Calcitonin 0.5 -1 unit/kg/24 hour if above measures fails
- Hemodialysis or Peritoneal Dialysis

3. Syndrome of inappropriate antidiuretic hormone secretion (SIADH)

SIADH refers to levels of ADH inappropriately high for the concurrent osmolality. This leads to persistent hypo-osmolality and water intoxication.

Cause of SIADH:
>Results from stress, infection, pain, surgery, mechanical ventilation, pulmonary, CNS lesions, lymphomas and leukemias

Clinical Features:
- Oliguria • Confusion • Weight gain • Seizures • Fatigue • Coma • Lethargy

Treatment of SIADH
- Fluid restriction. Hydrate with 0.9% Nacl limited to insensible water loses 500 ml/m²/24 hours   plus ongoing losses.
- In case of severe neurological involvement seizures, coma: hydrate with Hypertonic Saline 3% 150 ml/meter square over 1 hour plus Frusemide 1 mg/kg.

4. Oncology Emergencies by Anatomic Regions

A. Thoracic Emergencies

1. Superior Vena Cava Syndrome (SVS) and Superior Mediastinal Syndrome (SMS)
In pediatrics usually SVS and SMS occur together.

Etiology
- Intrinsic Causes: Venous thrombosis following introduction of catheter
- Extrinsic Causes: NHL, Hodgkin's Lymphoma, Teratoma, Germ Cell tumors

Clinical Features
- Plethoric, swollen congested face, eyes, neck and upper extremities
- Engorgement of Collateral Vessels
- Wet Brain Syndrome: Headache, Impaired Consciousness, Visual Changes, Syncope, Stupor and Seizures
- Cough, Wheezing, Hoarseness, Stridor, Dyspnea, Chest Pain, Orthopnea (Supine position worsens the symptoms)

Diagnosis
- X-Ray or CT Chest demonstrates a mediastinal mass
- Fine Needle Biopsy

Management
- For Thrombosis: Continuous Urokinase Infusion for 24 hours may be successful.
- Heparinization 100 mg/kg I/V push then 25 units /kg/hour by continuous IV
- For Mass Lesions: Radiotherapy
  Prednisolone

2. Pleural Effusion
Causes
- Hodgkin's and Non-Hodgkin's Lymphoma
- Wilms Tumor
- Neuroblastoma
- Osteogenic Sarcoma

Clinical Features
- Dyspnea
- Cough
- Chest Pain
- Decreased Breath Sounds, Dullness to percussion

Investigations
- X-Ray Chest
- Needle aspiration of fluid
- Usually exudates, may be transudate
- Fluid to be sent for biochemistry and cytology

Treatment
- Thoracocentesis may provide temporary relief
- Local palliative therapy to prevent recurrent effusions
- Local Radiation if mediastinal mass present
- Recurrent effusions will require pleural adhesion by tetracycline, bleomycin
- Pleurectomy.

3. Cardiac Problems

Myocarditis, Cardiomyopathy

Etiology
- Drugs (Doxorubicin, Daunomycin), radiation fibrosis or post BMT

Clinical Signs and Symptoms
- Heart failure, gallop rhythm, tachycardia and arrhythmias

Investigations
> Chest Radiography: large heart, venous congestion
> ECG: T wave
> Echocardiogram: decreased ejection fraction

Management
- Digoxin • Diuretics • Inotropic Drugs

4. Pericardial effusion

Clinical Symptoms and Signs
- Chest Pain
- Cough
- Respiratory Distress
- Tachycardia

Investigations:
- X-Ray Chest: large heart, water bottle type
- ECG: low voltage, ST changes
- Echo: echo free space displaced ventricular

Management
- Diagnostic Tap
- Therapeutic tap for tamponade
- Pericardiectomy

B. Abdominal Emergencies

The incidence of severe abdominal complications in children with cancer ranges from 5-50%.

1. Esophagitis: Most common GI problem in children receiving chemotherapy.

Causes
- Prolonged NG tube intubations
- Fungal Infection (candidiasis)
- Radiotherapy, certain forms of chemotherapy

Clinical Features
- Dysphasia, epigastric pain, mild hematemesis

Complications
- Ulceration
- Stricture
- Obstruction and perforation rare, when occurs may lead to mediastinitis

Diagnosis
- Oral Examination: monilial mouth lesions frequently present
- Esophagoscopy
- X-Ray Contrast Studies

Management
- Antacids
- Antifungal Drugs
- Strictures will need specific dilatation procedures.

2. Typhlitis
- Necrotizing colitis localized in caecum in setting of severe neutropenia in ALL and post BMT patients
- *Clostridium Septicum* and *Pseudomonas Aeruginosa* are most common causative agents

Clinical Features
- Right lower quadrant pain or mass
- Peritonitis, Perforation
- Septic Shock
- Mortality ranges from 50-100% in some series

Diagnosis
- Clinical Examination: right lower mass in severe neutropenic patient
- X-Ray abdomen: erect posture, pneumatosis intestinalis or bowel wall thickening
- Ultrasound abdomen: may show bowel wall thickening in region of caecum
- CT Abdomen: diffuse thickening of cecal wall
- Barium enema: severe mucosal irregularity, rigidity and loss of colonic haustrations

Treatment
- I/V Fluids
- NPO

- NG Tube Suctioning
- Broad Spectrum Antibiotics

Indications for Surgical Intervention
- Persistent GI Bleed
- Evidence of Perforation
- Clinical deterioration, uncontrolled sepsis from bowel wall infarction
- Surgery consists of removing necrotic portions of bowel and diversions via colostomy.
- More than 80% cases of typhlitis can be successfully managed without surgery.

C. Neurological Emergencies

1. Acute Alteration in Consciousness

Causes
- Bacterial CNS infections
- CVA (infarction, hemorrhage)
- Viral encephalitis
- Leukoencephalopathy
- Metastatic disease
- Liver failure
- Sepsis
- DIC
- Metabolic, Uremia

Clinical Features
- Confusion, stupor or coma
- Tentorial herniation from raised ICP caused by displacement of brain through tentorium. Presents with acute alteration in consciousness, Cheyne Stroke breathing, small reactive pupils that later becomes unequal and unresponsive to light; decorticate, decerebrate posture.
- Uncal Herniation: More rapid than Tentorial herniation, pupils asymmetrical dilated on side of lesion, motor response asymmetrical.

Emergency Management
- ABC
- CBC, electrolytes Urea, Creatinine,
- CT brain: To look for ventricle size, midline shift, and patency of saggital sinus
- LP: if no mass lesion found
- Dextrostix
- Coagulation Profile be corrected immediately
- Mannitol 20% 0.5-2 gram/kg/dose rapid I/V bolus
- Dexamethasone 1-2 mg/kg
- Head should be elevated at 30-45 degrees slightly extended in midline
- Hyperventilation
- Antibiotics and antiviral if indicated

2. Cerebro Vascular Accident

Children with cancer are at increased risk from CVA due to
- Direct or metastatic disease
- DIC
- Meningitis
- Platelet Resistant Thrombocytopenia.

Clinical features
- Impaired motor function and speech, seizures, obtundation

Diagnosis
- CT Scan of brain when child is stable, to look for hemorrhage and infarction
- LP: must be performed after excluding any mass lesion, CSF be need be sent for biochemistry, grams stain, c/s microscopy, for cytospin and for myelin basic protein
- MR Angiography

Treatment
- Usually supportive
- DIC if present should be vigorously treated.
- Saggital sinus thrombus: requires emergency radiation to prevent herniation and death
- Surgical debunking: life saving in patients with large area of radiation induced necrosis

3. Seizures
Etiology
- Metastasis
- Metabolic abnormalities
- CVA
- Treatment related sequel after chemotherapy (incrusting, radiation)
- CNS Infections

Investigations
- Blood Chemistry, Ca, Mg, Sodium, LFT, Renal Function
- CT Brain, LP if mass lesion ruled out on CT

Treatment
- Most seizures are self-limited, if unresolved use
- Diazepam 0.1-0.3 mg/kg/dose or Lorazepam .02 mg/kg over 2 minutes, if not controlled
- Phenytoin 15-18 mg/kg bolus, may cause cardiac depression, if Phenytoin ineffective
- Phenobarbital up to 10 mg/kg I/V every 20 minutes, if not controlled
- Paraldehyde 0.3 ml/kg in equal amount of mineral oil by retention enema

4. Spinal cord compression
Incidence and Etiology
5% of children with cancer develop spinal cord compression. 50% of them are caused

by sarcoma, the remainder by lymphoma, leukemia and neuroblastoma.
Mechanism: Direct extension or metastasis of epidural space via spinal foramina.

Clinical Features
- Back pain, urinary retention, localized tenderness, motor or sensory deficit, incontinence

Evaluation
- Thorough history and neurological examination
- X-Ray Spine: in 50% epidural disease may be missed
- MRI Spine: to detect epidural involvement

Treatment
- Dexamethasone:

    Should be started immediately, prior to diagnostic studies. For progressive disease give 1-2 mg/kg/day loading dose, followed by 1-1.5 mg/kg/day divided 6 hourly. For mild problem start with 0.25-1 mg/dose 6 hourly.
- Radiotherapy

    If epidural mass identified: treatment is aimed at rapid decompression, surgical intervention and local radiation
- Specific chemotherapy in addition to Dexamethasone and radiation

10.5 Child with bleeding disorder

Bleeding in a child can present as petechiae, purpura, ecchymosis (skin), mucosal bleeding (epistaxis, GIT, genitourinary), excessive bleeding with procedures (puncture sites) as well as intracranial hemorrhage.

Many children may only present as asymptomatic incidental abnormal coagulation screen detected during routine pre-surgical coagulation screening.

Process of normal hemostasis: This occurs in 3 stages:

1. Vessel Wall (Vasoconstriction)
2. Platelets (Adherence – Aggregation – Secretion) leading to a platelet plug formation, enough to stop bleeding from minor blood vessels as capillaries. Platelet disorders (in number or function) are characterized by bleeding from the minor vessels resulting in mainly petechiae and purpura and
3. Coagulation process that is required to control major bleeds.

Coagulation   (Coagulation Cascade): Consist of three parts:
  • Intrinsic Pathway
  • Extrinsic Pathway and
  • Common Pathway
The process ends in the formation of a soft fibrin clot. Factor XIII is then needed to stabilize this clot (Fibrin Stabilizing Factor)

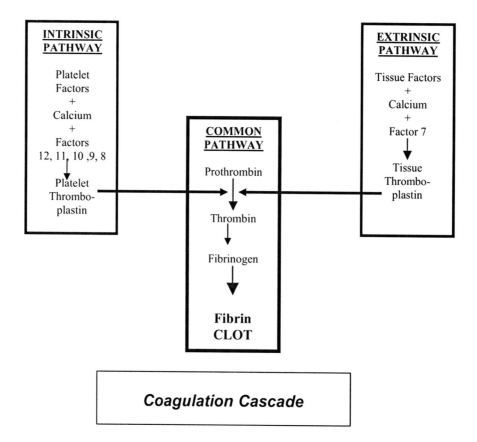

Coagulation Cascade

Clinical evaluation of a patient with bleeding disorder:

Important Points in History and Physical Examination:

- Severity and duration of Hemorrhage
- Age of onset of symptoms
- Recurrence
- Check if bleeding is mucosal in nature (consider platelet disorders)
- Frank bleeding, hematomas or hem-arthrosis suggest clotting factor deficiency.
- Nosebleeds and menorrhagia are common manifestations of V W Disease
- Family history of bleeding in males suggestive of X linked disease like Hemophilia
- A palpable purpuric rash with the typical lower extremity distribution suggest the vasculitis of Henoch-Schönlein Purpura.
- Acutely ill child with a purpuric rash suggest meningococcemia or bacterial septicemia.
- A purpuric rash that becomes necrotic suggest purpura fulminans due to viral or bacterial infection or deficiency of natural anti-coagulants (Protein C, S or Antithrombin).
- Organomegaly suggests an infiltrative process, either malignancy or storage disorder.
- A child with 1-2 weeks history of URTI followed by acute onset of skin bleed (petechiae, purpura, ecchymosis) with general well-being and no Organomegaly suggests Immune Thrombocytopenic purpura (ITP).

Key features of common childhood bleeding disorders:

1) Idiopathic Thrombocytopenic Purpura (ITP):

- Usually preceded by a history of URTI, 1-2 weeks prior to onset.
- Negative family history
- Acute onset of purpuric spots, sometimes nose or mucosal bleed, intracranial bleeding is rare (<1%)
- No Organomegaly (spleen tip may be palpable in less than 10% of cases)
- No lymphadenopathy
- 10% of the cases will have chronic course more than 6 months (in such cases rule out HIV, SLE or Lymphoma)

2) Acute Leukemia

- H/O fever, bone pains, infections

- Acute onset of skin bleeding, nosebleed or mucosal bleed
- Pallor and Hepato-splenomegaly
- Generalized Lymphadenopathy
- Other System Involvement: CNS Leukemia, Testicular Infiltrates, Joint Swelling etc.

3) Aplastic Anemia

- Preceding history of infection: Viral EBV, HBV
- H/O drug Intake (Chloramphenicol)
- Exposure to irradiation
- Exposure to toxins like Benzene
- Manifestations of BM failure include:
    - Anemia (pallor, easy fatigability, exertional dyspnea)
    - Neutropenia leading to serious bacterial or fungal infections
    - Thrombocytopenia (petechiae, purpura, ecchymosis mucosal bleed)

4) Hemophilia A or B (Factor VIII or IX Deficiency)

- X-Linked recessive inheritance
- Rarely can occur in female carriers through Lionization of the X-Chromosomes
- In all cases APTT is prolonged
- Can be classified into:
    #### i) Mild
    - Factor activity 6-30%
    - No spontaneous bleeding
    - No hemarthrosis except following significant trauma *(e.g.: post-circumcision)*
    - Bleeding episode anywhere including Intra cranial Hemorrhage

    #### ii) Moderate
    - Factor activity 1-5%
    - No spontaneous bleeding
    - Present with joint bleed after trauma

    #### iii) Severe
    - Factor activity <1%
    - Spontaneous recurrent joint bleed – with arthropathy and crippling
    - Need prophylaxis immediately after the first episode of joint bleed
    - Iliopsoas bleed may lead to severe grown pain and hypo-volemic shock On right side, this may be confused with acute appendicitis (psoas sign)

▪ U/S and CT are diagnostic

5) Von Willebrand Disease

• Most common hereditary bleeding disorder, found in 1-2% of general population
• Inheritance mainly autosomal dominant
• Three Types
    ▪Type I   Reduced V W F
    ▪Type II   Qualitatively Abnormal V W F
    ▪Type III   Absent V W F
• Mainly mucocutaneous bleeds, bruises, epistaxis, menorrhagia and post-operative
• Characteristically prolonged BT and APTT (may be normal particularly in Type I).
• V W Work-Up: Qualitative assay of VW antigen. VW activity (ristocetin co-factor activity), Factor VIII activity and level.

6) Henoch-Schonlein Purpura

• Acute Vasculitis Syndrome
• Rash in 100% of cases, initially urticarial and maculopapular then becomes purpuric and palpable, found mainly on lower extremities (extensor surface) and buttocks, less on upper extremities, trunk and very rare on the face.
▪ Arthralgia/Arthritis: 2/3rd of cases usually oligo-articular involving large joints
▪ Severe abdominal pain/Hemorrhage: 2/3rd of cases may be confused with acute abdomen, hematemesis and melena may occur
• Nephritis: Hematuria, proteinuria, edema ± hypertension seen in up to 20% that can develop into progressive renal disease.

Lab tests: bleeding tests are usually normal. IgA is reduced in 50% of cases.

7) Afibrinogenemia/Hypofibrinogenemia

Congenital: AR
• Present as Umbilical stump bleeding in newborn babies
• Mild → severe: mainly; mucosal bleeding ± IC Hemmorhagege
• 20% can present with hem-arthrosis
• In these patients replacement therapy can have thromboembolic Disease, so avoid raising fibrinogen levels more than 1 g/dl.
• Lab test: All tests are prolonged PT, APTT, and TT + full correction
• Tuberculin Test: Produces only erythema and not induration (no fibrin)
Acquired: Fibrinogen deficiency is associated with
    • Liver disease

- DIC
- HLH syndrome
- L Asparginase treatment *(impairs liver synthesis of fibrinogen)*
  Treatment: Each bag of Cryoprecipitate contains 250 mg of fibrinogen and raises the level by 0.1 – 0.2 g/L

8)   Congenital coagulation factor deficiencies:

Factor XIII Deficiency:

Autosomal recessive

50% of the Factor XIII activity resides in platelets. Bleeding is attributed to accelerated fibrin clot degradation.

- H/O Delayed separation of umbilical cord, delayed wound healing
- Umbilical cord bleeding
- Soft tissue Hemmorhagege, Subaponeurotic Hge, Hematoma and Hemarthrosis
  (Spontaneous I.C. Hemmorhage 25% of patients)
- Normal screening tests (PT, PTT, Platelet Count and Bleeding Time)
- Immunological assay of Factor XIII level

Treatment: Cryoprecipitate, Can be given once daily (long half life)

Factor II Deficiency: AR very rare – umbilical stump bleeding then mild bleeding

Factor V Deficiency: AR, Mild mucus membrane bleeding, epistaxis.

Factor VII Deficiency: AR, Severe <1U/dl causes bleeding like Hemophilia A.
I.C. Hemmorhage is common (20%), PT: Prolonged, APTT (N)

Acquired deficiency of Factors: Mainly seen with:
- Liver disease
- Vitamin K↓
- Warfarin Treatment

Factor X deficiency: Autosomal Recessive
- Can be severe → severe hemophilia like bleed
- PT + APTT → prolonged
- Factor X Assay

Factor XI deficiency (Hemophilia C): Autosomal recessive
- Milder bleeding than other: Hemophilia
- No spontaneous bleeding
- Most common bleeding is menorrhagia only aPTT is prolonged.

Factor XII Deficiency: Autosomal recessive
- Not associated with Hemmorhagic manifestations
- It mediates fibrinolysis → ↑ risk of Thrombosis
- Prolongation of APTT

Treatment of bleeding disorders: Replacement therapy and drug doses. (Also see section 10.8)

PPC 15-20 U/kg/dose OD for 4-5 days

Fresh frozen plasma 10-15 ml/kg/dose

Cryoprecipitate 5-10 ml/kg/dose.

Humate P: 40-60 u/kg loading, then 40 u/kg/12 hrs x 7 days

DDAVP parenteral 0.3 mg/kg (maximum dose 20 mg),

DDAVP Intranasal only 1.5 mg/ml preparation should be used

Tranexamic Acid dose 100 mg/kg/6 hrs for 3-4 days after tooth extraction *(N e v e r given in children with hematuria)*

10.6 Disseminated Intravascular Coagulopathy (DIC)

Definition: DIC is due to widespread activation of coagulation in the circulation, resulting in:
1. Consumption of some coagulation factors and platelets.
2. Fibrin deposition as thrombi.
3. Secondary fibrinolysis.

Etiology:

Acute

♠ Shock, burns, heat stroke

♠ Gastroenteritis + severe dehydration.

♠ Septicemia & severe infections.

♠ Incompatible blood transfusion.

♠ Acute pulmonary embolism.

♠ Acute liver failure.

♠ Cardiac arrest and post resuscitation.

Chronic

♠ Disseminated malignancy.

♠ Pancreatic carcinoma

♠ Promyelocytic leukemia.

♠ Renal vein thrombosis.

♠ Aortic aneurysm.

♠ Giant hemangioma.

♠ A-V fistula.

Pathogenesis:
   Widespread triggering of coagulation system can be initiated by:
   1. Endothelial damage in small blood vessels (e.g. trauma, toxic agent as endotoxins, or antigen-antibody complexes → damage of RBCs, leukocytes and
   Vessel wall → release thrombogenic substances).

   2. Release of thrombogenic substances that trigger the coagulation system (e.g. amniotic fluid, snake venom)
   This will result in:
   i.. Consumption of platelets and some clotting factors (I, II, V, VIII) → severe bleeding.
   ii. Vascular occlusion by fibrin clots → ischemia and necrosis in different organs.
   iii. Increased fibrinolytic activity leads to ↓fibrinogen and ↑ fibrin splitting products (FSP or FDP), which have anticoagulant effects.

Clinical Manifestations: DIC is always secondary to some other underlying disease and may   present as:
   1. Acute fulminant bleeding disorder or
   2. Chronic disorder with both hemorrhagic and thrombotic manifestations.
   3. Manifestation of underlying triggering disease (e.g. gastroenteritis + dehydration).
   4. Acute hemorrhagic manifestations (consumption of clotting factors & platelets)
      • Bleeding from puncture sites.
      • GI bleeding: Melena, hematemesis (coffee –ground vomitus).
      • Pulmonary hemorrhage.
      • Skin hemorrhages: Petechiae or ecchymosis.
   5. Ischemic manifestations and tissue necrosis (due to thrombosis).
      a. Skin: Gangrene
      b. Kidneys: Acute cortical necrosis.

    c. Mesenteric vessels → Ileus and intestinal obstruction.

    d. CNS → Disturbed consciousness, convulsions and paralysis.

6. Hemolytic anemia (due to extra corpuscular causes as toxic and/or mechanical destruction of RBCs as they pass through fibrin networks) → pallor, dark urine.

Laboratory diagnosis:
- Thrombocytopenia (usually severe).
- Prolonged bleeding time.
- Prolonged PT and APTT
- Deficiency of factors: I (fibrinogen), II (prothrombin), V and VIII.
- Increased fibrin degradation products (FDP or D-Dimers).

Treatment:
1. Correction and reversal of the primary process that caused the DIC.
2. Correction of infection, shock, hypoxia and acidosis.
3. Infusion of fresh frozen plasma, cryoprecipitate and / or platelets.
4. Heparin: 100 units/kg, 6 hourly to *decrease* the ongoing stimulus to coagulation. It is useful in significant arterial or venous thrombosis, meningococcemia, & pro-myelocytic leukemia). Monitoring by doing APTT is very important to avoid bleeding complications.
5. In newborn: Exchange transfusion with fresh blood.

10.7 Hypersplenism

Definition: Hypersplenism is a functional disorder of spleen characterized by:
1. Depression of one or more cellular blood element in peripheral blood despite of active formation in bone marrow
2. Splenomegaly
3. Correction of the above-mentioned findings after the splenectomy

Etiology:
1. Primary (no obvious cause as in idiopathic thrombocytopenic purpura).
2. Secondary: Splenomegaly secondary to a well defined disorders such as:
   - Hodgkin's disease
   - Chronic leukemia
   - Lymphosarcoma
   - Kalazar
   - Thalassemia

Mechanism:
1. Selective *sequestration* and *increased* destruction of formed blood cells in the spleen.
2. Inhibition of a normal or hyperactive bone marrow by an unknown hormone secreted by the spleen through prevention of growth & maturation of blood cells, or block to delivery of cells from bone marrow.

Manifestations:
1. Splenomegaly
2. Blood film: Neutropenia, thrombocytopenia and anemia (singly or in combination)
3. Bone marrow: normal or hyper cellular.

Treatment:
1. To treat underlying condition
2. Splenectomy is indicated in all cases with persistent pancytopenia.

10.8   Blood Components and Transfusion Therapy

The products used for therapy are: whole blood, packed red blood cells, granulocytes, platelets, and coagulation factors (fresh frozen plasma, cryoprecipitate and recombinant factor concentrates).

Blood components therapy requires:
- Proper anticoagulation of the blood.
- Screening for a variety of infectious agents.
- Blood group compatibility testing before administration

Indications for the use of various blood components:

1. Whole blood (WB):

Whole blood is indicated only when acute hypovolemia and reduced oxygen carrying capacity is encountered as in acute blood loss. The transfused volume varies greatly according to the clinical circumstances. The usual dose is 15 - 20 ml/kg.

Formula for calculation: Whole blood needed = 6 x W x D
W = Weight of child, D = Deficit (Desired – Present Hb).

2. Packed Red Blood Cells (PRBC):

Packed cells are the most frequently transfused blood component. They are given to treat chronic anemia, to increase the O_2 carrying capacity of blood and to maintain satisfactory tissue oxygenation. Each unit contains 250 -300 ml of RBCs /unit.
The transfusion is indicated if the underlying cause is irreversible or if the anemia exists with low oxygen carrying capacity. Transfusion may be indicated if Hb. is < 7 g%. The aim is to increase Hb to 10 g%. Regular transfusions are required in Thalassemia major, Fanconi anemia, congenital dyserythropoietic anemia and in hyper-hemolytic states of G6PD and sickle cell disease.
The usual dose for a top up transfusion is 10-15 mL/kg.
or Packed cells Transfusion (ml required) = 4 X Weight X Deficit

3. Platelet concentrates:

Platelet concentrate is indicated for the support of children with quantitative (e.g. severe thrombocytopenia) and qualitative (e.g. thrombasthenia) disorders in which there is a risk of life threatening bleeding (Intracranial bleed, this mostly occur when platelet count drops to < 10). The ideal goal of platelet transfusion is to raise the platelet count to > 50 X 10^9 platelets /L in children and > 100 X10^9 platelets/L for neonates. Platelet concentrate contains 5 -7 X10^{10} platelets /unit. The usual dose is 0.1 unit /kg. Platelet transfusion is generally avoided in conditions with rapid destruction of platelets like ITP and Hypersplenism unless there is a possibility of a life threatening bleeding.

4. Fresh frozen plasma (FFP);

Plasma, the liquid portion of whole blood, is separated from cells and frozen within 6 hours of collection to make "fresh frozen plasma (FFP)" This contains coagulation factors II, V, VII, IX, X and XI in physiological amounts. FFP also contains the naturally occurring Antithrombin III.

Uses: Multiple factor deficiencies: FFP is indicated when there are multiple factor deficiencies associated with bleeding   e.g. Liver disease. In patients with liver disease and abnormal coagulation FFP is used prior to invasive procedures like Liver biopsy.

In single factor deficiency: FFP should only be used if no virus safe fractionated product is available; currently this applies to Factor V Factor XI and factor X deficiencies

In DIC without bleeding, blood products are not indicated, if the patient is bleeding a combination of platelets, FFP and cryoprecipitate is indicated

Reversal of warfarin effect: FFP is recommended if there is major bleeding in a patient on Warfarin therapy.

5. Cryoprecipitate:

Cryoprecipitate is the cold insoluble remnant of one unit of FFP thawed between 2° C and 6° C. It contains factor I (fibrinogen), factor VIII, vWF and factor IX,

Cryoprecipitate is indicated in patients with afibrinogenemia, hypofibrinogenemia, dysfibrinogenemia and factor VIII deficiency.

The usual dose is 1 bag/5 kg body weight.

6. Recombinant factor concentrate:

Recombinant clotting factor concentrates are also available for factors VIII and IX. They are indicated in severe hemophilia A and B. The usual dose of factor VIII is 20 -50 Unit/kg and for factor IX 0.7 Unit/kg.

Typical Transfusion Reactions:
- *Febrile reactions:* Occurs in 1:10 transfused patients. Fever, chills and urticaria occur at the end of transfusion, usually because of sensitization to WBC HLA antigens. May be prevented by filtering of blood products to remove white cells.
- *Allergic reaction*: Fever, urticaria and anaphylactoid reaction, Occur often because of sensitivity to donor's plasma proteins.
- *Circulatory overload*, especially in the presence of chronic cardiopulmonary deficiency. Can be prevented by diuretic therapy (Frusemide 1-2 mg/Kg IV given pre or midway during the transfusion)

Management of Transfusion Problems
1. Stop the transfusion
2. Return the blood or blood component to the blood bank with a fresh sample of patient's blood to retype and cross match.
3. Immediate supportive measures: Intravenous rehydration, to support blood pressure and maintain high urine flow.
4. Check immediately for hemoglobinemia, hemoglobinuria, and Hyperkalemia.
5. Check for jaundice and anemia later on

Long –term Complications of Transfusions:
- Iron overload.
- Alloimmunization to red and white blood cells or platelets and plasma proteins.
- Graft – versus-host disease.
- Transfusion–associated infectious disease transmission (e.g. hepatitis B or C, HIV, CMV, Epstein Barr virus, parvovirus, malaria, syphilis and Brucellosis etc).

11

Nephrology

11.1   Hematuria (Red Urine)

Definition:
>5 RBC per high power field in sediment from 10 ml of centrifuged freshly voided urine.

Classifications:
> **Microscopic:** when urine color is clear.
> **Macroscopic** (gross): when urine is smoky, brownish, cola or red to pink color. It is
also   important to establish if hematuria is from upper or lower renal system.

Causes:
- **Asymptomatic microscopic hematuria**; found in 0.5- 2% of school age children
- **Exercise induced**
- **Infections**; Bacterial UTI, TB, Adenovirus, Schistosomiasis
- **Glomerular** hematuria is usually associated with cast, proteinuria or hypertension, e.g. Post infective glomerulonephritis, Hemolytic uremic syndrome, Focal segmental and membrano-proliferative glomerulonephritis and IgA nephropathy
- **Congenital**: Renal cysts, hydronephrosis or diverticula, cystic disease
- **Genetics**: Alport syndrome, infantile Polycystic disease of the kidneys
- **Calculi** or hypercalcemia, hypercalciuria
- **Vascular**: Henoch Schonlein Purpura, S L E or Polyarteritis Nodosa.
- **Hematological**: Sickle cell disease , bleeding disorders and renal vein thrombosis
- **Tumors**
- **Chemical cystitis and drugs induced**
- **Trauma**
- **Factitious**

Drugs known to cause Hematuria
- Antibacterial; Ampicillin, Penicillin, Sulphonamide, Methicillin, Kanamycin & Polymyxin
- Anticoagulants
- Non steroidal anti-inflammatory; Indomethacin, Aspirin,
- Other drugs; Amitriptyline, Cyclophosphamide, colchicines and Chlorpromazine
- Heavy Metals; Lead, Gold, Copper & phosphorus

Hematuria must be differentiated from causes of colored urine
- Hemoglobinuria
- Myoglobinuria
- Alkaptonuria
- Porphyria
- Food & Food coloring agents
- Drugs: Rifampicin, Deferoxamine, Phenothiazines, Pyridium and Phenindione

Diagnostic approach:
1.   Hemostix: Bed side testing: Changes the color from yellow to green. The test could be positive for hematuria, hemoglobinuria or myoglobinuria. It could be falsely positive in presence of peroxidase activity of some bacteria causing urinary tract infections. False negative test occurs if the patient is taking reducing agent e.g. ascorbic Acid (Vitamin C)

2. Urine microscopy:
3. **Presence of > 5 red cells/cubic mm. Glomerular hematuria is usually associated with proteinuria and red blood cell casts. In lower urinary tract bleed; red blood cells are usually non-deformed, pink- red and without casts.**
4. Urine Biochemistry for proteinuria and hypercalciuria
5. Renal Biochemistry to exclude renal impairment and hypercalcemia
6. Renal ultrasound for morphological renal abnormalities

Algorithm for diagnosis of Hematuria

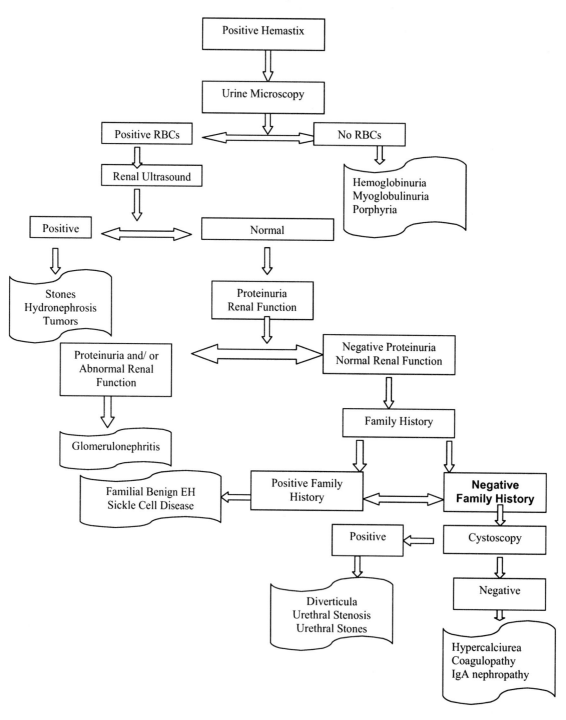

Common causes of Recurrent / persistent Hematuria:

1. Familial Benign Essential Hematuria (FBEH)

•Familial persistent hematuria without proteinuria, may progress to renal failure and hearing defect.
•Hematuria can be microscopic, continuous, persistent, with or without episodes of gross hematuria.
•Transmitted as autosomal dominant condition, sporadic cases have been reported.

Pathology: Normal light microscopy and immunofluorescence of the renal biopsy
Although electron microscopy shows diffuse extreme attenuation of the Glomerular basement membrane (100-200 nm), the structure and contour of GBM is normal.
Normal immunohistochemical studies of GBM.

2. Sickle Cell Nephropathy

Hematuria occurs in both homozygous (HbSS) and heterozygous (HbAS) sickle cell disease. Hematuria could be gross and painless. Hematuria commonly arises from the left kidney more than the right kidney. In papillary infarction hematuria is associated with sever pain. Renal medullary sickling, vascular obstruction & RBC extravasations are the main contributing factors

3. Alport Syndrome

An inherited progressive nephritis characterized by ultra-structural changes of the GBM & sensorineural deafness. Males are severely affected than females, Frequency 1:5000, Onset: Either Juvenile or Adult onset. 14% of pediatric group present before 1st year & 72 % before 6 years

Either microscopic and/ or macroscopic hematuria may occur. Macroscopic hematuria usually occurs 2 days post respiratory tract infections and last for 1-10 days.
Proteinuria, hypertension & renal failure occur progressively with age. 40% may develop Nephritic Syndrome.

Non-Renal Manifestations of Alport Syndrome:
Progressive sensori-neural deafness:
Children have normal hearing at birth, but deafness is usually evident by the age of 15 years.
Ocular Defect:
Anterior Lenticonus, Subcapsular cataract and Retinal changes including the fovea.

Pathology:
Light microscopy may show mesangial proliferation, segmental sclerosis, hyalinosis & interstitial foam cells. Immunofluorescence is usually negative but granular deposits of C3 & IgM may occur in the glomeruli. Advanced cases shows immunoglobulin deposits along GBM. Irregular thickening of GBM, splitting & splinting of the Lamina densa characterizes the ultra structural picture on electron microscopy.

11.2 Glomerulonephritis (GN)

Classification of Glomerular injury:

1. **Primary**; when there is no extra renal manifestations
   - Immune mediated
     - Post infectious acute glomerulonephritis
     - Membranoproliferative GN
     - IgA nephropathy
     - Membranous nephropathy
   - Unknown etiology
     - Minimal Change Nephrotic Syndrome
     - Focal Segmental Glomerulosclerosis

2. **Secondary** GN associated systemic diseases
   - Systemic immune mediated diseases
         Systemic Lupus Erythematosus, Scleroderma
         Mixed Connective Tissue diseases
   - Vasculitis
         Henoch-Schonlein Purpura
         Poly arteritis Nodosa
         Wegner's granulomatosis
   - Systemic infections
         Sub Acute Bacterial Endocarditis (SABE)
         Shunt Nephrosis
         Syphilis, malaria and Hepatitis

3. **Hereditary** disorders
   - Familial Nephritis (Alport Syndrome)
   - Sickle cell anemia
   - Congenital Nephrotic Syndrome

4. **Miscellaneous** etiology
   - Diabetes Mellitus
   - Amyloidosis
   - Lymphoma

Acute Post Streptococcal Glomerulonephritis (APSGN)

Acute GN is a post infective immune mediated disorder characterized by sudden appearance of one or more of acute nephritic features:
    Hematuria, RBC casts in the urine (Coffee or Smokey urine)
    Edema,
    Hypertension
    Features of Renal failure (Oliguria, Azotemia)

Etiology and Patho physiology
APSGN follows infection with certain nephritogenic strains of Group A β hemolytic streptococci (type 12 and 49 after throat infections and type 49 and 57 after pyoderma)

In response to the nephritogenic organisms, the excess amount of antigen antibody complex derived from antigen stimulation, traverse the basement membrane and result in complement activation, neutrophil stimulation, release of lysosomes and induce inflammatory response which damage the glomeruli, obliterate capillary lumen and reduce glomerular filtration rate leading to sudden oligurea, fluid retention, hypertension, acidosis, hyperkalemia and hyperphosphatemia.

APSGN can occur sporadically or epidemically. Incidence is decreasing in developed world due to improvement in overcrowding and hygiene. Epidemic APSGN occurs mainly in developing countries.

Other organisms known to cause post-infective GN may be:
1. Bacterial:
    - Staphylococcus species
    - Pneumococci
    - Meningococci
    - Klebsiella
    - Salmonella
    - Mycoplasma
2. Viral Causes
    - Coxsackie virus
    - Echo virus
    - Epstein Barr virus
    - Hepatitis B virus
    - Influenza virus
    - Mumps
    - Rubeola virus

Pathology:
Changes are diffuse involving all the glomeruli. Light microscopy shows evidence of inflammation with increased cellularity and proliferation of neutrophils within the mesangium. Basement membrane is usually normal. Electron microscopy shows sub epithelial and sub endothelial deposition of antigen antibodies complex, which are defined by immuno-fluorescence as IgG and C3.

Clinical Picture:
M: F 2:1
Typical age is school age between 5-15 years.
The clinical picture is characterized by:
Sudden onset of edema, hypertension, hematuria
Varying degree of renal failure
Pharyngitis and impetigo may be present: Pharyngitis is more common Microscopic hematuria and proteinuria occurs in 30 % of patient during the prodromal illness. The latent period is 7-14 days after pharyngitis up to 2 weeks after impetigo.
85% of patients will have edema and 30-50 % present with gross hematuria. Hypertension is common but 5% may develop hypertensive encephalopathy. Constitutional symptoms like fever, lethargy, abdominal pain, anorexia and headache, may occur.
Oliguria is frequent but some patients may complain of frequency and dysuria.

Congestive heart failure may occur secondary to extra cellular volume expansion, hypertension and acidosis.

Differential diagnosis of Acute Nephritis
• Post streptococcal AGN
• Post-infectious AGN (due to infectious agents other than group A β – hemolytic streptococci)
• Sub acute bacterial endocarditis
• Henoch-Schonlein purpura
• IgA nephropathy
• Hereditary nephritis
• Systemic lupus erythematosus
• Systemic vasculitis

Investigations;
Urine: High urine osmolality, proteinuria and hematuria with red blood cells, white blood cells and red blood cells casts.
Plasma: Blood urea nitrogen is elevated
GFR is seldom below 50%.
Metabolic acidemia
Hyperkalemia, Hyponatremia and hyperphosphatemia occur in sever cases.

Immunological features are hypocomplementemia (**Low C3 and C4** levels).
Serological test are positive for streptococcal infections, ASO titer >200 iu/L post pharyngitis and anti hyalouridnase and anti deoxyribonuclease after both pharyngitis and pyoderma.
Microbiological test: Throat swab may be positive for streptococci

Treatment:
1. Monitoring of physical and hemodynamic status
   • Daily body weight as evidence of fluid retention
   • Intake and output chart
   • BP
2. Penicillin V orally for 10 days to eliminate Streptococcal disease
3. Edema and oligurea
   • Fluid restriction = Urine out put + insensible fluid loss (400 ml/ m² body surface area/day), observe for polyuric phase and increase fluid accordingly
   • Avoid pulmonary edema, if occurs treat with oxygen, Frusemide, Dialysis
   • Acute renal failure: see the section of ARF
4. Hypertension
   • Mild: Loop diuretics, Fursomide 1-2 mg /kg
   • Moderate Preferably ACE Inhibitors, Lisinopril
   • Severe   Labetalol infusion
5. Diet
   • Restrict sodium and potassium intake
   • Protein restriction in case of azotemia

Prognosis: 90% of APSGN recover without significant alteration of renal function
- Oliguric phase resolve in 2 weeks followed by polyuric phase
- Gross hematuria resolves in 2-3 weeks
- Hypocomplementemia resolve in 4 weeks
- Proteinuria resolve in 2-6 months
- Microscopic hematuria may take up to 12 months

0.5-2 % patients may progress rapidly to extensive renal scarring, crescent formation and progressive renal damage (Rapidly progressive Glomerulonephritis)

Follow up of patient is required up to 1 year to check signs of CRF or Hypertension.

11.3 Proteinuria

Definition:

Passage of more than 150 mg of protein in 24 hours urine (0.15 gm/ 24 hours) Albumin is the largest fraction of protein in normal proteinuria (< 30 mg / 24 hours or 0.03 g/ 24 hours). The remainder is Tamm-Horsfall protein, which is a mucoprotein of no known function

Method of detections:

1. Urine dipsticks, a semi quantitative test that detects albumin and is reported as follows:
   - 0 = Negative
   - 1+ trace
   - 2+ $\cong$ 100 mg/dL
   - 3+ $\cong$ 300 mg /dL
   - 4+ $\cong$ 2000 mg /dL
2. 24 hours (12 hours in pediatrics) quantitative assessment

Classification:

Non pathological proteinuria; asymptomatic and not associated with edema
- **Postural (Orthostatic)** proteinuria is the excretion of normal or increased amount (up to 10 folds) of protein in the urine, in erect posture, not associated with hematuria, abnormal creatinine clearance or complement levels. Dipstick for protein is negative in first urine after night sleep.
- **Febrile proteinuria**; fever > 38.3° C (101° F) may cause 2+ of proteinuria
- **Exercise proteinuria** after vigorous exercise, doesn't exceed 2+, and is rare in females

Pathological proteinuria:
- **Tubular:** Could be acquired or inherited, not associated with edema
  Passage of low molecular weight protein $\cong$ albumin, amount does not exceed 1gm /24 hours. Detected by urine electrophoresis for low molecular weight proteins.
- **Glomerular:**
  Selective proteinuria is the passage of albumin and lower molecular weight protein through basement membrane. It is pathognomonic for Minimal Change Nephrotic Syndrome

Persistent asymptomatic proteinuria:

Proteinuria in an apparently healthy child, usually < 2 gm per 24 hours, without hematuria, for minimum of 3 months. Found in 6 % school-age children.

Causes of Proteinuria:
- Nephrotic syndrome due to various causes
- Pyelonephritis
- Hereditary nephritis
- Fanconi syndrome

Investigations for proteinuria:

Urine microscopy and culture

Renal Ultrasonography
24 hours urine protein collection
Random urine protein to Creatinine ratio
Creatinine clearance
Serum protein, albumin, and complement levels

11.4   Nephrotic Syndrome

Definition:

A clinical state of varying etiologies characterized by edema, heavy proteinuria (>1G/meter square/day), hypo-albuminemia (<25 G/L) with or without hyper-cholesterolemia.

Basic defect is an increased permeability of the glomerular capillary basement membrane leading to protein leak from the kidneys. Nephrotic syndrome can be primary, when the pathology is within the kidney, or secondary, when it occurs as part of a recognized systemic disease.

Histological classifications: of glomerular lesions associated with primary and secondary Nephrotic syndrome are classified as:

- Minimal-lesion Nephrotic syndrome

- Diffuse mesangial hypercellularity

- Focal Glomerulosclerosis

- Membranous glomerulonephritis

- Membranoproliferative glomerulonephritis.

Secondary causes as part of a recognized systemic disease
- Post infectious:

    o   Group A beta-hemolytic streptococci

    o   Syphilis

    o   Malaria

    o   Tuberculosis

    o   Viral infections (e.g., Varicella, hepatitis B, HIV type 1 and infectious mononucleosis)

- Collagen vascular disease (e.g., SLE, rheumatoid arthritis, polyarteritis Nodosa)

- Vasculitis; e.g. Henoch-Schonlein Purpura

- Renal vein thrombosis

- Diabetes mellitus

Hereditary Causes

- Congenital Nephrotic Syndrome

- Hereditary nephritis (Alport Syndrome)

340

- Sickle cell disease

- Nail Patella Syndrome

Miscellaneous causes

- Amyloidosis

- Malignancy (e.g., leukemia, lymphoma, Wilms tumor, pheochromocytoma)

- Hypersensitivity to various toxic agents (e. g, bee sting, poison ivy and oak, snake venom)

- Medications (e.g., Probenacid, Fenoprofen, Captopril, Lithium, Warfarin, Penicillamine, mercury, Gold, Trimethadione, paramethadione)

- Heroin use

Investigations at initial presentation:
1. Full blood count
2. Renal profile - urea, electrolyte, Creatinine
3. Serum albumin
4. Urinalysis and Culture
5. Quantification for urinary protein excretion (spot urine protein to creatinine ratio or 24 hour urine protein estimation)

Other investigations if the clinical features are atypical / or in the presence of poor prognostic features:
1. ASOT
2. Serum complement (C3, C4) level
3. Antinuclear factor / anti DS DNA
4. Others as indicated

Renal biopsy:
Not indicated for idiopathic nephrotic syndrome in children prior to starting corticosteroid therapy.
Main indications for biopsy are:
1. Steroid resistant nephrotic syndrome defined as failure to achieve remission despite 4 weeks of adequate corticosteroid therapy.

2. Presence of atypical features to suggest other renal diseases e.g. Persistent hypertension, gross hematuria as per the discretion of the pediatric nephrologist.

Minimal change Nephrotic syndrome (MCNS)

A clinical state characterized by heavy proteinuria, hypo-albuminemia, edema, hyper-cholesterolemia, and normal renal function.

MCNS is the most prevalent of persistent glomerular injury in children with an incidence of 1-2 new cases / 100,000 children below 16 years / year.

Commonest age group is 2-3 years; males are commonly affected than females. 2/3 of children present before 5 years and 5-10% present after 10 years of age.

Pathophysiology:

Filtration of low molecular weight anionic plasma proteins across the glomerular basement membrane is normally prevented by a negatively charged filtration barrier, which consists of proteoglycan molecules of heparan sulfate. In patients, the concentration of heparan sulfate mucopolysaccharide in the basement membrane is lower, therefore large amounts of protein cross the barrier leading to hyper-albuminuria, hypo-albuminemia and edema.

In the Nephrotic state, levels of almost all serum lipids are elevated due to two pathogenic processes:
(1) Hypo-proteinemia stimulating generalized protein synthesis in the liver, including the lipoproteins and
(2) Diminution of lipid catabolism caused by reduced plasma levels of lipoprotein lipase.

Pathology:

According to the International Study of Kidney Diseases in Childhood (ISKDC), the histological classification and incidence of various types of Nephrotic syndrome are:

- Minimal-change Nephrotic syndrome: accounts for 85% of all cases

- Focal segmental Glomerulosclerosis (FSGS) occurs in 9.5%

- Mesangium proliferation occurs in 2.5%

- Membranous nephropathy or other etiologies occurs in 3.5%

The structural changes believed to be responsible for causing proteinuria are:
Damage to the endothelial surface, causing loss of the negative charge

(1) Damage to the glomerular basement membrane
(2) Effacement of the foot processes.

The foot processes are firmly attached to the visceral surface of the glomerular basement membrane. The space between the bases of the foot processes form the filtration slits, and this space constitutes the site for the convective forces that govern the filtration through the visceral epithelium.

Pathophysiology:

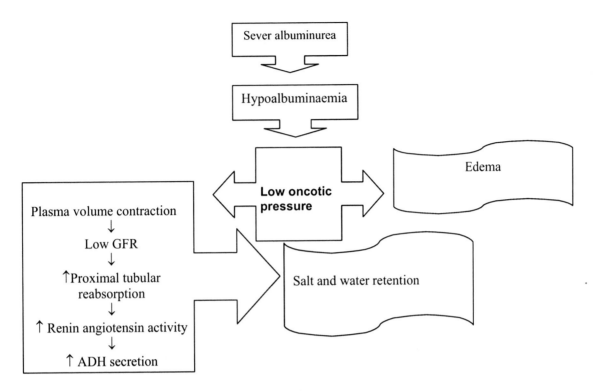

Clinical picture:
Sudden occurrence of edema of the face and legs. Scrotal edema, ascites and pleural effusion may occur (anasarca). The picture is usually preceded by passage of frothy urine. Oliguria may develop later. Children with MCNS are usually hypovolemic with normal blood pressure. Proteinuria is highly selective. 25 % of cases may have microscopic hematuria but gross hematuria is unusual.

Complications:

(1) Hypovolemia may present with abdominal pain, vomiting and diarrhea, secondary to mesenteric vessels hypo perfusion, dizziness, tachycardia, hypo tension, sluggish peripheral circulation and shock especially after vigorous diuretic therapy.

(2) Urinary immunoglobulin and complement factor B losses lower the patient's resistance to infections and increase the risk of serious sepsis. Pneumo coccal peritonitis, Haemophilus influenzae infection, Gram-negative sepsis and Staphylococcus cellulitis. Other precipitating factors for infections include edema, impaired lymphocyte function and use of steroids and immunosuppression drugs for the treatment

(3) Loss of antithrombin III and plasminogen via urine and the simultaneous increase in clotting factors, especially factors I, VII, VIII, and X, increases the risk for arterial thrombosis, venous thrombosis, and pulmonary embolism, which occurs in 5% of children with Nephrotic syndrome.

(4) High glomerular permeability causes the excretion of vitamin D–binding protein and complexes in the urine, leading to

- Malabsorption of calcium and development of bone disease (e.g., osteitis fibrosa cystica) because of enhanced parathyroid hormone production
- Osteomalacia because of impairment in mineralization.

(5) Other protein like transferrin and thyroid binding protein may also be lost

Investigations:

Heavy Proteinuria as demonstrated by:
- Presence of 40 mg/m²/hour or 50 mg /kg/day protein in 12- 24 hours urine collection.
- Spot urine collection for <u>Urine protein, urine Creatinine ratio</u>
  Urine albumin and urine Creatinine ratio
- Low selectivity protein index = (IgG: Transferrin Excretion ratio) < 0.1

Normal serum sodium, potassium, chloride and blood urea levels
Hypoalbuminemia, hypo-proteinemia and hyper-cholesterolemia
Hypocalcemia and hypomagnesaemia
Normal complement level
Increased hematocrit (Hct.) levels reflecting the degree of Hypovolemia and hemoconcentration
Blood culture in febrile children

Indication for Renal biopsy in childhood Nephrotic syndrome:
- A typical clinical picture
  - (1) Presentation before the age of 2 years or after 12 years age
  - (2) Presence of gross hematuria
  - (3) Presence of persistent hypertension
  - (4) Hypocomplementemia
  - (5) Nitrogen retention
- Steroid dependant and steroid resistant Nephrotic syndrome

Management:

Bed rest if gross edema present
Diet: Low salt, normal protein and calories intake
Fluid intake: Normal
Diuretics: Can be dangerous by aggravating Hypovolemia, may be given with salt free albumen if indicated
Albumin: May be used in hypo perfusion states, 0.5 to 1G/Kg IV, over one hour
Infections: Peritonitis and skin infections are the likely complication and should be treated adequately
Steroid (Prednisolone) is the mainstay of treatment:
Management aims to induce and maintain complete remission without serious adverse effects of therapy.
Standard International study of kidney disease course (ISKD) recommends following regimen:
- Induction dose: 60 mg / m²/day for 6-weeks
- Followed by maintenance dose of 40-mg/ m² on alternate days for 6 weeks.

Recently on review of randomly controlled trials it was noted that shorter course is associated with higher rate of relapses, Treatment of initial presentation for 6 months substantially reduces the relapse rate

Treatment definitions:

Remission: Albustix 0 to trace for 3 consecutive days

Relapse: Albustix 2+ or more for 3 consecutive days, having previously been in remission

Steroid resistant: Failure to achieve remission with prednisolone 60 mg / m²/day for 4 weeks.

Steroid dependence: 2 relapse on steroids or within 2 days of stopping steroids

Frequent relapse: 2 relapse in a month

Indication of immunosuppressive therapy:

- Steroid resistant Nephrotic syndrome
- Steroid dependant Nephrotic syndrome
- Frequent relapses in a Steroid Sensitive case

Prognosis:

93 % of MCNS become free of proteinuria in 8 weeks of steroid therapy, but 80 % of children with steroid sensitive Nephrotic syndrome will relapse once or more, of those 50 % relapses occur frequently or will become steroid dependent.

Early relapse after initial treatment and short duration of remission increases the risk of frequent relapses.

Response to steroid is associated with good long-term prognosis for renal function and resolution of the disease. Frequency of relapses improve with time, 50-70% of children being relapse free at 5 years and 85% relapse free at 10 years follow up.

Parents should be taught to monitor urine protein by dipsticks

Parents should be warned about immunocompromised state, avoiding live vaccines for 6 weeks after completion of steroid treatment and possibility of adrenal crises if treatment stopped suddenly.

Summary of Treatment

1. Initial episode:

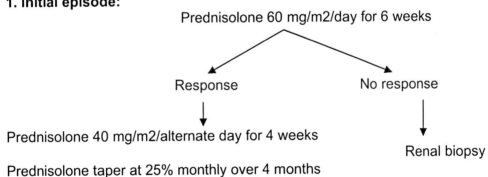

Prednisolone 60 mg/m2/day for 6 weeks

Response   No response

Prednisolone 40 mg/m2/alternate day for 4 weeks

Renal biopsy

Prednisolone taper at 25% monthly over 4 months

2. Relapse:

Prednisolone 60 mg/m2/day till remission

Then 40 mg/ m2/alternate day for 4 weeks and discontinue

3. Frequent relapses:

Reintroduce as for (2), then taper and keep alternate day Prednisolone at 0.1 – 0.5 mg/kg/dose for 6 months

4. Relapse while on Prednisolone treatment:

As for (3) if not steroid toxic,

Consider Cyclophosphamide if steroid toxic

5. Post cyclophosphamide relapse:

As for (2) and (3) if not steroid toxic.

If steroid toxic, refer to Pediatric nephrologist to consider second course Cyclophosphamide or Cyclosporine therapy

Congenital Nephrotic Syndrome

It is an Autosomal recessive disease with a poor prognosis.

Clinical presentation occurs early with edema or incidental observation of proteinuria during early infancy. Recurrent infection is the usual cause o death and early renal failure occurs within the first 2 years of life. Recently, Finnish type of this disease is known to be caused by mutations in the gene known as *NPHS1*. This gene codes for a cell adhesion protein called nephrin, which is synthesized by podocytes. Dysfunction of Nephrin and another podocyte protein called podocin are associated with the development of proteinuria.

11.5   Acute Renal Failure

Definition:

Acute Renal Failure is a sudden decrease in renal function accompanied by retention of nitrogenous waste products and disturbance of water and electrolyte balance.

Oliguria is a reduction in urine output less than 300 ml/m^2 surface area per day or < 0.5 ml/kg/hr in children and <1 ml/kg/hr in infants.

Etiology:

Pre-Renal Failure
- Hypovolemia, dehydration, shock, CHF, Nephrotic syndrome
- Peripheral Vasodilatation (e.g.: sepsis)
- Impaired Cardiac Output

Parenchymal Renal Failure
- Acute Glomerulonephritis
- Acute tubular necrosis
- Hemolytic Uremic Syndrome
- Acute Pyelonephritis
- Acute Interstitial Nephritis
- Tumor lysis syndrome
- Hemoglobinuria, Myoglobulinuria
- Uric acid nephropathy

Post Renal Failure
- Reflex Nephropathy
- Obstructive Uropathy
- Neurogenic Bladder
- Posterior urethral valve

Investigations:
- Blood:
    - FBC, Blood film to look for anemia, leucopenia and thrombocytopenia
    - Renal profile
    - Blood gas
    - Serum Albumin, Ca, P, Uric acid
- Urine:
    - Dipstick: Protein, Specific gravity, blood
    - Microscopy
- Imaging: Renal ultrasound
- Other investigations depending on cause and situation

Complications:
- Hypertension
- CHF and Pulmonary Edema
- Hyperkalemia
- Hyperphosphatemia
- Metabolic Acidosis

Diagnostic Criteria:

Children:

	Pre- Renal	Intrinsic ARF
U. Osmolality	>500	<350
Urine Sodium	<20	>40
Urine/Plasma Urea	>8	<3
Urine/Plasma Creatinine	>40	<20
Renal Failure Index	<1	>1
Fractional excretion of Sodium	<1%	>2%

Neonates:

	Pre-Renal	Intrinsic ARF
U. Osmolality	>400	<400
Urine Sodium	30 ± 20	60 ± 35
Urine/Plasma Urea	>8	<3
Urine/Plasma Creatinine	30 ± 10	10 ± 4
Renal Failure Index	<3.0	>3.0
Fractional excretion of Sodium	<2.5%	>2.5

Diagnostic fluid challenge:
In acute phase of renal failure when it is not clear if renal shutdown is pre-renal or due to intrinsic renal disease, a fluid challenge of 20-30 ml/kg over 30 minutes with I.V. furosemide 2-5 mg per kg is given to see if urine is produced to indicate the reversible nature of pre renal shut down.

Renal Failure Index: $RFI = \dfrac{U.\,Na \times P.cr.}{U.\,Cr.}$

Fractional Excretion of Filtered Sodium
$$F.\,Ex.\,Na = \dfrac{U\,Na \times P\,cr}{P\,Na \times U\,cr} \times 100$$

Estimation of GFR (Schwartzman Formula)
$$\dfrac{49 \times Height\,(cm)}{Plasma\,Creatinine\,(\mu mol/L)}$$

Treatment:

1. **Fluid Balance**
    i) **In cases of ARF with intravascular depletion (Pre-Renal Failure)**
        Prompt fluid resuscitation is required.
        20-ml/kg body weight of isotonic fluids (normal Saline) should be given over

1 hour, which could be repeated if necessary.
Urine output should be increased within 4 hours.

ii) **ARF with volume overload**

Fluids should be restricted and diuretics should be given. Intravenous Frusemide has a rapid onset of action. Dose should start as 2 mg/kg/dose tid, but may be increased to 0.5 mg/kg/hr as infusion.

iii) **ARF with pulmonary edema** will require peritoneal dialysis

iv) **Monitor urine output, weight, BP, CVP**

2. **Acid Base Balance**

If severe acidosis is present (pH <7.2) or is contributing to Hyperkalemia, Sodium Bicarbonate should be infused using the following calculations:

*Mmol of Bicarb. Required = (Desired – observed Bicarb.) x Weight kg x 0.6

Only half the calculated value is given over 1 hour as 4.2% (Half diluted solution of 8.4% NaHCO3).

3. **Hyperkalemia:**

Serum K+ concentration > 6.0 mmol/l (neonates), and > 5.5 mmol/l (children). Cardiac toxicity generally develops when plasma K+ > 7 mmol/l.

Regardless of degree of hyperkalemia, treatment should be initiated in anyone with ECG abnormalities.

- 12-lead **ECG** to look for hyperkalemic changes:

      i. Tall peaked T waves

      ii. Prolonged PR interval

      iii. Widened QRS complex

      iv. Flattened P wave

      v. Sine wave (QRS complex merges with peaked T waves)

      vi. Ventricular Fibrillation or asystole

- If ECG is abnormal or plasma K+ > 6 – 7 mmol/l, connect patient to cardiac monitor and give the following in sequence:

- Nebulized salbutamol 2.5 – 5 mg stat, (onset of action 30 mints)
- IV 10% Calcium gluconate 0.5 – 1.0 ml/kg (1:1 dilution) over 5 – 15 mints (Immediate onset of action)
- IV dextrose 0.5 g/kg (2 ml/kg of 25%) over 15 – 30 mints, then IV insulin 0.1 unit/kg (onset of action 30 mints) * insulin may not be necessary.
- IV 4.2% Na bicarbonate 1 mmol/kg over 10 – 30 mints, (onset of action 15 – 30 mints) NaHCO3 not considered useful unless metabolic acidosis is responsible for hyperkaliemia.
- Calcium polystyrene sulphonate (Calcium Resonium) 0.25g/kg oral Or rectally 4 times/day (maximum 10g/dose) [give rectally (NOT orally) in neonates   0.125 – 0.25g/kg 4 times/day] OR
- Sodium polystyrene sulphonate (Resonium) 1g/kg oral or rectally 4 times/ day (maximum 15g/dose)
- IV Frusemide 1 – 2 mg/kg (onset of action 15 – 30 mints) Useful in chronic hyperkalemia due to heart failure, hyperaldosteronism.

Asymptomatic hyperkaliemia (no ECG changes) – give calcium or sodium polystyrene sulphonate. Dialysis may be necessary to remove large amounts of potassium.

4. **Hyponatremia:**
    - Usually dilutional from fluid overload.
    - Treat if symptomatic or serum Na < 120 mmol/l (correct to 125).
      Aim to bring up serum Na level to 120 to alleviate symptoms, then correct over 24– 36 hours.
    - Na deficit (mmol Na) = 0.6 x body weight (kg) x (125 – serum Na)
    - Infuse deficit over several hours
    - Dialyze if above measure fails.
    - If asymptomatic treat with fluid restriction.

5. **Hypocalcaemia:**
    - Treat if severe or symptomatic, and / or if NaHCO3 is required for Hyperkalemia
    - Give IV 10% Calcium gluconate 0.5 ml/kg over 30 – 60 minutes with continuous ECG monitoring.

6. **Hyperphosphatemia**
    - Low phosphorus diet
    - Phosphate binders e.g. calcium carbonate (CaCO3) PO with main meals

7. **High uric acid:** Uric acid can precipitate in kidneys to further aggravate renal failure
    - Use Allopurinol
    - Urinary alkalinization

8. **Nutrition**
    Goals in managing nutrition:
    - i. Maintaining adequate caloric intake
    - ii. Avoiding excessive protein intake
    - iii. Minimizing phosphorus and potassium intake
    - iv. Reducing fluid intake (if applicable)

    Energy requirements during critical illness depends on basal requirements and Hyper-metabolism, the prediction of which can be determined by the following:
    Average energy requirements are same as daily fluid requirements are:

Weight (kg)	kcal/kg/day
0 – 10:	100 Kcal / Kg
10 – 20:	1000 + 50 K cal/kg
> 20:	1500 + 20/kg

    - Total parenteral nutrition via central line if enteral feeding is not possible; use concentrated dextrose (25%), lipids (10 – 20%) and protein (1.0 – 2.0g/kg/day).
    - If oliguric and caloric intake insufficient because of fluid restriction, start dialysis earlier.

9. *Hypertension: See relevant page on treatment of hypertension*

10. **Drugs:**
   Avoid using Nephrotoxic drugs
   Adjust doses or interval of amino glycoside, Cephalosporins and some penicillin according to creatinine clearance and drug levels.

11.6 Chronic Renal Failure

Definition: Persistent retention of blood urea nitrogen for more than 3 months duration

Classification: Based on GFR (glomerular filtration rate. Normal 80-120 ml. /1.73 m²/ minute)

Mild:	GFR >50 ml /1.73 m²/ minute
Moderate:	GFR 20-50 ml /1.73 m²/ minute
Severe:	GFR 10-20 ml /1.73 m²/ minute
End Stage RF:	GFR < 10 ml /1.73 m²/ minute

Causes:

Reflex nephropathy secondary to recurrent urinary tract infections during childhood contributes to 12-20 % of all end stage renal failure cases in adulthood

1. Intrinsic/Parenchyma renal diseases:
   - Chronic pyelonephritis
   - Reflex nephropathy
   - Chronic Glomerulonephritis
   - Inherited glomerulonephritis; Alport syndrome
2. Vascular renal diseases
   - Renal artery stenosis
   - Renal artery thrombosis
   - Renal vein thrombosis
3. Congenital and inherited renal diseases
   - Cystic diseases of the kidneys
   - Renal agenesis
   - Dysplastic kidneys
4. Obstructive uropathy

Clinical Picture:

- A symptomatic
- Oliguric renal failure in chronic glomerulonephritis with progressive symptoms
- Polyuric renal failure in obstructive, reflex nephropathy and tubular renal failure

Symptoms of chronic renal failure:

Symptoms do not develop until at least 70% of the renal functions are lost

- Anorexia, poor appetite and fatigability
- Nocturia
- Edema
- Hypertension
- Ecchymosis, epistaxis and mucous membrane bleeding.
- Growth failure
- Convulsions

Complications:

- Congestive cardiac failure secondary to fluid retention, hypertension and acidosis
- Anemia secondary to nutritional and Erythropoietin deficiency

- Renal osteo-dystrophy secondary to deficiency of vitamin D, hypocalcemia and secondary hyper-parathyroidism and hyperphosphatemia
- Hyperkalemia +/- arrhythmia
- Recurrent infections
- Growth failure and delayed puberty

Management:
1. Clinical evaluation
   - Check for Hypertension, edema, anemia
   - Intake / Output Chart
2. Investigations:
   - Urine microscopy for hematuria
   - Urine biochemistry for proteinuria
   - Chronic / Iron deficiency anemia
   - Biochemical renal function; Renal and bone profile, serum uric acid
3. Dietary management
   - Low protein diet: 1.2-1.5 gm/ kg
   - Calories 25 % above normal
4. Fluid, electrolyte and acid base management:
   - Oliguric renal failure: Fluid intake should be equal to urine output + insensible water loss (400 ml/Meter square body surface area)
   - In Polyuric renal failure, no fluid restriction
   - Limited Na, K, and phosphate intake according to blood level
   - Phosphate chelation by calcium carbonate tablets
   - Sodium bicarbonate to correct acidosis 2-5 mmol/kg/day
   - Diuretics therapy for edema
5. Prevention of complications
   - Antihypertensive as indicated
   - Vitamin D and calcium supplements
   - Hematonics and Erythropoietin supplements
   - Growth hormone therapy
6. **Dialysis**: Indications:
   1. Excess fluid retention/ pulmonary edema
   2. Uncontrolled hypertension
   3. Uncontrolled osteodystrophy
   4. Uncontrolled electrolyte imbalance
   5. Sever nitrogen retention (Uremia)

   Types of dialysis
   1. Peritoneal dialysis
      - Simple and well tolerated by children
      - Can be done at home by cycling dialysis or Continuous Ambulatory peritoneal dialysis (CAPD)
      - Recurrent peritonitis may result in dialysis failure
   2. Hemodialysis
      Hemodialysis is difficult in children because of difficulty in getting the vascular access (A-V fistulae). The hemodynamic effects are poorly tolerated by children leading to hypo tension, blood loss

1. **Renal Transplant** Is the optional therapy for chronic renal failure
2. Psychosocial care: CRF necessitate multi-disciplinary approach and extensive psychosocial support for the child and his family. Counseling should be entertained from diagnosis till transplant

11.7   Hypertension in children

Introduction:

In childhood, blood pressure (BP) normally rises with age, It varies with height, sex and age. Children, even very young babies, can develop high blood pressure. **The American Heart Association recommends that all children age 3 and older have yearly blood pressure measurements.** Early detection of high blood pressure will improve health care of children. High blood pressure is a major risk factor for heart disease and stroke in adulthood.

Definitions: (Refer to the Tables of BP centile readings in appendices section)

- **Normal blood pressure**: BP < 90th percentile for gender, age, and height.
- **Pre hypertensive**: Systolic and/or diastolic blood pressure (BP) between 90th and 95th percentile for gender, age, and height.
- **Hypertension**: Systolic and/or diastolic blood pressure (BP) > 95th percentile for gender, age, and height.
- **Sever hypertension**: BP >97th percentile for the child age, sex and height
- **Malignant hypertension**: Hypertension with organ failure (heart/ kidney/eye or CNS)
- **Accelerated hypertension**: A recent significant increase over baseline blood pressure that is associated with target organ damage.
- **Hypertensive encephalopathy**: is hypertension with change in the level of sensorium / convulsions.
- **Hypertensive emergency**: is a condition in which elevated blood pressure results in target organ damage (CNS, CVS and the kidneys).

Recognition of systemic hypertension in children and adolescents requires careful blood pressure measurement using **proper technique**. Blood pressure measurements are taken using a stethoscope and an arm cuff (Sphygmomanometer). Cuff bladder size is very important in accurate measurement of BP. The bladder of cuff should cover 2/3 of arm length and ¾ of mid arm circumference. A *small cuff always gives inappropriately high reading.*
BP should always be measured in sitting position and when child is not crying or too irritable. Sleeping BP is more reliable.

Ambulatory blood pressure monitoring (ABPM) is a test in which a portable device that takes blood pressure readings regularly is worn by the patient for an extended period (usually 24 hours). ABPM can identify children with 'white coat' hypertension, thus avoiding unnecessary diagnostic testing and treatment in these children.

Classification:

1. **Primary or essential** hypertension is more common in adolescents
2. **Secondary** hypertension with underlying cause is commoner in infants and children.

Causes of secondary hypertension:

1. Secondary transient hypertension in association with underlying disease
   - Acute glomerulonephritis
   - Hemolytic Uremic Syndrome
2. Secondary sustained hypertension

- Renal hypertension
    i. Renal Parenchymal disease. E.g. reflex nephropathy, chronic glomerulonephritis, Polycystic kidney disease, renal dysplasia
    ii. Reno vascular disease, e.g. Vasculitis, renal artery stenosis, renal artery thrombosis
    iii. Renal tumors

- Coarctation of the aorta
- Catecholamine-excess hypertension
    iv. Pheochromocytoma
    v. Neuroblastoma
- Corticosteroid excess hypertension
    vi. Congenital adrenal hyperplasia
    vii. Conn's and Cushing disease

Risk factors for hypertension in childhood
- Family history of high blood pressure in parents
- Childhood obesity
- Low birth weight
- Elevated salt intake

Clinical Features:

Symptoms:
Vary according to the underlying cause. Essential hypertension could be silent. Commonest features are:
- During infancy; congestive heart failure, failure to thrive, vomiting and irritability
- Headache is the most common presenting symptom beyond infancy, nausea, vomiting, tiredness, irritability, polyuria, polydipsia, growth retardation
- Features of malignant hypertension; visual impairment, lower motor neuron facial palsy, convulsions, loss of consciousness and hemiplegia.

Signs:
- Papilledema
- Absence of femoral pulse (Coarctation of aorta)
- Signs of congestive heart failure
- Signs of chronic renal failure

Investigations:
1. Urine microscopy for evidence of glomerulonephritis
2. Urine biochemistry for proteinuria
3. Renal biochemistry for acute or chronic renal insufficiency
4. Plasma cortisol Renin and aldosterone, urine and plasma catecholamines if clinical picture suggests
5. Electrocardiogram (ECG) for evidence of left ventricular hypertrophy
6. Echocardiography for Coarctation of aorta, evidence of LVH
7. Imaging
    - Renal Ultrasonography
    - Micturating Cysto urogram

- Radio nuclear imaging; Tc- dimercaptosuccinic acid (DMSA) or Tc- diethylen etriaminepentaacetic acid (DTPA) scanning
- Doppler study or MRI angiography for renal artery stenosis
- CT abdomen for pheochromocytoma and Renal tumors.

Treatment:

Most children with pre hypertension or mild essential hypertension will improve with modification of their life style; weight reduction, sodium restriction and exercise Drug therapy is indicated in moderate to severe secondary hypertension. Treatment Goals is reduction of systolic and diastolic pressure to < 90-95th percentile for gender, age, and height depending on the etiology and severity of the hypertension.

Primary hypertension
- Diuretics
- Angiotensin converting enzymes (ACE) inhibitors
- Calcium Channel Blockers
- β- Adrenergic blockers, e.g. Propranolol, Atenolol

Hypertension associated with proteinuria or/ and renal insufficiency:
- Angiotensin converting enzymes inhibitors (ACE) when hypertension is associated with proteinuria, e.g. Captopril, Enalapril and Lisinopril
- Diuretic for acute glomerulonephritis, in presence of congestive cardiac failure
- Vasodilator for acute glomerulonephritis, e.g. Hydral azine, Nifedipine and minoxidil.
- α- Adrenergic blockers for catecholamines excess hypertension, e.g. Phenoxy - benzamine, Phentolamine, Prazosin and Labetalol

Intravenous Labetalol is also useful in hypertensive emergency; doses should be titrated according to response

11.8   Urinary tract infection

Definition: Presence of actively multiplying organisms within the urinary tract.

Prevalence:

1 – 2% in girls
0.8 – 1% in boys
5% of girls below 18 years have had at least one episode of UTI in their life.

Etiology:
- Escherichia Coli
- Klebsiella
- Proteus
- Pseudomonas

Clinical manifestations:
- Asymptomatic
- Non-Specific: Failure to thrive, PUO, Secondary bed wetting, Prolonged jaundice in newborn,
- Pyrexia
- Bladder Symptoms; Dysuria, frequency and urgency
- Recurrent Abdominal or Supra-pubic Pain
- Hematuria

Clinical signs:
- Minimal
- Febrile
- Abdominal Tenderness
- Enlarged tender Kidneys
- Hypertension
- Sepsis

Diagnosis:

Urine Analysis: By dipstick or microscopy to look for:
WBC, RBC, Cast and Nitrates
Urine culture
Method of collection is very important
- Urine bag collection is highly associated with false positive growth
- MSU (Mid stream urine) / CCU (Clean catch urine)
- Catheter sample is most reliable
- Supra pubic collection is reliable in small infants

Significant culture result means $>10^5$ Colonies/ml of single organism especially when associated with presence of >10 pus cells

False +ve results are due to contamination of sample from gut or skin bacteria on perineum because of inadequately cleansed skin, bag specimen, delay in sending urine to lab leading to multiplication of contaminated bacteria.

False –ve. Results are due to prior use of antibiotics, over hydration and antiseptic use

CBC
> ‣ Increased WBC, Neutrophils
> ‣ Increase inflammatory parameters (ESR & C-RP) indicate pyelonephritis

Renal profile: Urea and Creatinine

Blood culture: to look for associated Sepsis

Management:
Management of UTI is not simple because of following difficulties:
- Asymptomatic bacteria
- Non-specific symptoms.
- Easy contamination of normal urine due to difficulties in sample collection
- Differentiation of lower from upper UTI
- Need to rule out underlying urinary tract anomalies
- Long term consequences like recurrent UTI, VU reflux, reflux nephropathy and renal damage leading to silent Chronic renal failure

Treatment of an acute episode of UTI:

Principles:
- Establish diagnosis early, don't use antibiotic prior to urine collection
- Prompt antibiotics treatment in full dosage and proper duration.
- If the child is sick, do not wait for culture results, just perform microscopy for pus cells and bacteria and commence treatment.

Choice of drugs:
Depends upon the organism and resistance pattern in the community.

Duration
Full dosage for 7-10 days.
There is no evidence that 14 days therapy decrease the recurrence rate or eradication.

Supportive care:
Fluids
Nutrition
Antipyretic
Avoid non steroidal analgesic, nephrotoxic drugs and contrast medium.

Further management:
Prophylaxis by low dose antibacterial is necessary after treatment of acute infection to keep urinary tract free from infection until preliminary investigations have been carried out to identify the cause of infection.

Recurrence:
50%   in 1 year
75%   in 2 years

Radiological investigations:

Every child who has documented UTI should have further work-up to prevent from progressive renal damage by observing the status of the kidneys, urinary tract and to know the underlying cause, including:

- Obstruction
- Renal Scarring
- Vesico Ureteric Reflux
- Other anomalies, etc

Decision about which technique to use is based on availability and experience of skills.

Imaging techniques:

1) **X-Ray KUB region:** Simple, but not usefull except for: Spina bifida or calculi

2) **Ultrasound examination:**
- To diagnose morphological disorders; hydronephrosis, hydroureter
- To assess renal size, volume and position
- Simple non-invasive, no radiation hazards

Disadvantages of Ultrasound:

No information about renal function, inflammation, renal scarring or reflux

On its own it does not exclude renal pathology

3) **Radio nuclear scan:**

A. **DMSA (Dimercaptosuccinic acid) for the study of renal structure**
- Provides functional images of the kidney
- Shows renal scarring
- Renal size and persistent focal defect
- Immediate study demonstrate infective renal involvement, repeat DMSA confirms permanent changes
- Low dose radiation 20-25%

B. **DTPA (Diethylin triamino penta acetic acid) for Renal functions**
- To evaluate renal blood flow, uptake and urinary excretion
- Estimate relative renal functions
- When combined with diuretics this can identify obstructive uropathy.
- Indirect Radio nuclear cystography (IDRC) to follow patients with VUR
- Sometimes difficult to differential between obstruction and dilatation.

C. **Micturating (Voiding) Cysto-urethrogram MCUG:**
- Indicates bladder structure, function and capacity
- Residual urine volume, bladder neck
- Intra renal reflux
- Vesico urethral reflux their grading and severity
- Post-urethral valves
- But the technique requires radiation and urinary catheterization

D.) Intravenous Pyelogram (IVU/IVP) :
- Comprehensive overview of renal anatomy
- Functional assessment in mild renal impairment
- Poor sensitivity to detect posterior renal scarring
- Available generally and easily explainable

E.) Urodynamic studies:
- Especially for neuropathic bladder
- To study function, measure detrusor activity
- Bladder pressure
- Urine flow

Patient Follow-up:
- Urine Culture monthly for 3 months, then every 3 months for 1-2 years, Repeat if symptomatic.
- Growth Assessment: Height, Weight and BP on every clinic visit
- Renal Function: Blood Urea and Creatinine in chronic cases
- Imaging: DMSA, DTPA, IVU - MCUG

Long term management: To prevent renal scars in high risk children:
- Children under age 2 years
- Recurrent pyelonephritis
- Pyelonephritis with urinary anatomic abnormality

Indications for inpatient admission:
- Sick or toxic children
- Risk of renal scar
- Febrile children under 1 year old

Long term antibiotic prophylaxis: The purpose is to prevent re-infection and further scarring.

Indications
1. Until all investigations have been carried out
2. Frequent and troublesome symptomatic recurrence
3. VUR grade I-III
4. If kidney is already scarred
5. First year of life – growing kidney
6. Post urethral implantation

Duration
1. If kidneys are not at risk, 6 months or less, longer if repeated infections
3. In VUR continue as long as reflux persists.
4. In Scarred kidney continue until the kidney are fully-grown.

Follow-up
Frequent recurrence of infection with resistant organisms during prophylaxis suggests dysfunctional voiding problems, which may require further studies of urinary function.

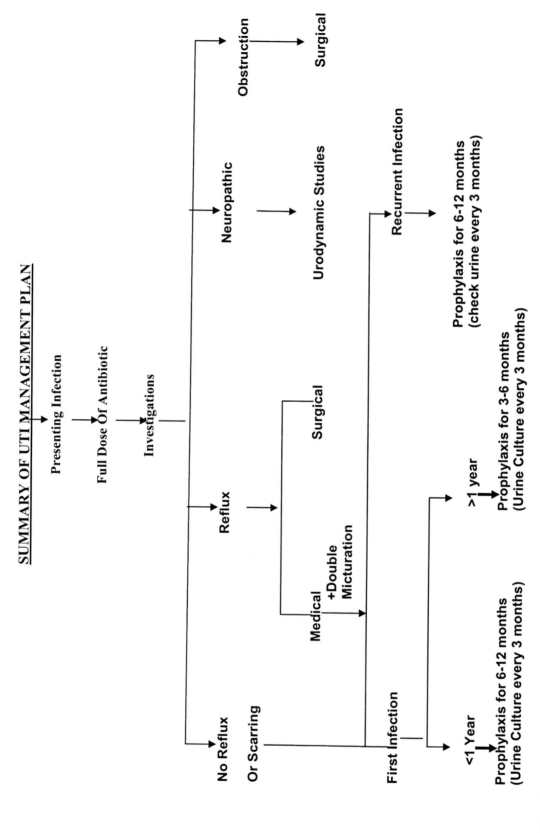

SUMMARY OF UTI MANAGEMENT PLAN

Presenting Infection → Full Dose Of Antibiotic → Investigations

No Reflux Or Scarring

Reflux

Medical +Double Micturation / Surgical

First Infection

<1 Year
Prophylaxis for 6-12 months
(Urine Culture every 3 months)

>1 year
Prophylaxis for 3-6 months
(Urine Culture every 3 months)

Neuropathic → Urodynamic Studies → Recurrent Infection → Prophylaxis for 6-12 months (check urine every 3 months)

Obstruction → Surgical

NB: Recurrence during Prophylaxis → Re-Investigate → Full dose of antibiotics and continue Prophylaxis for 6-23 months

12

Endocrine System

12.1 Diabetes Mellitus

Definition:
Diabetes mellitus is a clinical syndrome caused by relative or absolute insulin deficiency and/or insulin resistance and is characterized by sustained hyperglycemia and derangement of lipid and protein metabolism.

Classification (WHO 2000): It is based on etiology not on type of treatment.

> Type 1 (IDDM)
> Type 2 (NIDDM)
> - Obese
> - Non-obese
> - MODY
> IGT (Impaired glucose tolerance)
> Gestational Diabetes
> Neonatal Diabetes

Type 1 Diabetes is with evidence of Immunological pancreatic beta-cell destruction.

Type 2 Diabetes is caused by defects in insulin secretion and/or insulin resistance

MODY:
- Usually affects older children & adolescents.
- Not rare as previously considered
- Has specific mode of inheritance (AD)
- Not associated with immunologic or genetic markers
- Insulin resistance is present

Transient Neonatal Diabetes
- Observed in both full term & preterm babies
- Caused by immaturity of islet cells
- Polyuria & dehydration are prominent
- Baby looks well & feeds vigorously
- Highly sensitive to insulin
- Disappears in 4-6 weeks

Type 1 Diabetes Mellitus
The model of etiology of type 1 DM resembles that of Rheumatic fever. An immunologic reaction triggered by an environmental factor in a genetically susceptible subject leading to islet cells destruction and insulin deficiency.

Genetic factors: Multifactorial predisposition
- HLA markers & DQ57 Aspartate theory
- Ethnic differences
- Familial clusters
- Association with chromosomal defects and many hereditary disorders
- Association with blood group A (Kidd-locus)

Role of autoimmunity
- Presence of islet cell antibodies & anti GAD antibodies.
- Circulating immune complexes
- High autoimmune antibodies & Ig A and low interferon level.
- Cell Mediated Immune reactions in b-cells:
  - Lymphocytic infiltration
  - Immunofluorescence antibodies

Environmental factors
- Seasonal variations
- Migrant population studies
- Epidemiologic data
- Low concordance rate in identical twins (50%)
- Experimental animal models

Suspected causative agents
Viruses
  - Coxsackie B4, Reoviruses, EMV, EBV
  - Rubella, Mumps & Measles
Dietary toxins
  - Nitrosamine
  - Cyanide
  - Aflatoxin

Other modifying factors
1. **Insulin counter-regulatory hormones:**
   - Glucagons
   - Cortisol,
   - Catecholamine
   - Thyroxin,
   - GH & somatostatin
   - Sex hormones
2. **Emotional stress**

Impaired glucose tolerance (IGT):
- IGT is present when the blood glucose level (fasting, random or PP) is below the WHO defined diabetic cut-off levels, but are higher than the normal levels.
- Studies showed that 50% of subjects with IGT develop NIDDM while 30% revert to normal & 20% remained with IGT.

Other causes of Hyperglycemia

1. Pancreatic diseases
   - Hereditary relapsing pancreatitis
   - Cystic fibrosis
   - Beta-thal major
   - Hemochromatosis
   - Alfa-antitrypsin deficiency

2. Endocrine disorders
- Cushing syndrome
- Acromegaly
- Pheochromocytoma

3. Chromosomal defects
- Down syndrome
- Turner & Noonan syndrome
- Klinefelter syndrome

4. Genetic conditions
- Achondroplasia
- Prader-Willi syndrome
- Laurence-Moon syndrome

5. Metabolic
- Hyperlipidemias type III, IV & V
- Porphyrias

6. Neuromuscular disorders:
- Muscular dystrophy & myotonia
- Hereditary ataxia
- Lipodystrophy

7. Others
- Progeria syndromes
- Sickle cell anemia

8. Drugs
- Diuretics & antihypertensive
- Counter-regulatory hormones
- Psychotropic drugs
- Others: INH, Phenytoin and Indomethacin

Clinical Presentation
- Classical triad of polyuria, polydipsia & weight loss, if unrecognized child may present with DKA.
- Anorexia is more common than Polyphagia, which could be mistaken for Anorexia nervosa in teenage girls.

Diagnosis
- In symptomatic children a random blood glucose level > 11 mmol/l (200 mg/dl) is diagnostic. Refer child urgently to hospital for treatment
- OGTT is not required for diagnosis unless NIDDY or IGT is suspected.

Clinical course
- Diagnosis & initiation of insulin
- Period of metabolic recovery:
  - Hepatomegaly
  - Peripheral edema
  - Hair loss
  - Variation in visual acuity
- Honey-moon period
- Total insulin dependency

Honeymoon period:
- Observed in 50-60% of early diagnosed patients
- Due to compensatory efforts of remaining b-cell to increase insulin production temporarily
- Patient may be symptom free or require minimal insulin for about 3-12 months, if not recognized, hypoglycemic complications result. Honey moon eventually ends bringing insulin requirements at steady level

Treatment Goals
- Prevent death & alleviate symptoms
- Achieve biochemical control
- Maintain growth & development
- Prevent acute complications
- Prevent or delay late-onset complications

Treatment Elements
- Education
- Insulin therapy
- Diet regulation
- Exercise
- Monitoring

Educate child & care givers about:
- Diabetes
- Insulin injections
- Glucose monitoring and record keeping
- Life-saving skills, Recognition of Hypoglycemia & DKA
- Meal plan
- Sick-day management

Insulin treatment
Insulin types: Animal types (porcine & bovine) were used before the production of human-like insulin (semi-synthetic & DNA-recombinant types), recently more potent insulin are produced (e.g. insulin Lispro).

Insulin Action
Insulin decreases blood sugar by inhibiting hepatic glycogenolysis & gluconeogenesis and stimulating glucose uptake, utilization & storage by the liver, muscles & adipose tissue. Insulin being an anabolic hormone stimulates protein & fatty acids synthesis.

Insulin Types
- Short acting (neutral, soluble, regular)
  - Peak 2-3 hours & duration up to 8 hours
- Intermediate acting:
  - Isophene (peak 6-8 h & duration 16-24 h)
  - Biphasic (peak 4-6 h & duration 12-20 h)
  - Semi Lente (peak 5-7 h & duration 12-18 h)
- Long acting (Lente, ultra Lente & PZI) Peak 8-14 h & duration 20-36 h

Accepted insulin regimens
a. Twice daily: either NPH alone or NPH + Soluble insulin
b. Thrice daily: Soluble insulin before each meal and NPH only before dinner
c. Intensive 4 times/day: Soluble insulin before meals + NPH or PZI at bed time
d. Continuous s/c infusion using pumps loaded with Soluble insulin
e. Long acting insulin analog (Glargine or Lantos) at night along with two injections of short acting insulin (Lispro or Aspart) given at main meal times

Insulin availability
- Insulin is available in different concentrations 40, 80 & 100 U/ml
- WHO now recommends U 100 to be the only used insulin to prevent confusion
- Special preparation for infusion pumps is soluble insulin 500 U/ml.

Insulin Doses
Doses vary from person to person, depending on diet, lifestyle, and body weight.
- Total daily dose vary from 0.8 -1.5 units per kg of body weight.
- Frequent changes to the insulin dose may need to be made during adolescence or periods of rapid growth.
- A totally insulin-dependent **adult** needs approximately 0.7 - 1.0 units of insulin per kg of body weight per day

Insulin Syringes & Pens
- Syringes come in three sizes - 30, 50 and 100 units. Choose one large enough to hold the total number of units of insulin your child needs for each injection. Short needles (8 mm) are now available.

- **Reuse:** Studies have shown that syringes can be reused once without increased risk of infection. Do not touch the needle or clean with an alcohol swab. Usually after one day of use the needle is no longer as comfortable to use. If you are reusing syringes, clean after each injection to eliminate the traces of insulin from the barrel.

- **Injection Aids** are available to help overcome the fear of injecting the needle. Most devices hold the syringe and have a spring action that injects the needle through the skin. Ask your Health Care Team for more information.
  Sharing: Never use another person's syringe or needle.
  Disposal: The proper disposal of syringes is important to prevent injury to others. A needle clipper can be used to clip the needle off the barrel of the syringe. The syringe can then be thrown into regular garbage. You can also dispose of the entire syringe, with the needle attached into a puncture-resistant container such as a 'bleach/javel' (opaque) bottle with cap.

Insulin Pens
Pens offer an alternate method of preparing an insulin injection. Someone who is uncomfortable preparing a syringe, perhaps because of poor eyesight, may prefer pens. Pens are easier to carry around by teenagers.

Insulin is stored in a cartridge inside the pen. A needle is screwed onto the end of the pen at the time of each injection.

Insulin mixing is not required (as needed with the syringe); however, one pen will inject the long-acting insulin and a second pen will inject the short-acting insulin. As a result, you may need two injections before breakfast and two injections before supper.

368

Insulin Injections – Technique

Insulin must be injected into the fat layer that is just under the skin. The injection can be done on specific sites on the body. It is recommended that insulin be injected at the same site and same time of day for one week. For instance, inject the right thigh in the morning before your child is dressed, and the right arm at suppertime. The following week, switch to the left side. Rotation of the injection sites prevents hardening of the skin and changes in the absorption rates of the insulin.

Injection:

1) Once the syringe is prepared with insulin, wipe the chosen injection site with an alcohol swab and allow the skin to dry.
2) Gently pinch up the skin (optional), and inject the needle at a 90° angle.
3) Once needle has pierced the skin, release the skin if you are pinching, inject the insulin at a steadily, count to ten for the insulin to absorb and then withdraw the needle.

Insulin is absorbed differently from different sites e.g. highest from abdomen, arm and thigh and lowest from buttock

Insulin Pump

Insulin pump is a device about size of a "pager" fitted with an insulin cartridge. A catheter is inserted into the fatty tissue (usually abdomen) by a needle, the needle is then removed. Insulin is delivered through a narrow length of tubing through the catheter into the fatty tissue. The catheter need be changed every two to three days. The pump is programmed to deliver a "basal rate" of insulin every few minutes over twenty-four hours. Extra insulin is given as "boluses" for meals and snacks. The insulin pump is designed to mimic normal insulin release by the pancreas.

Although use of insulin pump means more freedom around food intake and activity, it is not for everyone. It requires good knowledge of carbohydrate counting and frequent testing of blood sugars. The child must be old and responsible enough to bolus insulin safely with meals. Pumps are also expensive, and not always covered by insurance. Sometimes using the "multiple injections" regime for insulin delivery can be an acceptable and cheaper alternative.

Insulin adverse effects
- Hypoglycemia
- Lipoatrophy / Lipohypertrophy
- Obesity
- Insulin allergy, Insulin antibodies

Diet Regulation
- Balanced diet with strict avoidance of simple sugars.
- 50-60% of calorie requirement should be obtained from complex carbohydrate.
- Distribute carbohydrate load in preferably 3 meals & 2 snacks
- Encouraged low salt, low saturated fats and high fiber in the diet.

Exercise
- Decreases insulin requirement by increasing insulin sensitivity & glucose utilization.
- It can precipitate hypoglycemia in the unprepared diabetic patient.

Monitoring
- Compliance (check records)
- HbA1C levels every 2 months
- Growth & development
- Well being, life style, School & hobbies

Practical Problems
- Injection sites & technique
- Insulin storage & transfer
- Mixing insulin
- Insulin & school hours
- Adjusting insulin dose at home
- Sick-day management
- Recognition & Rx of hypo at home

Complications
  Acute:
    Diabetic Keto Acidosis
    Hypoglycemia
  Late-onset:
- Retinopathy
- Neuropathy
- Nephropathy
- Ischemic heart disease & stroke
- Arthropathy & limited joint mobility
- Cutaneous lesions
- Impotence
- Associated autoimmune diseases

Dawn phenomenon: Early morning hyperglycemia due to counter effect of insulin by nocturnal growth hormone secretion. Managed by increasing evening dose of insulin.

Somogyi phenomenon: Nocturnal or early morning hypoglycemia leading to release of insulin counter regulatory hormone leading to a false morning hyperglycemia which may be wrongly interpreted as due to lack of nocturnal insulin dose. The actual treatment should be to reduce the night time insulin dose or to split the dose.

Important causes for poor diabetic control on insulin:
- Poor compliance
- Onset of puberty with rapid change in weight and emotional stress
- Obesity
- Infection
- Lipoatrophy at insulin injection sites leading to poor insulin absorption
- Improper Insulin storage

Advances in the Management
- Better understanding of diabetes allows more rational approach to therapy.
- Primary prevention could be possible if the triggering factors are identified.
- Chronic diabetic complication can be prevented by strict glycemic control.

Future Promises
- Final cure of IDDM is by successful islet cell transplantation.
- Primary prevention by a vaccine or drug will be offered to at risk subjects identified by genetic studies.
- Gene therapy will also be explored.

12.2 Diabetic Ketoacidosis

This is an acute life threatening condition. It may occur at presentation in a newly diagnosed patient or as a complication in a known diabetic patient due to following precipitating factors:

> Infection
> Social & psychological stress
> Erratic insulin dosing or ineffective insulin
> Poor treatment compliance

Clinically this present as an acute metabolic decompensation with exaggeration of diabetes symptoms + symptoms related to ketosis & dehydration (Abdominal pain, vomiting, severe dehydration, acidotic breathing, drowsiness & coma)

Ketoacidosis is a serious acute complication of diabetes mellitus. Always consult with a more senior doctor on-call as soon as you suspect Diabetic Ketoacidosis (DKA) even if you feel confident of your management.

Remember:	Children Can Die From DKA

Possible causes for death are:

Hypokalemia	This is preventable
Aspiration Pneumonia	This is preventable
Cerebral Edema	This is unpredictable and occurs more frequently in younger children and new diabetics. It has a mortality rate of around 80%. It occurs due to a rapid osmotic shift.

1. Emergency Management in A&E Dept.

1.1 General Resuscitation: A, B, C

• **Airway:** Ensure that the airway is patent and if the child is comatose, Insert an airway and contact the Anesthetist on-call.

• **Breathing:** Give 100% oxygen.

• **Circulation:** Insert an IV Cannula, take blood samples (see below) and start resuscitation.
If **shocked** (tachycardia, poor capillary filling, and hypotension) give 20-30 ml/kg 0.9% Saline as quickly as possible and repeat as necessary.

If drowsy keep NPO and if comatose or recurrent vomiting, insert N/G Tube, aspirate and leave on open drainage.

1.2   Diagnosis
Clinically Ketoacidosis is recognized by:
I)   **Symptoms**
          a) Thirst
          b) Polyuria & Polydipsia
          c) Abdominal Pain ± Vomiting
ii)   **Signs**
          A. **Acidosis:** (acetone smell of breath and
              Kussmaul breathing) Acidosis can lead
              to:
                   • Cerebral Depression
                   • Negative Inotropism
                   • Insulin Resistance and
                   • Peripheral Vasodilatation

          B. **Dehydration:** Estimation of dehydration as %. A recent clinic
              Weight may be available and will be more accurate when compared
              with present weight. Alternatively, a growth chart should be consulted to
              find the reference weight of a child of that age (the 50th percentile).
                   • 5%   Dry tongue, thirst, but generally well
                   • 10%   Above signs plus sunken eyes, decreased urine
                                   output, marked thirst, generally unwell.
                   • >10%   the above plus cool peripheries, capillary refill >2 sec,
                                   decreased BP & acidotic breathing.

          C. **Drowsiness or Coma**
          D. **Signs of infection**

1.3   Investigations
     A)   **Side Room**
               1)   BM: High or very high (usually > 15 mmol/L)
               2)   Urine: Glucose high or very high (3-4%)
                              Ketones high or very high (3-4+)
     B)   **Laboratory**
               1) Blood glucose: usually >15 mmol/L
               2) U & E, Creatinine, Bicarbonate
               3) ABG or CBG
               4) FBC
               5) Urine for glucose and ketones
               6) Blood/Urine/Stool/Throat Swab and CSF cultures <u>may</u> be indicated
               7) Chest X-Ray (if lower respiratory tract infection is suspected)

2.   General Management:
The nurse should keep a flow chart for fluid balance, clinical assessment, tests,
insulin regimen and progress.

2.1   Fluids Therapy
It is **essential** that **all** fluids given are documented carefully, particularly the fluid,
which is given in the emergency room, as this is where most mistakes occur.

• Fluid Volume

Once circulating blood volume has been restored, calculate fluid requirements as follows:

Total Fluid Requirement = Maintenance + Deficit

Deficit (Liters) = % Dehydration x Body Weight (kg)

To avoid over zealous fluid replacement, which may be a risk factor for cerebral edema, calculate deficit fluid as if the patient is no more than 10% dehydrated.

Maintenance Values

A) Calculate preferably using Weight

> First 10 kg x 100 ml per Kg
> Between 11-20 kg x 50 ml per Kg
> > 20 kg x 20 ml per Kg

•Add maintenance and deficit volume and give evenly over the next 36 hours:

> **Hourly Rate = Maintenance + Deficit**
> **————————————**
> **36**

• If the serum sodium is > 150 the deficit should be replaced over 48 hours. Because of the risk of cerebral edema, it is essential that sodium levels fall gradually.

2.1.1 Replacement Fluids

Irrespective of initial sodium level use 0.9% Sodium Chloride (Normal Saline), changing to 0.45% saline with 5% dextrose when blood glucose drops <12 mmol/L. Add potassium supplements as indicated.

Allow oral fluids in small amounts when child is not nauseated

2.2 Insulin Management

• Use only regular or Lispro Insulin
• Continuous IV Infusion is recommended
• Put 50 units Human Actrapid in 49.5 ml Sodium Chloride 0.9% Saline
 (1 unit/ml) and using a syringe pump runs at 0.1 unit/kg/hr initially.
• Check blood sugars every hour initially and then 2 hourly when stable.
 When blood glucose drops to 12 mmol/L, change IV fluids to 5% dextrose
 Dextrose/o.45% Saline as noted above.
• If blood sugar level drops to < 10 mmol or falls >4 mmol/hr decrease the
 Insulin Infusion to 0.05 u/kg/hr.
• When the child is fully conscious and acidosis is corrected (PH > 7.3) change to
• Continue with IV Fluids until the child is drinking well and able to tolerate food.
 The child can then usually return to his normal insulin and diet. Discontinue Insulin infusion
 30-45 minutes after the first subcutaneous injection to avoid rebound hyperglycemia.
• For newly diagnosed diabetic children, start the regular regimen as follows:

Total Daily Dose	**= 0.5 u/kg/day**
Morning Dose	**= 3/4 of Total Dose (Children <7 yr of age)** **= 2/3 of Total Dose (Children > 7 yr of age)**
Evening Dose	**= 1/4 or 1/3 of total daily dose depending on age.**

Morning dose is composed of 70% intermediate acting insulin (NPH), and 30% soluble insulin (Actrapid), while evening dose consists of 50% NPH & 50% Actrapid insulin.

Remember: **Insulin requirement during DKA is higher than the usual because of acidosis and infection causing insulin resistance.**
Insulin regimen should be reviewed every 4 hours.

2.3   Other Treatment

2.3.1   Potassium
Total body potassium is always low in DKA but serum level may be low, normal or high.
Supplementation should begin as soon as circulation is secured & patient has voided. Be   cautious if serum potassium level is >5 Mmol/l. Potassium should be added as 20 mmol per 500 ml bag till the child is acidosis free. If the serum potassium level is <2.8 or >5.6 mmol/L, the ECG should be monitored.

2.3.2   Bicarbonate
• Acidosis is correctable by fluids and insulin alone in most patients.
• If pH < 7.0 then 8.4% Sodium Bicarbonate 1 ml/kg as an infusion over 45 minutes may be used, preferably in ICU settings.
• Hazards of bicarbonate treatment:
  - Hypokalemia
  - Sodium overload
  - Rebound alkalosis
  - Paradoxical ↓ in CSF pH
  - ↓ Enzyme activity
  - ↓ Tissue oxygenation

2.3.3   Antibiotics: If indicated, after appropriate screening.

3   Ongoing Management:

3.1   Each urine sample should be checked for glucose and ketones. (Urinary catheterization should be avoided but is useful in the child with impaired consciousness).

3.2   Documentation of fluid balance is of paramount importance. All urine needs to be measured accurately and tested. All fluid input must be recorded.
If massive diuresis continues fluid input may need to be increased. If large volumes of gastric aspirate is obtained it should be replaced with 5% Dextrose/0.45% saline plus 10 mmol/l KCL.

3.3   Monitor the level of consciousness hourly by using **Glasgow Coma Scale.**

3.4   Check biochemistry, blood pH and laboratory blood glucose 2 hours after the start of resuscitation and then at least 4 hourly. Review of fluid composition and rate according to each set of electrolyte results.
Acidosis may not correct in the presence of inadequate hydration or occult infection.

On occasions, the measured level of acidosis may appear to worsen transiently as resuscitation is carried out because acidotic products are brought into the circulation.

3.5 Bedside blood glucose levels should be checked hourly whilst on an insulin infusion. If the blood glucose falls by >5 mmol/hour consider reducing the rate of insulin infusion. If this fails, slow down IV Fluid replacement, so that rehydration takes place over 48 rather than 24 hours.

3.6 A cardiac monitor should be used if potassium is below 2.8 or above 6.0 (as a bedside guide to potassium levels).

4. Cerebral Edema:

4.1 Signs and Symptoms Include
- Headache, Confusion, Irritability, reduced conscious level
- Seizures, small pupils/rapidly varying pupillary size, increasing BP, slowing pulse
- Papilledema (not always present acutely)
- Possibly respiratory impairment

4.2 Management of Cerebral Edema
Cerebral edema in DKA indicates a very poor prognosis and should be prevented or managed very carefully by following measures:
- The child should be moved to ICU (if not there already).
- Elevate the head side of the bed
- Give Mannitol 0.5 g/kg stat (= 2.5 ml/kg Mannitol 20% over 15 minutes),repeated doses of Mannitol (above dose every 6 hours) should be used to
- Reduce rate of fluids to half immediately and recalculate to 2/3 maintenance and replace deficit over 72 rather than 24 hours.
- IV Dexamethasone and Barbiturates are useful
- Arrange for intubation and if necessary hyperventilation to reduce blood pCO_2.
- Intracerebral pressure monitoring may be required.

Summary of Diabetic Keto-acidosis Management

EMERGENCY RESUSCITATION
ABC
• Give 100% oxygen
• If shocked consider plasma expansion
  (10 ml/kg of 4.5% Albumin or 25 ml/kg 0.9% saline)
• Insert N/G Tube as necessary

INITIAL ASSESSMENT
• Confirm diagnosis
• Assess degree of dehydration
• Look for signs of acidosis
• Determine level of consciousness
• Look for a precipitating cause

INVESTIGATIONS:
• Urine Glucose, ketones
• BM and Lab Blood Glucose
• UE, Creatinine, Bicarbonate
• Astrup (Blood Gas)
• FBC, Blood Culture, CXR as needed

SODIUM BICARBONATE
• Consider bicarbonate if blood pH is < 7.0
• 8.4% Na HCO3 1 ml/kg over 30 minutes
• Better under ICU settings

FLUIDS THERAPY
• Use sodium chloride 0.9% (normal saline)
• Rate/hr = $\dfrac{\text{Maintenance + Deficit}}{36}$
• Deficit (Liters) =% Dehydration X Body wt
• Maintenance = first 10 kg of wt x 100 ml
  Between 11-20 kg x 50 ml
  Any wt >20 x 20 ml
• Replace over 48 hours if initial sodium level is >150 mmol/L

POTASSIUM
• Add potassium if peripheral circulation is good and child is passing urine.
• Put 20 mmol potassium in each 500 ml bag till child is out of acidosis.
• If initial k level >5.5 mmol withhold & use Cardiac monitor.

INSULIN
• Add 50 units of soluble insulin (Human Actrapid) to 49.5 mls of Normal Saline (=1 unit/ml) and run at 0.1 units/kg/hour
• When BM is <12-mmol/l change IV Fluids to 5% Dextrose in 0.45% saline.
• When child is alert without acidosis change to 4 hourly sub cutaneous Insulin injections.

12.3 Disorders of Thyroid Gland

Anatomy

- Derived from pharyngeal endoderm at 4th week of gestation
- Migrate from base of the tongue to cover the 2nd & 3rd tracheal rings.
- Blood supply from ext. carotid & subclavian arteries and blood flow is twice the renal blood flow/g tissue.
- Starts producing thyroxin at 14 weeks gestation.

Physiology

- Maternal & fetal glands are independent with little trans-placental transfer of T4.
- TSH doesn't cross the placenta.
- Fetal brain converts T4 to T3 efficiently.
- Average intake of iodine is 500 mg/day. 70% of this is trapped by the gland against a concentration gradient up to 600:1

Thyroid Hormones

- Iodine & tyrosine form both T3 & T4 under TSH stimulation. However, 10% of T4 production is autonomous and is present in patients with central hypothyroidism.
- When released into circulation T4 binds to:
  - ✓ Globulin   TBG   75%
  - ✓ Prealbumin   TBPA   20%
  - ✓ Albumin   TBA   5%
- Less than 1% of T4 & T3 is free in plasma.
- T4 is de-iodinated in the tissues to either T3 (active) or reverse T3 (inactive).
- At birth T4 level approximates maternal level but increases rapidly during the first week of life.
- High TSH in the first 5 days of life can give false positive neonatal screening

Thyroid Stimulating Hormone (TSH)

- Is a Glico-protein with Molecular Wt of 28000
- Secreted by the anterior pituitary under influence of TRH
- It stimulates iodine trapping, oxidation, organification, coupling and proteolysis of T4 & T3
- It also has trophic effect on thyroid gland
- T4 & T3 are feed-back regulators of TSH
- TSH is stimulated by a-adrenergic agonists
- TSH secretion is inhibited by:
  - o Dopamine
  - o Bromocreptine
  - o Somatostatin
  - o Corticosteroids

Conversion of T4 to T3 is decreased by:

- Acute & chronic illnesses
- b-adrenergic receptor blockers
- Starvation & severe PEM
- Corticosteroids
- Propylthiouracil
- High iodine intake (Wolff-Chaikoff effect)

Total T4 level is decreased in:
- Premature infants
- Hypopituitarism
- Nephrotic syndrome
- Liver cirrhosis
- Protein Energy Malnutrition
- Protein losing enteropathy
- Drugs: Steroids, Phenytoin, Salicylate, Sulfonamides, Testosterone

Total T4 is increased with:
- Acute thyroiditis
- Acute hepatitis
- Pregnancy
- Drugs: Estrogen, clofibrate and Iodides

Functions of Thyroxin
- Linear growth & pubertal development
- Normal brain development & function
- Energy production
- Calcium mobilization from bone
- Increasing sensitivity of b-adrenergic receptors to catecholamine

Common thyroid disorders in children:

Goiter

It simply means enlargement of thyroid gland that is usually stimulated by TSH or by goitrogens.

Kilpatrick grading of Goiter
- Grade 0:   Neither visible nor palpable
- Grade 1:   Not visible, but palpable
- Grade 2:   Visible when neck is extended & on swallowing,
- Grade 3:   Visible in neutral position
- Grade 4:   Large goiter

Goitrogens

Food: Soybeans, Millet, Cassava, and Cabbage
Drugs: Anti-thyroid, Cough medicines, Sulfonamides, Lithium, Phenylbutazone, PAS, Oral hypoglycemic agents

Simple Goiter
- Enlargement of thyroid gland with normal function & without pathologic changes.
- Gland is homogenously enlarged without nodules.
- Usually seen in areas with mild iodine deficiency where iodized salts are not routinely used and is easily treated with iodine supplements.
- Also common in teenage girls and pregnant women due to the goitrogenous effect of sex hormones. It disappears spontaneously and no treatment is required.

Hypothyroidism

Epidemiology
- Neonatal screening reveals incidence that varies between 1-5/1000 live births
- The most common cause of preventable mental retardation in children
- Both acquired & congenital forms are linked to iodine deficiency
- Diagnosis is easy & early treatment is beneficial

Etiology
Congenital
- Hypoplasia & mal-descent
- Familial enzyme defects
- Iodine deficiency (endemic cretinism)
- Intake of goitrogens during pregnancy
- Pituitary defects
- Idiopathic

Acquired
- ✓ Iodine deficiency
- ✓ Auto-immune thyroiditis
- ✓ Thyroidectomy or RAI therapy
- ✓ TSH or TRH deficiency
- ✓ Medications (iodide & Cobalt)
- ✓ Idiopathic

Congenital Hypothyroidism
- Primary thyroid defect: usually associated with goiter.
- Secondary to hypothalamic or pituitary lesions: not associated with goiter.
- 2 distinct types of clinical presentations:
    - ✓ Neurological with MR-deafness & ataxia
    - ✓ Myxedematous with dwarfism & dysmorphism

Clinical features
- Gestational age > 42 weeks, Birth weight > 4 kg
- Open posterior fontanel
- Nasal stuffiness & discharge
- Macroglossia
- Constipation & abdominal distension
- Feeding problems & vomiting
- Non pitting edema of lower limbs & feet
- Coarse features, Dry, pale & mottled skin, Umbilical hernia, Hoarseness of voice, low hair line & dry, scanty hair, Hypothermia & peripheral cyanosis
- Decreased physical activity
- Prolonged (>2/52) neonatal jaundice
- Growth failure, Retarded bone age
- Stumpy fingers & broad hands

Neurological manifestations
- Hypotonia & later Spasticity
- Lethargy
- Ataxia
- Deaf ± Mutism
- Mental retardation
- Slow relaxation of deep tendon jerks

Skeletal abnormalities:
- Infantile proportions
- Hip & knee flexion
- Exaggerated lumbar lordosis
- Delayed teeth eruption
- Under developed mandible
- Delayed closure of anterior fontanel

Occasional features
- Overt obesity
- Speech disorder
- Impaired night vision
- Edema & Anasarca
- Decreased bone turnover
- Decreased factors VIII, IX & platelets adhesion
- Decreased GFR & hyponatremia
- Increased levels of CK, LDH & AST
- Psychiatric manifestations

Associations
- Autoimmune diseases (Diabetes Mellitus)
- Cardiomyopathy & CHD
- Galactorrhea
- Muscular dystrophy + pseudohypertrophy (Kocher-Debre-Sémélaigne syndrome)

Diagnosis
- Early detection by neonatal screening
- High index of suspicion in all infants with increased risk
- Overt clinical presentation
- Confirm diagnosis by appropriate lab and radiological tests

Laboratory tests
- Low (T4, RI uptake & T3 resin uptake)
- High TSH in primary hypothyroidism
- High serum cholesterol & carotene levels
- Anemia (normo, micro or macrocytic)
- High urinary creatinine/hydroxyproline ratio
- CXR: cardiomegaly
- ECG: low voltage & bradycardia

Imaging studies
- X-ray films can show: Delayed bone age or epiphyseal dysgenesis, Anterior beaking of vertebrae, Coxa vara & coxa plana
- Thyroid radio-isotope scan
- Thyroid ultrasound
- CT or MRI

Treatment
- Life-long replacement therapy
- 5 types of preparations are available:
  - L-thyroxin (T4)
  - Triiodothyronine (T3)
  - Synthetic mixture T4/T3 in 4:1 ratio
  - Desiccated thyroid (38 mg T4 & 9 mg T3/grain)
  - Thyroglobulin (36 mg T4 & 12 mg T3/grain)

- L-Thyroxin is the drug of choice. Start with small dose to avoid cardiac strain.
- Dose is 10 mg/kg/day in infancy. In older children start with 25 mg/day and increase by 25 mg every 2 weeks till required dose.
- Monitor clinical progress & hormones level

Prognosis
- Depends on:
  - Early diagnosis
  - Proper diabetes education
  - Strict diabetic control
  - Careful monitoring
  - Compliance
- Is good for linear growth & physical features even if treatment is delayed, but for mental and intellectual development early treatment is crucial.
- Sometimes early treatment may fail to prevent mental subnormality due to severe intra-uterine deficiency of thyroid hormones.

Hyperthyroidism

This is usually caused by autoimmune disease involving a multi-nodular goiter.
Excess TSH from the pituitary or T4 from a solitary thyroid nodule is less common.
Thyrotoxicosis is seven times more common in girls than boys and generally occurs in the pre-pubertal period. A family history of thyroid problems or other autoimmune diseases is common.

Clinical Features
- Behavioral problems, hyperactivity & agitation
- Tall stature, weight loss, diarrhea
- Tachycardia & Palpitations
- Intolerance to heat & Excessive sweating
- Goiter is occasionally present with bruit

- Tremors
- The term "Graves' disease is used when eye signs are present. These include proptosis, lid lag, lid retraction & ophthalmoplegia.

Diagnosis

- Levels of free T4 & free T3 are low while TSH level is very low or undetectable.
- TSH level does not increase following TRH injection.

Treatment

- Beta-blockers (Propranolol) control the acute symptoms and anti-thyroid drugs (Carbimazole, Methimazole or Propylthiouracil) suppress the overactive gland.
- If medical treatment fails Thyroidectomy or radioactive iodine therapy is necessary.

Thyroid Cancer

- Extremely rare in childhood
- May develop as a complication of a "cold" non-functioning nodule.
- Pathology is adenocarcinoma
- Treatment by surgery & radiotherapy.

12.4 Short stature

Children who have growth failure over a significant period of time develop short stature. This is defined as absolute height which is <3 SD below the mean for the age and sex or and or a linear growth velocity consistently < 5 cm per year from 2 to 12 years of age.

The key to the initial evaluation of short stature is a careful history and determination of the anthropometrics parameters over a length of time

History:

Whenever possible, obtain the original birth records to document length, weight, and Head circumference at birth

> Assessing the heights of both parents is absolutely essential: .
> Generally, men over report their height, and women underreport their weight.

Ideally, measure the height of each parent in the clinic for optimal calculation of the mid-parental target height, according to 1 of several formulae, among which the author prefers the following:

Target height in cm for a girl = [mother's height in cm + (father's height in cm - 13)] divided by 2.

Target height in cm for a boy = [(mother's height in cm + 13) + father's height in cm)] divided by 2

1. Document pubertal timing in first-degree relatives.
   - Determine the age at onset of menarche for the child's mother and the age of adult height attainment for the father.
   - These 2 milestones usually can be recalled by most parents and have proven reliable predictors of pubertal timing and tempo in parent-child pair studies of puberty.
2. Review of symptoms by organ system provides additional clues to the etiology underlying short stature.
   A. Gastrointestinal
   - Diarrhea, flatulence, or borborygmi (frequent, discomforting, or even audible peristalsis) suggest malabsorption.
   - Vomiting can suggest an eating disorder or a central nervous system (CNS) disorder (e.g., dysgerminoma).
   - Consider dietary intake and composition. In particular, ask about intake of carbonated beverages, juices, and other casual intake.
   - Pain or abdominal discomfort suggests inflammatory bowel diseases.

   B. Cardiac disease: Signs include peripheral edema, murmurs and cyanosis.

   C. Chronic infections: Poor wound healing and opportunistic infections are signs of potential immune deficiency.

   D. Pulmonary
   - Sleep apnea can be a cryptic cause of short stature.
   - Other chronic diseases that may result in short stature include severe asthma associated with chronic steroid use and cystic fibrosis (CF).

   E. Neurologic
   - Visual field deficits often herald pituitary neoplasm
   - Vomiting, early morning nausea, polyuria, or polydipsia often is associated with masses of CNS.

F. Renal
- Polyuria and polydipsia are important symptoms of hypothalamic and/or pituitary disorders and chronic renal disease.

G. Social
- Participation in sports requiring weight control (e.g., wrestling, crew, gymnastics) may uncover anorexia nervosa or bulimia induced by the patient, peers, or coaches.
- Growth often is impaired in refugees and in children emerging from foster care or certain international adoption settings.
- The growth pattern with adequate nutrition in a loving environment over time is critical to distinguish pathologic GF from normal variant short stature in such patients.

Physical Examination: Endocrinologists rely heavily upon accurate and reliable height assessment.
- Measure **standing height.**
- For children who cannot stand or recline completely (e.g., those with spina bifida, those with contractures), arm span provides a reliable alternative for longitudinal assessment of long bone growth.
  - Ascertain **arm span** by facing the child against a flat firm surface (usually the wall), fully extending the arms, and measuring the maximal distance between the tips of the middle fingers.
  - If this positioning is impossible physically, a flexible tape measure may be rolled along the dorsal aspect of the arms and upper back to determine arm span.
- Documenting **growth velocity** over time complements the initial height assessment.
  - Calculate growth velocity as the change in standing height over at least 6 months (for children) or in length over at least 4 months (for infants).Growth velocity less than **4-5 cm/yr between ages 3-10 yrs** is abnormal. During the first three year of life, rapid shifts in growth rate occur ,at puberty may see decline in growth rate just before adolescent growth spurt
  - Poor linear growth is defined as linear growth velocity more than 2 SDs below the mean for gender, genetic composition, and chronologic age.
- Weigh all patients.
- In infants, determine the fronto-occipital circumference.
- With suspicion of short-limb dwarfism, the **sitting height** can be obtained by measuring the upper body segment, or crown to pelvis, as the child sits upright on a platform-mounted stadiometer (or on the floor with a wall-mounted stadiometer).
  - Alternatively, the lower segment can be determined by measuring from the superior midline brim of the symphysis pubis to the floor, with the child standing (feet placed together).
  - The **upper-to-lower segment ratio** (US/LS) should be close to 1.
  - The ratio is greater than 1 in children with shortened limbs, as it is in individuals with hypochondroplasia or achondroplasia.
- Palpate for thyroid enlargement and firmness, which can be associated with Hashimoto thyroiditis, the most common cause of acquired hypothyroidism.
- Test visual fields for signs of pituitary and/or hypothalamic tumors, initially by gross confrontation.

- Inspect fourth metacarpals, which are shortened in persons with pseudo-hypo-parathyroidism.
- Inspect mucous membranes for ulcerative stomatitis, typical of Crohn disease and various trace mineral and vitamin deficiencies.
    - Pretibial ulcerations are seen with Crohn disease and ulcerative colitis.
    - Rectal tags and clubbing with Crohn's disease.
- Confirm the history with direct measurements whenever possible. For example, measure both biologic parents' heights during the clinic visit.
- Both the arm span and US/LS ratio can be informative regarding the cause of short stature. Patients with short limb dwarfism usually have an US/LS ratio less than 0.4.
- Arm span also detects a decrement in growth, which otherwise is indiscernible in a child with myelomeningocele.
- Carefully examine the midface dysmorphic features.
    - Associated anomalies of midline structures, such as the pituitary gland, are common in patients with major midline facial anomalies like bifid uvula or a single central maxillary incisor tooth.
    - Growth hormone deficiency or panhypopituitarism should be considered as a cause of short stature in such patients.

Types of Short stature (Classification):

There are many classifications for short stature, the classical one whichone, which used in many text bookstextbooks are to divide them into to three groups:

1. Short and thin (Non endocrine, Nutritional)

2. Short and obese (Endocrine)

3. Short and dysmorphic (syndromic)

The following classification is easy to follow:
- **Non endocrine causes** of short stature divided into 3 major categories as follows:
    - **Constitutional delay** of growth and sexual development
    - **Familial** short stature
    - **Chronic diseases:** malnutrition is the leading cause of short stature worldwide.
- **Genetic causes** of short stature are as follows:
    - Down syndrome (trisomy 21),
    - Ullrich-TTurner syndrome (45,XO)

Systemic causes of growth failure in children (partial list):

Gastrointestinal
Protein or caloric deprivation
Inflammatory bowel disease - Crohn disease, ulcerative colitis
Cystic fibrosis
Gluten intolerance
Protein-losing enteropathy

Endocrine (< 15% of cases)
Thyroid: Hypothyroidism, Primary - Hashimoto thyroiditis, Pendred syndrome
Pituitary: Growth Hormone deficiency
Pancreatic: Poorly controlled type 1 diabetes mellitus - Mauriac syndrome
Hypothalamic: Chronic hypernatremia - Hypothalamic adipsia, diabetes insipidus
Adrenals: Cushing syndrome, iatrogenic glucocorticoid administration, Addison disease

Genetic (known defect)
Down syndrome (trisomy 21)
Silver-Russell syndrome
Hypochondroplasia
Shwachman-Diamond syndrome

Pulmonary:
Cystic fibrosis
Severe poorly uncontrolled asthma
Chronic obstructive pulmonary disease
Restrictive lung disease

Cardiac
Hypoxemia
Congestive heart failure

Renal
Chronic renal insufficiency
Renal failure
Renal tubular acidosis

Psychosocial dwarfism
Chronic neglect
Starvation

Lab Studies:

Initial work up is limited to CBC, ESR, Urine analysis and renal profile to rule out occult anemia, renal diseases, UTI and chronic inflammatory diseases.

Further Investigateions are needed if:

Growth rate is abnormal,

Height is significantly below the genetic potential or less than 3rd percentile for age. or specific symptoms of systemic disease are present

> **Disproportionate failure in weight gain should direct investigations to conditions associated with under nutrition**

- Laboratory studies to look for the major causes of poor linear growth in children include the following:
    - o **Karyotype** by G-banding
        - The 45, XO pattern defines patients with Ullrich-Turner syndrome.
        - Because 10% of patients with Ullrich-Turner syndrome possess a mosaic Karyotype (e.g., 45, XO; 46, XX), counting at least 30 cells reduces the possibility of missing a patient with mosaic Turner Syndrome.
    - o Cautionary note about measuring serum levels of **Growth Hormone**:
        - Beyond the first months of life, endogenous GH is secreted in a pulsatile fashion. These intermittent peaks are greatest after exercise, and during deep sleep, therefore, **measuring a single, random serum GH value is of no use** in the evaluation of the short child.
        - Beyond the neonatal period, values obtained during the daytime are unlikely to be detectable.
        - While a random serum GH value greater than 10 mg/dl generally excludes GHD, a random low serum GH concentration does not confirm the diagnosis and requires to be confirmed by stimulation technique using Arginine or Clonidine.
        - **Insulin-induced hypoglycemia** is the most powerful stimulus for GH secretion; however, this test also carries the greatest potential for harm A safer **provocative testing** of GH is by using Arginine or Clonidine stimulation under the supervision of a pediatric endocrinologist.

    - o **Complete blood count** for hematological disease
    - o **ESR** for inflammatory bowel disease
    - o **Anti endomysial IgA and IgG**, transglutaminase IgG, and antigliadin IgG titers for gluten enteropathy (antiendomysialanti endomysial IgA is more sensitive, and IgG is more specific).
    - o Serum total **thyroxin (total T4) and thyrotropin (TSH)** levels to test for hypothyroidism
    - o **Sweat chloride** testing: Consider in short patients with a history of meconium ileus or pulmonary symptoms to exclude CF.
    - o Serum transferrin and pre-albumin concentrations for under nutrition

Imaging Studies:

- Antero-posterior radiograph of left hand and wrist to assess **bone age**. The more retarded the bone age ,greaterage, greater the likelihood of organic disease, particularly long standing hypothyroidism and the greater potential for catch up

- Bone age also useful to distinguish constitutional (bone age < chronological age) from genetic /familial short stature (BA = CA) growth delay

Treatment:
Treat underling cause of short stature.
In case of growth hormone deficiency subcutaneous growth hormone is given daily till the fusion of epiphyseal growth plate occurred

12.5 Ambiguous Genitalia

Definition:
Appearance of Genitalia which does not permit gender assignment in a child.
This includes infants with bilateral cryptorchidism, hypospadias with bifid scrotum, clitoromegaly, posterior labial fusion, phenotypic female appearance with palpable gonad (with or without inguinal hernia), and infants with discordant genitalia and sex chromosomes.

This is a neonatal emergency.
The commonest cause of AG is congenital adrenal hyperplasia (CAH)

There are two major concerns in dealing with such patients:
- 1. Underlying medical issues
  - Dehydration, salt loss (adrenal crisis),
  - Urinary tract infection,
  - Bowel obstruction
- 2. Decision on assigning sex of rearing and consequent psychosocial issues
  - Avoid wrong sex assignment and
  - Prevent gender confusion

Evaluation: Ideally, baby/child with parents should be brought to a competent team of experienced paediatric endocrinologist, surgeon, psychiatrist and geneticist.

History:
- Parental consanguinity.
- Obstetric: previous abortions, stillbirths, and neonatal deaths.
- Pregnancy: drugs taken, exogenous androgens and endocrine disturbances.
- Family History: Unexplained neonatal deaths in siblings and close relatives
  - Infertility, genital anomalies in the family
  - Abnormal pubertal development
  - Infertile aunts
- Symptoms of salt wasting in the first few days to weeks of life.
- Increasing pigmentation
- Progressive virilisation

Physical Examination:
- Dysmorphism (Turner phenotype, congenital abnormalities)
- Cloacal anomaly
- Signs of systemic illness
- Hyperpigmentation
- Blood Pressure
- Appearance of external genitalia
  - Size of phallus, erectile tissue
  - Position of urethral opening (degree of virilisationvirilization)
  - Labial fusion / appearance of scrotum
  - Presence / absence of palpable gonads
  - Presence / absence of cervix (per rectal examination)
  - Position & patency of anus
  - Psychosocial behaviour (in older children)

Investigations:

- Karyotypinge
- Ultrasound examination for uterus, vagina & urinary system
- Genitogram for female internal organs
- To exclude salt losing type of CAH

    Serial electrolytes after second of life
    Urine Na, K at the time of presentation
    ACTH stimulation test
    Serum 17-Alfa Hydroxyprogesterone (taken after the first day of life)
    Cortisol, Testosterone, Renin, Androstenedione
    24 - hour urine for pregnanetriol
    Testosterone, LH, FSH
- LHRH stimulation test (stimulated LH, FSH at 0', 30', 60')
- hCG stimulation (testosterone, DHT at Day 1 & 4)
- Androgen receptor study (may not be available)
- DNA analysis for SRY gene (sex-determining region on the Y chromosome)

Trial of Testosterone enanthate 25 mg IM monthly 3x doses to assess the response of the androgen receptor and the ability to convert testosterone to DHT.
This is done to demonstrate adequate growth of the phallus and is essential before a final decision is made to raise an ambiguous child as a male.

Algorithms Approach to Ambiguous Genitalia

Management:
Goals
- Preserve fertility
- Ensure normal sexual function
- Phenotype and psychosocial outcome concordant with the assigned sex

General considerations;

- Admit to hospital. Salt losing CAH which is life threatening must be excluded.
- Urgent diagnosis
- Do not delay decision on sex assignment
- Do not register the child until final decision is reached
- Protect privacy of parents and child pending diagnosis
- Counseling of parents that Intersex condition is biologically explainable.
- Encourage bonding

Gender Assignment:

Gender assignment and sex of rearing should be based upon the most probable adult gender identity and potential for adult function. Factors to be considered are:

- Underlying diagnosis
- Fertility potential
- Adequacy of the external genitalia for normal sexual function. A minimum phallic length of 2 cm is essential when considering male sex of rearing.
- Endocrine function of gonads. Capacity to respond to exogenous androgen.
- Parents' socio-cultural background, expectations and acceptance
- Psychosocial development in older children.

Decision about sex of rearing should only be made by an informed family after careful
evaluation, documentation, and consultation.

Gender Reinforcement:

- Appropriate name
- Upbringing, dressing
- Treatment and control of underlying disease e.g. CAH
- Surgical correction of the external genitalia as soon as possible

• Assigned female –

46,XX, 46,XY, Gonadal dysgenesis, True hermaphroditism
Requires removal of all testicular tissue and vaginoplasty after puberty
In girls, bilateral inguinal hernia is rare (femoral hernia is the rule). Always suspect the presence of gonads in such cases.

• Assigned male - 46XY

- Orchidopexy
- Remove all Mullerian structures
- Surgical repair of 'hypospadias'

12.6 Intersex disorders

Intersex or Hermaphrodites means discrepancy between gonadal morphology and external genitalia

Ambiguous genitalia means abnormality in external genital appearance not allowing sexual identification

Classification: based on the differentiation of the gonad following variations may be encountered:

1. Female pseudohermaphrodite - two ovaries
2. Male pseudohermaphrodite - two testes
3. True Hermaphrodite - ovary and/or testis and/or ovotestis
4. Mixed gonadal dysgenesis - testis plus streak gonad
5. Streak gonadal dysgenesis - bilateral streak gonads (dysgenetic gonad resembling ovarian stromal tissue. No germ cells.)

Pathophysiology:

The internal ducts and external genitalia may vary in development, since the presence of apparently male or female gonads does not necessarily correlate with the patient's gender identity. Chromosomal sex determines gonadal sex, which determines the phenotypic sex. **The type of gonad present determines the differentiation/regression of the internal ducts (i.e., müllerian and wolffian ducts) and ultimately determines the phenotypic sex.**

Gender identity is determined not only by the phenotypic appearance of the individual but also by the brain's prenatal and postnatal development.

Steps in sex differentiation:

Determination of genetic sex

Egg (23,X) + Sperm (23,X) = 46,XX genetic girl

Or

Egg (23,X) + Sperm (23, Y) = 46, XY genetic boy

The gonadal ridges can be easily recognized by 4-5 weeks of gestation. At that time, they already include the undifferentiated germ cells, which will later develop into either eggs or sperm. The formation of gonadal ridges similar in both sexes is a prerequisite step to the development of differentiated gonads. This organization of cells into a ridge requires the effects of several genes, such as SF-1, DAX-1, SOX-9, etc. If any one of these genes is non-functional, there is no formation of a gonadal ridge and therefore no formation of either testes or ovaries.

By 6-7 weeks of fetal life, fetuses of both sexes have two sets of internal ducts, the **Müllerian (female) ducts and the Wolffian (male) ducts.** The external genitalia at this stage appear to be female and include a genital tubercle, the genital folds, urethral folds and a urogenital opening

Determination of Gonadal Sex

XX fetus = ovary (with no SRY)

OR

XY fetus = testes (with SRY located on the Y chromosome)

Determination of Internal Ducts

Male's testes produce Müllerian inhibitory substance (MIS) that inhibits female organ

393

development. Testes also produce androgens that enhance male development (epididymis, vas deferens, and seminal vesicle).

High local testosterone levels appear to be necessary for Wolffian duct differentiation because maternal ingestion of androgens does not cause male internal differentiation in a female fetus, nor does this differentiation occur in females with congenital adrenal hyperplasia (CAH).

Female organs develop due to lack of MIS and testosterone.

External genitalia

The external genitalia of both sexes are identical in the first 7 weeks of gestation

Over the next 8 wks differentiation is moderated by testosterone, which is converted to 5-DHT by the action of an enzyme, 5-alpha reductase, present within the cytoplasm of cells of the external genitalia and the urogenital sinus.

Diagrammatic representation of development of external genitalia:

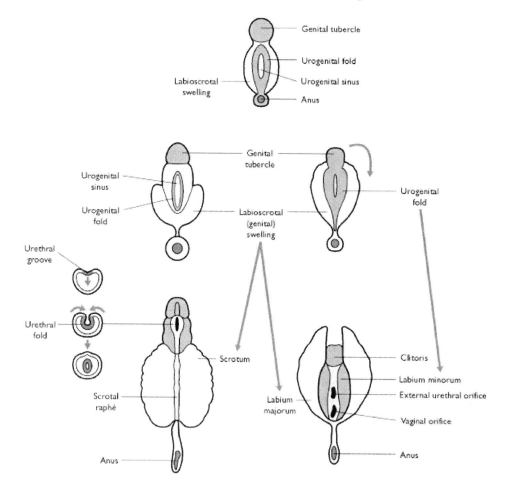

Clinical Evaluation:

History:

* A family history of genital ambiguity, infertility, or unexpected changes at puberty may suggest a genetically transmitted trait
* Recessive traits tend to occur in siblings, while X-linked abnormalities tend to appear in

males scattered sporadically across the family history
* History of early death of infants in a family
* Maternal drug ingestion is important
* History of maternal virilization may suggest an androgen-producing maternal tumor

Examination:
* External genitalia examination
* Note the size of the phallus, it may represent clitoromegaly or hypospadias.
* Note the position of the urethral meatus.
* Labioscrotal folds may be fused at the midline, giving an appearance of a scrotum.
* Rugose scrotal or labioscrotal folds with increased pigmentation suggest the possibility of increased corticotrophin levels as part of adrenogenital syndrome

Gonadal examination:
* Documentation of palpable gonads is important. Although ovotestis has been reported to descend completely into the bottom of labioscrotal folds, in most patients, only testicular material descends fully.
* If examination reveals palpable inguinal gonads, diagnoses of a gonadal female, Turner syndrome, and pure gonadal dysgenesis can be eliminated.
* Impalpable gonads, even in an apparently fully virilized infant, should raise the possibility of a severely virilized female pseudohermaphrodite with CAH.

Rectal examination:
May reveal the cervix and uterus, confirming internal müllerian structures.

Female pseudohermaphrodite

The causes include CAH (in 60% cases) or due to the effect of maternal androgen use
21-Hydroxylase deficiency: Accounts for 90% of CAH patients, 75% of patients have salt-wasting nephropathy. The disease is due to autosomal recessive mutation located on chromosome 6. Prenatal diagnosis can be done by noting an elevated amniotic fluid 17-hydroxyprogesterone during the second trimester or by HLA typing of amniotic cells.
Postnatal diagnosis is confirmed by an elevated serum level of 17-OHP taken after the second or third day of life to avoid false positive results due to normally high levels earlier.
Maternal androgens: Progestational agents or androgens are used during the first trimester of pregnancy, After the first trimester, these drugs cause only phallic enlargement without labioscrotal fusion. Ovarian tumors can also produce virilization of a female fetus.

Male pseudohermaphrodite

Caused by Isolated deficiency of Mullerian Inhibitory Substance or due to LH deficiency/resistance, Leydig cell agenesis, Leydig cell hypoplasia, Deficient testosterone biosynthesis, androgen insensitivity (causing testicular feminization syndrome) or 5-alpha-reductase deficiency

True hermaphrodite

In these cases both ovarian and testicular tissues are present usually as an ovotestis, a palpable gonad is present in 61% of patients; of these, 60% are found to be an ovotestis

13.1 Neurological Examination of Children

The examination of CNS is different for Newborn, infant and older children, this being due to the maturing nervous system. That is why some abnormal findings like up going planters may not be abnormal in small infants. The neurological examination in children from 5 years and above is as easy, like adults. The examination is also easy under one year but 1 year to 4 years requires special techniques; it may have to be done piecemeal requiring several sittings. The aim of examination is to find the site of lesion. In the history one must identify accurate onset and course of illness in order to limit the list of differential diagnosis.

The examination starts by close observation of the child while history taking allowing a free movement and activity of the child without interruption, this give the child an opportunity to demonstrate his skills freely, which may not be possible to perform voluntarily. Examine wherever the child is comfortable. You may need several sittings. You may need to examine in sleep/sedation. Leave the difficult procedures like hammers/tuning forks and gag reflex to the last. Sensations though an important part of neurological examination cannot be tested in detail below 5 years of age.

Examination of Infant (1 month to 1 year):

Head:
Observe the shape and size (circumference) of Head.
Look for the, fontanelle, and better note down the measurements.
Palpate for sutures.
Look at the face and see if there are any particular dysmorphic features.
.
Examination of Cranial nerves: Is done by Colored toys etc.

Olfactory nerve testing is not possible at this age.

The **visual following** of toys tests vision, eye movements, and nystagmus. Use a bright pen torch for pupillary reaction. One can check gross visual acuity from a distance.

Observe for Jaw deviations on opening of mouth or yawning or crying and also note any wasting of masseters and temporalis muscles. This tests motor part of the **5th nerve**. With a fine and sterilized wick of cotton Conjunctival/ corneal reflex is tested (5th sensory or afferent and 7th nerve efferent or motor part).

Facial deviation on smiling/crying or eye closure difficulty helps to note weakness of **7th nerve**.

Hearing (**8th nerve**) can be tested by toy, loud clap and calling name or by proper **distraction test**. The auropalpebral reflex (to observe eye closure on loud clap) tests 8th afferent and 7th nerve efferent.

9th and 10th nerves are tested together and indirect things help in localization. The Secretions drooling, feeding difficulties, choking suggest tenth nerve dysfunction and gag reflex differentiates bulbar weakness from pseudo bulbar palsy. A poor or no response on touching posterior pharyngeal wall and hanging palate suggests 10th nerve dysfunction.
Head deviations, neck retractions, and wasted sternomastoid are seen in **11th nerve** lesions.

Tongue wasting, Fasciculations, deviation suggest weakness of **12th nerve**. While observing the fasciculation normal undulations of tongue have to be kept in mind. Fasciculation are commonly seen in Spinal muscular atrophy most of the times and occasionally in posterior fossa tumor.

Co-ordination:
Tested by approach to toys. Reaching for toy and taking to mouth (all these can be done when the child is with mother/mother's lap). Make the child to sit and look for trunk ataxia.

Motor system/ musculoskeletal:
The examination is grouped under Inspection, Tone, Power and Reflexes..
Inspection: Look for posture, abnormal movements, wasting, shortening, contractures, pseudohypertrophy, fisting etc.
Tone: One can check tone by flexing and extending, shaking, and rolling limbs across joints.
Power: MRC grades are difficult but one can make an approximate guess about the grades. Approach to objects, holding of toys pull and kicking response should be observed carefully.
Traction test performed in supine position, head and trunk are lifted by pulling both arms up, normally the head should come in line with trunk but in a hypotonic child you will not a marked head lag.

Vertical suspension is performed by lifting the child vertically while holding him at axilla. It assesses the tone and power of the proximal joints at the shoulder level. If there is hypotonia or severe weakness the child appears to slip through the examiners hand.

Reflexes:
Lying on mothers lap or wherever the child is comfortable. Put the limbs almost in semi-flexed posture.
Superficial reflexes: abdominal, cremasteric and planters.
Neonatal reflexes: Most of the neonatal reflexes disappear by 6 months of age. Their persistence suggests delay in maturation and anything, which damages brain.
Sensations: definitely difficult in children. Never pinch a child to test sensation without permission from parents or explanation. Most of the time parents have noted loss of sensation or else ask them to pinch for you. You could tickle to note the sensation. For pain ask mother to demonstrate it.

Examination of 1 to 4 years old children

While history taking is on, observe for abnormal movements, preference of hands, vision – on response to objects/toys, see him playing,
Examine him in sitting, standing and even in mother's lap.
Observe for co-ordination and other cerebellar signs.
For examination of gait, ask parents to accompany or stay at the other end.

Examination of >4 years old children

The neurological examination is like adults, with some help from parents for higher functions.

Higher mental functions: Observe for appearance, behavior, speech, and comprehension of spoken speech, orientation to time, place and person

Memory: look for attention, immediate memory, recent memory and past memory

Abstract/Judgment.: by giving idioms or problems.

Cranial nerves:

Olfactory, (1st): Exclude rhinitis or nose block, explain what you are performing, initially eyes open and then, eyes closed and each nostril separately. Use coffee or Soap. Avoid scents or irritating agents.

Optic nerve: Visual acuity, Field of vision, Color vision, Funduscopy.

3rd, 4th and 6th.: Check eye movements, Pupillary reflex (optic nerve –afferent and 3rd efferent.)

Trigeminal (5th) nerve: Motor: observe jaw opening/closure. Opening jaw against force, wasting of masseters and temporalis muscle. Sensory part is tested by checking the sensations on the face. Corneal reflex is tested by fine cotton wick.

Facial (7th) nerve: UMN: Lower half of face is involved therefore patient can wrinkle forehead by asking him to follow a toy upward. Bells phenomenon is absent and EMG is negative.

In **LMN** type: Complete half, deviations of face to normal side, Bells phenomenon (eye balls move up on eye closure), wasting is seen, EMG is neurogenic type.

8th (auditory) nerve: Loud speech. Each ear tested separately, whisper, Clock, tuning fork test. Auro-palpebral reflex: Closure of eyes on clapping noise (afferent 8th and efferent 7th).

9th (glossopharyngeal) and 10th (vagus): Phonation. Uvula deviation/fall. Oral secretions (Drooling), Gag reflex. (Afferent 9th and efferent 10th). Differentiate bulbar from pseudo bulbar palsy.

11th Accessory nerve: Head deviation/tilt, wasting of sternomastoid. Force against resistance to sides and lifting of shoulders. Neck flexion.

12th (hypoglossal) nerve: Deviation of tongue on protrusion to the weaker side (contrast to facial weakness). Rapid side to side & to/fro movements of the tongue and on force against cheek.

Motor system: To examine neck muscles, Upper and lower limbs, check deep tendon reflexes and the superficial reflexes. Check for co-ordination/cerebellar signs by finger nose test, finger-to-finger approach, quick supination and pronation, heel–knee-shin test, Deep tendon reflexes are pendular or hung up jerk is observed in cerebellar diseases.

Gait is examined by walking normally on a straight line, followed by toe and heel walking and asking to make a quick turning around.

Interpretation:

The aim of neurological examination is to localize the site of lesion. One needs to determine if the lesion an upper motor neuron or lower motor neuron? For **UMN**, one has to further locate if it is at the level of cortex, white matter, basal ganglia, brainstem, cerebellum, or spinal cord. For **UMN** the diagram below give you a quick and mathematical approach to the site of lesion.

For **LMN** one has to further locate the lesion if it involves anterior horn cell, spinal roots, peripheral nerves, neuromuscular junction or muscles. Keep in mind the joints and tendon diseases may also mimic weakness.

Cortex (1): Asymmetrical weakness, seizures, mental memory changes, and speech involvement.
White matter (2): Gait problems, deficit more than cortex, visual dysfunction.
Internal capsule (3): Dense hemiplegia, hemi anesthesia, hemianopia.
Basal ganglia (4): Abnormal movements, rigidity.
Brainstem (5): Cranial nerves one side and weakness opposite/ bilateral cranial nerves and bipyramidal signs. Unconsciousness.
Spinal cord (6): LMN at the site of lesion, UMN below. Bilateral signs. Level from the Sensory / motor / reflex. Bladder and bowel involvement.

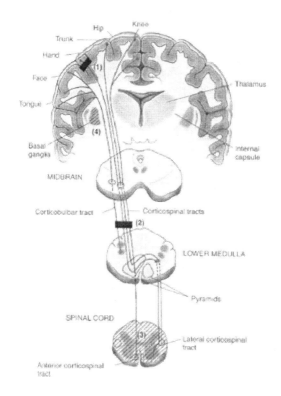

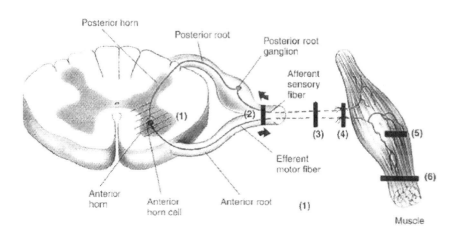

Differentiation of various LMN lesions:

	AHC (1)	N/R (2/3)	Muscle (5)	NMJ (4)
Symmetry	Asymmetrical.	Distal	Proximal	Cranial nerves
Wasting	+	+	- or Symet.	—
Pseudohypertrophy	-	-	+	-
Fasciculations	+	+/-	-	-
DTR	-	-	+	+
Sensations	N	Lost	N	N
CK	N	N	High	N
NCV	N/ V	V	N	N
EMG	Neurogenic	Neurogenic	Myopathic	Decremental
Biopsy	Neurogenic	Neruo/inflam	Myo/dys/infl	EM

AHC- Anterior horn cells, CK- Creatinine kinase enzyme, EMG- Electromyogram NCV- Nerve conduction velocity, NR- Nerve root, NMJ- Neuro muscular junction,

Asym- asymmetrical, Symet- symmetrical, + yes, - No, N – normal, ^^- raised, V-reduced, neuro- neurogenic, inflam- inflammatory, myo- myopathic, EM- electron microscopy.

13.2 Approach to a floppy infant

Normal tone is dependent upon the intactness of the spinal reflex arc, which is under several supra-spinal influences (Corticospinal tract, reticulospinal tract, cerebellospinal tract). The corticospinal tract and the cerebellospinal tracts are important for the maintenance of normal muscle tone.

Clinical Features:
Muscle tone is defined as the normal resistance felt in the resting muscle. Clinically It is determined by three methods:
- Flexing and extending at the joints passively
- Rolling of an extended limb and
- Shaking of the limb.

Floppiness stands for decreased tone or hypotonia. It manifests in certain postures:
- Typical hanging jaw
- Frog like posture while child is laying supine
- Head lag on traction and
- Child slipping through hands on vertical suspension

Etiology:

Floppiness or hypotonia is a constellation of signs not diagnostic of any particular site of lesion. It is more often seen in **lower motor neuron lesions**; however one must not forget that the upper motor neuron lesions can also produce hypotonia, especially during the acute phase of CNS insult (cerebral/spinal shock). **Central hypotonia** is also seen in hypotonic cerebral palsy and cerebellar disease.
While examining a child with hypotonia, always look for the dysmorphism and laxity of joints, as certain syndromes like downs syndrome and Ehler Danlos syndrome can present with severe hypotonia.
Exaggerated deep tendon reflexes, up-going planters are features of upper motor neuron lesion and intact normally elicited reflexes suggest muscle disease. The rest of the findings will differentiate site of lesion (see chapter on neurological localization).

Investigations: Depend on the site of lesion. However following investigations are done in all.

> Serum creatine kinase
> Nerve conduction velocity
> EMG if indicated
> Chromosomal study in a Dysmorphic child
> Specific tests are done depending upon the suspected diagnosis.

13.3 Acute flaccid paralysis

The term stands for sudden onset of hypotonic weakness due to varying etiology. The weakness may be due to lesion in lower or upper motor neuron, joints, ligaments or bones leading to painful walk or limp.

Under **WHO program** of polio eradication, any acute flaccid paralysis case have to be identified and referred to the designated hospital to rule out polio as underlying cause. All cases mimicking polio caused by whatever etiology need to be referred from all over the country to a designated centre (SQU in Oman) to be examined and investigated to exclude polio. Every suspected case need to undergo a thorough neurological and laboratory testing. In addition to neurophysiology work up two stool samples have to be collected (as early as possible, preferably within twenty four hours), sent to the central viral laboratory (Darsait laboratory) for polio virus isolation. This program was started in Oman in 1990. The last case of poliomyelitis was seen in Oman in 1994, however in September 2005, two cases of poliomyelitis were seen from Salalah. These were two brothers living in Yemen and were un-immunized for polio.

Clinical presentation and Differential Diagnosis:
Please refer to the chapter on floppy child

Investigations: Depend upon the site of lesion; however following investigations are done on all cases:

> Sickling test
> Serum creatine kinase
> Nerve conduction velocity
> EMG if indicated
> Two stool specimens within one week of illness (preferably 24 hours apart) for virus culture mainly poliovirus.

Counseling:
Parents need explanation for transfer to SQUH and need for particular set of investigations. The parents have to be informed about their anxiety about diagnosis of poliomyelitis. They might have been told about this diagnosis in peripheral referring hospital.

13.4 Ataxia and Movement disorders

Ataxia is defined as disturbance in fine control of posture and movements.

Control of Balance and sites of involvement:
The cerebellum and its major input system, from the frontal lobes and the posterior column of spinal cord, normally control the posture and movements. Any cause that disturb this axis, results in ataxia. The cerebellum has two lobes (hemispheres) and central vermis. The two lobes have three components, neocerebellum, paleocerebellum, and archicerebellum.

Lesion of **vermis** produces truncal ataxia and titubations. The child cannot sit unsupported and shakes from side to side.
In lesions of **cerebellar hemispheres** there is tendency to fall towards the side of lesion with dysmetria and hypotonia on the same side.
Other features of cerebellar disease are ataxic **gait,** a wide-based, lurching and staggering. The **speech** is scanning i.e. there is increased separation of syllables.
There will be limb and ocular **dysmetria**, finger nose and finger-to-finger ataxia and **intention tremors**.
Frontal lobe lesion may produce signs and symptoms similar to those of Cerebellar disease.

Differentiation between Cerebellar and Sensory ataxia: The sensory ataxia is due to loss of sensory input to the cerebellum because of peripheral nerve or posterior column disease. The gait is wide-based, high stepping. The patient often looks at the feet to know their position on ground and in space. Position and vibration sense is also impaired. The in coordination tends to increase on closing the eyes. (Positive **Rhomberg's test**). The speech is normal.

Etiology:
Ataxia may be **acute, chronic or recurrent**. The recurrent may start initially acutely.

A. Acute ataxia:
> Post infectious
> Drug ingestion
> Miller Fisher syndrome
> Myoclonic encephalopathy
> Neuroblastoma
> Brain stem encephalitis
> Trauma/ hematoma
> Vertebrobasilar occlusion
> Rarely hemorrhage in brain tumor.

Post-infectious cerebellitis:
Acute ataxia occur in children who were previously healthy, it starts with dizziness, nausea and vomiting followed by nystagmus, intention tremor, imbalance and staggering gait. It is usually seen in children between 2 to 7 years with a very sudden onset. It is thought to be due to an autoimmune response to the viral agent e.g. Varicella, infectious mononucleosis or other viral infections (polio, mumps, Coxsackie, herpes, simplex or ECHO viruses). Symptoms are non – progressive

for a couple of days or weeks and then subside. (Recovery may take 3 weeks to 5 months). It is usually a self-limiting disease and the recovery is usually complete. It is a diagnosis of exclusion. Ataxia is maximum at the onset. Clear sensorium is there and nystagmus if present will be mild. Pure ataxia of trunk and limbs with mild nystagmus is usually associated with complete recovery on the other hand marked nystagmus, tremor of head, irritability, is likely to be followed by persistent neurological sequel. No treatment is required; sometimes a short course of steroids may be given.

Accidental drug ingestion:

Incidence is highest between 1 and 4 years of age.

Overdose of hypnotics, tranquilizers, toxic doses of anticonvulsants especially Phenytoin and carbamazepine may cause ataxia and nystagmus.

Acute intoxication with glue, solvents, petrol sniffing, alcohol ingestion and antihistamines may also cause ataxia.

It is diagnosed on the basis of history and urine examination for drug metabolites and blood for toxic analysis.

Management usually involves care for ABC, intravenous fluids and occasionally dialysis.

Encephalitis (brainstem) / Viral encephalitis of posterior fossa:

Clinical features are cranial nerve dysfunction and ataxia.

Course is variable from complete recovery to considerable neurological impairments. For diagnosis: Lumber Puncture shows mononuclear leucocytosis and normal to high proteins. Evoked auditory potential will be prolonged. EEG is normal

B. Recurrent ataxia: Uncommon, usually seen in:
Migraine
Metabolic disorders:
>   Pyruvate metabolism disorder/ Pyruvate dehydrogenase deficiency
>   Hartnup's disease
>   MSUD (Maple Syrup Urine Disease).

C. Acute ataxia with prolonged or intermittent course:
>   Myoclonic Encephalopathy
>   Neuroblastoma syndrome (Dancing eye dancing feet syndrome)
>   Brain Tumors
>   Multiple sclerosis
>   Metabolic disorders

D. Chronic or progressive ataxia:
>   Brain tumors
>   Congenital malformations
>   Hereditary ataxias like ataxia telangiectasia, Friedreich ataxia

Ataxia telangiectasia is a disorder of DNA repair affecting nervous and immune systems. This condition is inherited as Autosomal recessive mode and defect is located to chromosome 11. The clinical features are progressive truncal ataxia that begins during the first year. There may be delay in motor development and oculomotor dyspraxia. The intellectual development is normal at first but lags with time. Telangiectasia on bulbar conjunctiva develops after 2 years of age and some time as late as 10 yrs. Subsequent deterioration with many requiring wheelchair in early adolescence. Chronic sino-pulmonary infection due to low IgA. IgE, IgG are also very low and may be absent. IgM may be elevated. Due to chromosomal breakage, increased incidence of neoplastic complications esp. ALL is there. Elevated serum alpha-fetoprotein serves as tumor marker. These patients have an increased WBC sensitivity to irradiation, which can be used diagnostically, and to identify heterozygotes carriers.

Friedreich ataxia: The most common inherited ataxia. It is caused by unstable trinucleotide repeat sequence on chromosome 9. The size of the triplet expansion correlates with an earlier age at onset and more rapid progression. The onset is usually between 2-16 yrs. Initial feature is ataxia or clumsiness in 95%. Over time there is steady deterioration with most patients confined to wheelchair by 20 yrs. Dysarthria, areflexia, dysdiadochokinesia develop in almost all patients. Extensor plantar responses in 90%, joint position and vibration sense absent in the feet in 90% and in hand in 30%. Pes cavus, scoliosis, cardiomyopathy, optic atrophy and diabetes may also present. The Management is symptomatic.

Movement disorders

They are stereotyped movements caused by extra pyramidal dysfunction, they disappear in sleep, EEG is normal and there is no associated loss of consciousness.
These movements may be at rest or on action and could be controlled by force

Chorea

Rapid and coarse movements affecting proximal part of limb, the movements are repetitive but not stereotyped or rhythmic. The movement migrates from site to site and from limb to another.
It has no specific form.
Milking sign: Alternate tightens and loosens of the grip is a sign to be found in these patients and to be learned by experience.
The tongue is difficult to maintain in protruded position.
Pronation of hands on raising the arms above head.
The chorea may be of one side (hemi chorea).

Etiology:
> Sydenham's chorea (rheumatic fever)
> Drug induced
> Genetic conditions: Huntington disease, Ataxia telangiectasia, benign familial chorea, and Autosomal dominant form
> Systemic disorders: Hyperthyroidism, SLE and Pregnancy

Athetosis

This is slow writhing movement of the limbs, more distal, if without chorea it is almost always due to prenatal brain injury, asphyxia or kernicterus.

Ballismus

Is a rare but high amplitude violent flinging of a limb from the shoulder or the pelvis. In children it is almost always associated with chorea and is seen in SLE and Sydenham's chorea.

Tardive dyskinesia

Is a complex syndrome characterized by buccolingual masticatory movements; lips smacking, puckering, and chewing. The usual causes are the psychotropic drugs, e.g. Phenothiazines, haloperidol, obsessive-compulsive psychosis, theophylline and antiemetics.

Dystonia

Is a sustained muscle contraction. It may be of the limbs and spine or whole body (also called focal, segmental and generalized). Commonly seen in children in post hypoxic ischaemic encephalopathy. It can be seen in genetic condition called Dystonia muscularis deformans.

Myoclonus

Encompasses several involuntary movements characterized by rapid muscle jerks. It may be single muscle, a group of muscles or whole body. Myoclonus can be seen in anxiety, sleep, or be exercise induced. This may be a familial essential type or be epileptic. It can be symptomatic due to drugs, basal ganglia degeneration, post injury, metabolic: hepatic and renal failure

Tics

Are simple or complex stereotyped repetitive movements (motor tics), or verbal tics that are brief, and purposeless. These movements can be suppressed voluntarily.
A combination of motor and vocal/verbal tics is called Tourette syndrome.

13.5 Febrile Seizures (convulsions)

Definition:

International League against Epilepsy (ILAE) defines the febrile seizures as seizure associated with fever in absence of a CNS infection or electrolyte imbalance in a child between 6 months to 6 years (median, 18 months) age. Normal or Abnormal neurological examination before seizure is not a criteria anymore.

Simple Febrile Seizure is generalized, brief and usually single.
Complex febrile seizure: if seizures are:
1) Focal or Partial
2) Prolonged (more than 15 minutes)
3) If multiple during same episode of fever (prior neurological status is not a consideration) and
4) If there is a febrile Status
About ten percent of all febrile seizure are complex in nature

Epidemiology:

This is the most common and quite worrisome problem from parent's perspective.
2-4 % of Pediatric population in USA & Europe (AAP 1996).
Children with family history of FS or children with developmental delay are more at risk for first febrile seizure:

Evaluation of a child with Febrile Seizure:

History: Important to differentiate from shivering, breath holding attack.
Note child's previous development, family history, drugs history.
One must always keep Neurologic infection in mind (Chances of underlying Meningitis in febrile seizure is 2-5%). Meningitis presents with fever and a seizure in 10 % children.
Examination: Usually has no neurological deficit. Always look for source of infection and rule out intracranial infection.

Investigations: Correlate with clinical examination.

- CBC, Electrolytes, Bone profile, Blood sugar, Urine and Blood culture etc.
- Lumbar Puncture: AAP 1996 guidelines suggest to strongly consider LP for a child with first febrile fit below 12 months, make a careful assessment in a 12-18 months while LP is not routinely needed above 18 months if meningeal signs are not present.
- Consider LP if child is lethargic, first complex febrile seizure, If given prior antibiotics. Or if any clinical sign of meningitis/encephalitis is found.
- EEG: Not recommended in a simple febrile seizure, EEG Has more chances of abnormality in complex febrile seizures or in a child with family history of epilepsy, Pre-existing neurodevelopmental abnormality or deficit. EEG has no predictive value. Slowing of waves is seen in 86 % within 24 hrs. 33% at 3 to 7 days and it turns normal usually by 7 to 10 days.
- Imaging (CT/MRI): Recommended for Pre-existing neuro deficit, neuro-cutaneous features, micro/ Microcephaly, prolonged postictal deficit and recurrent complex febrile seizures.

Pathophysiology:

Is not clear. Sudden spike of high temperature is more likely to cause the seizure, Immune complexes may be responsible.

Recurrence:

1/3rd patients will have a second attack, 1/3rd of 1/3rd (10-11%) have 3rd attack, The recurrence is more likely if there is a family h/o febrile seizures or of epilepsy, Below 18 months age, Child with features of complex febrile seizures. Higher the peak of fever, lower is the recurrence (myth of high temp more the recurrence is wrong).

Risk of subsequent Epilepsy: is 2 to 10%, **Definite risk factors are**:

Neurodevelopmental abnormality
Complex febrile seizures
Family history of epilepsy.
More than one complex feature
Family history of febrile seizures
Gender and Ethnicity.

Genetics: Febrile seizures are considered to be Multifactorial in nature, Several gene locations have been described, Autosomal dominant, 8q, 19p, positive family history more recurrence (20 % if one parent and 33% if both parents) and negative family history less recurrence, Monozygotics 56%, Dizygotic 14%

Management of seizures at Home:

Parental education and proper counseling and explanation with the leaflet etc.

At home proper recovery position and advice for not inserting any object in the mouth. Lower the temperature by removing clothes, **tepid sponging**, and use of fan. Consider rectal antipyretics/ diazepam. The dose of diazepam is 0.5m/kg and not to exceed 10mg maximum dose. Also to advice parents about proper care of respiration. In case the seizure does not stop in maximum ten minutes, plan for hospitalization.

Management in hospital:

A B C.
Intravenous diazepam (rectal if no IV access).
If status, treat as Status Epilepticus

Prevention of febrile seizures:

Intermittent therapy: Antipyretics and Diazepam.

Daily therapy: Sodium Valproate or occasionally barbiturates in frequently recurring cases.

Prevention of epilepsy:

No relation with treatment of febrile seizures.
Antiepileptics do not prevent epilepsy (Berg and Shinnar 1997)
Rarely afebrile seizures, neurodegenerative disorders, mitochondrial disorders may have onset with febrile seizure.

Counseling:

Majority have benign course and grow out it, (brain damage, epilepsy usually do not occur in typical cases). Counselling is given to educate parente on how to manage if there is another seizure next time.

13.6 Epileptic child

Definition:

Seizure or Convulsion: Is a paroxysmal/ episodic time related abnormal motor, sensory or behavioral abnormality that results from abnormal electrical activity in the brain.

Epilepsy: Is the occurrence of two or more unprovoked seizures more then 24 hours apart.

Incidence:

This is one of the common neurological problems in children. Incidence of single seizure is 5% but the incidence of epilepsy is only 0.5%.

Common facts about Epilepsy:

Whenever we encounter a child with epilepsy one has to be sure it is epilepsy only and has to be differentiated from other movement disorders mimicking it, like breath holding spasms, benign positional vertigo, night terrors, nightmares, syncope etc

If there is available eyewitness it will be most useful. If available, a video may be very useful. These days' mobile phones with camera are available; parents may manage to record an attack. In doubt, always wait and investigate. Take a detailed history of seizure (prodrome, ictus, postictal, day or night); write in detail description of attack, age of onset, frequency, Neuro-deficit family history etc. The diagnosis of epilepsy is based on history, history, history and history.

Examination is usually normal in majority but look for neuro-cutaneous markers (café au-let spots), focal neurological signs, associated developmental delay or regression and signs of other systemic diseases.

EEG may helps in localization, classification and ascertaining particular types of seizures (Hypsarrhythmia, absence seizures etc), however normal EEG does not exclude epilepsy as is the case in 40-50 % cases.

Classification:

ILAE 1981 Classification
(based on seizure type and accompanying EEG)

- Partial - Simple
        Complex
        - Partial seizure with secondary
            generalization

- Generalized - Absence
                - Atypical absences
                - Myoclonic
                - Tonic-clonic
                - Tonic or Clonic
                - Atonic
- Unclassified

The **international classification** of Epileptic seizures was first adopted in 1970 and revised in 1981. It was based on description of seizure and electrophysiological features:

1. Partial (focal, local) seizures: When the onset is focal in nature. Partial seizures are further divided into:

   A. Simple partial seizure: No loss or impairment of consciousness.
   1. With motor symptoms
   2. With somatosensory or special sensory symptoms
   3. With autonomic symptoms
   4. With psychic symptoms

   B. Complex partial seizures: With impairment of consciousness
   1. Beginning as simple partial seizure and progressing to impairment of consciousness.
      (a) With no other features
      (b) With features as in **A1-4 above**
      (c) With automatisms
   2. With impairment of consciousness at onset
      (a) With no other features
      (b) With features as in **A1-4 above**
      (c) With automatisms

   C. Partial seizures with secondary generalization

2. Generalized seizures: They are bilaterally symmetrical and are associated with loss or impairment of consciousness.
Generalized seizures (convulsive or non-convulsive) involving both hemispheres, consciousness is always affected and there are bilateral motor/EEG manifestations. This is further divided in to:
   A. Absence seizures
      1. Typical
      2. Atypical
   B. Myoclonic seizures
   C. Clonic seizures
   D. Tonic seizures
   E. Tonic-clonic seizures
   F. Atonic seizures

3. Unclassified epileptic seizures
   Inadequate data not fitting above description
   Some neonatal seizures, rhythmic eye movements, chewing, swimming etc
   Need for the revised classification

After ILAE 1981, refinements were introduced at subsequent meetings of the commission in 1986, 1987 and 1988, following three major categories were further devised:

Idiopathic: Without underlying cause, hereditary predisposition, age related onset, not associated with structural, nervous or mental disorders, normal inter-ictal EEG background, and favorable response to AEDs

Cryptogenic: Hidden cause

Symptomatic: Not genetic, poor control, prognosis related to underlying cause

Certain epilepsies are age related, such as

• West syndrome (infantile spasms under one year, mental retardation and Hypsarrhythmia)

• Lennox-Gastaut syndrome (1-5 years, mixed epilepsy and mental retardation)

• Landau-Kleffner syndrome (3-15 yrs, Acquired epileptic aphasia, Partial or generalized seizures, Behavioral and psychomotor disturbances)

Situation-related seizures

• Febrile seizures/convulsions

• Isolated seizures or isolated status epilepticus

• Seizures in metabolic or toxic event Alcohol, drugs, eclampsia, uremia, etc.

Mechanism of epileptogenesis:
Exactly unknown, De novo hyper excitable neurons,
Channelopathies: Glycine in hyperekplexia, excess of Excitatory neurotransmitters, glutamate / aspartate or lack of Inhibitory – GABA. There may be triggers like old cerebral scar, hamartoma, AV Malformation. Abnormal Kindling, Immature brain and genetic factors like BFNC, JME may come into play.

Diagnosis:

EEG:
An abnormal EEG should always be present during seizure episode but the seizures don't occur in EEG lab and the EEG done in interictal phase is normal in 40% of cases. The yield may be improved by provocation test using: sleep deprivation, photic stimulation, hyperventilation or by continuous video EEG recordings

Imaging (MRI, CT, U/S, PET, SPECT Scans of brain): Not routinely done in children with epilepsy. It is indicated when there are:
      Partial seizures or persistent focal discharges on EEG
      Postictal weakness or neuro deficit
      Neuro-cutaneous disorders
      Extremes of age.
In big institutes of neurology where imaging is performed in epilepsy, 20% scans are abnormal, and 1% could identify surgical cause.

Differential Diagnosis of Seizures

Neonates and infants
- Jitteriness and benign myoclonus
- Apnoea
- Gastro-oesophageal reflux
- Shuddering attacks
- Benign paroxymal torticollis
- Hyperekplexia

Young children
- Breath holding spells
- Reflex anoxic seizures
- Parasomnias
- Benign paroxysmal vertigo
- Paroxysmal choreoathetosis
- Tics and ritualistic movements
- Rage attacks

Childhood and Adolescents
- Vasovagal syncope
- Migraine
- Narcolepsy
- Panic attacks
- Pseudoseizures

Any Age
- Endocrine, metabolic and toxic causes
- Drug-induced dystonia
- Cardiac dysrhythmias

Management:

Which anti-epileptic drug:
After making the diagnosis one has to decide the type of an ideal antiepileptic drug. An ideal drug (long acting, minimal side effects, simple kinetics, minimal drug interactions, available oral and IV form, effective against all types of seizures)
Each child is evaluated individually; one must know drug- dose related and idiosyncratic side effects. Titrate the drug dose and increase gradually until seizure is controlled or side effects appear before embarking on second drug. Never stop drug suddenly

Choice of Anticonvulsants:

Seizure type	First line	Second line
A. Partial Seizures		
Simple partial Complex partial Secondarily generalized	Carbamazepine Valproate	Lamotrigine Topiramate Phenytoin Phenobarbitone Clonazepam
B. Generalized Seizures		
Tonic-clonic Clonic	Valproate	Lamotrigine Topiramate Clonazepam Carbamazepine Phenytoin Phenobarbitone
Absence	Valproate Ethosuximide	Lamotrigine Clonazepam
Atypical absences Atonic, tonic	Valproate	Lamotrigine Topiramate Clonazepam Carbamazepine Phenytoin
Myoclonic	Valproate Clonazepam	Topiramate Phenobarbitone Piracetam Lamotrigine*
	(* May cause seizure aggravation in SMEI and JME)	
Infantile Spasm	ACTH or Prednisolone Vigabatrin (in TS)	Nitrazepam / Clonazepam Valproate

Antiepileptic drugs in children, doses and side effects

Drug Name	Initial dose mg/kg/day	Maintenance dose mg/kg/day	Blood level mcg/ml	Half life in hours	Common side effects/ Warning signs
Carbamazepine	5	10-35	4-12	14-27	Ataxia, rash, Neutropenia
Clonazepam	0.01	0.1-0.3	Not reliable	20-40	Sedation, salivation

Clorazepate	3.75 mg bd	15-60mg per day	N/r	20-60	Sedation,
Ethosuximide	10-15	15-40	N/r	30-40	Neutropenia
Felbamate	15	15-45	40-80	20-23	Hepatotoxicity, Aplastic anemia
Gabapentin	10	30-60	Not yet	5-7	Sedation, ataxia
Lamotrigine	0.2-0.6	5-15	....	12-25	Neutropenia
Levetiracetam	15	45	Not yet	5	Sedation,
Oxcarbazepine	10	20-40	Not yet	9	Same as carbamazepine
Phenobarbital	3-5	5-10	15-40	35-73	Sedation, hyperkinesias
Phenytoin	5-10	5-10	10-25	24	Gum hyperplasia, dark pigmentation, hirsutism
Primidone	5	10-25	8-12	8-22	As Phenobarbital
Tiagabine	4 mg/day	4-32 mg/day	Not yet	16	Sedation, ataxia
Topiramate	1	1-9	Not yet	18-30	Weight loss, glaucoma
Valproate sod.	10	40(60)	50-100	6-15	Hepatotoxicity, hair loss
Vigabatrin	40-60	60-80	Not yet	Days	Visual field defects
Zonisamide	1.5	6	Not yet	24	Sedation

Lennox-Gastaut syndrome and other syndromes

Is a drug resistant epilepsy syndrome of childhood.
Commonly used drugs are Sodium valproate, Benzodiazepines, Topiramate, Levetiracetam, Lamotrigine, and Surgical management.

Benign childhood epilepsies with Centro-temporal spike BCECTS/ Rolandic seizures:
One of the common type of seizure of childhood accounts for 10-40 % of seizures in childhood. The seizures occur in sleep and can be partial or generalized. The onset may be around 3 year's age and usually resolved by puberty. The common drug used is Carbamazepine and Sulthiame.
98 percent become seizure free after treatment

Neonatal seizures (Also see section 2.8)

The seizures in neonatal age are Subtle, Generalized tonic, Multi-focal clonic, Focal, Myoclonic.
Phenobarbital, Benzodiazepines, Lamotrigine, Phenytoin, Sodium Valproate can be used

singly or in combination.
Pyridoxine dependency seizures and a trial with this should always be kept in mind
Pyridoxine is given as 5-50 mg/kg/day, life long if there is response.

Ketogenic diet, Immunoglobulins, Steroids: In Ketogenic diet 3:1 to 4:1 fats to carbohydrates/ proteins, Ketone bodies have to appear in urine.
Useful in Myoclonic seizure, syndromes >other seizure.
Usually tried in specialized centers.
There are risks associated with the diet therapy in form of brain edema, electrolyte imbalance and worsening of seizures.

Surgical treatment
Resistant cases, (failure to medical treatment)
Temporal lobectomy, Non temporal lobe resection, Hemispherectomy, Callosotomy.

Follow up monitoring:
CBC: (carbamazepine, Lamotrigine)
LFT, AMYLASE: (Sodium valproate)
Renal function tests: (topiramate),
Ophthalmology check: (Vigabatrin and topiramate),
Weight monitoring: (topiramate, valproate, and carbamazepine)
Drug levels: Not performed routinely and done if seizure are uncontrolled, Multiple antiepileptic drugs or drug interacting with the AEDs, to check for compliance Switching over drugs and while Withdrawing drugs when there are multiple drugs.

Guidelines for discontinuation of treatment in seizure free patients:
Longer the duration of treatment, better prognosis
Successful drug withdrawal seizure free 2-5 yrs (3.5 yrs)

Prognosis of epilepsy:
Depends on type of seizure, Age of onset, associated neuro-deficit and underlying cause,

Parents counseling:
> **Compliance:** Need to **treat for at least 2 years seizure-free period** and then to taper off over 3 - 6 months. **Do not stop the medication** by themselves. Sudden withdrawal of drugs may precipitate breakthrough seizures or possibly status epilepticus attack.
> In photosensitive patients **TV** should only be watched in a brightly lit room. Avoid sleep deprivation and alcohol.
> Use shower instead of bath, do not lock bathroom.
> No **cycling** in traffic, no climbing sports and no unsupervised swimming
> Allow **driving** only in well-controlled epilepsy (seizure-free for at least 1 year, off or on treatment) or purely nocturnal seizures.
> Inform **school** about disease and drugs.

13.7 Status Epilepticus

Prolonged seizure of **more then 30 minutes** duration or seizures recurring without regaining consciousness in between, though any prolonged seizure of >10 minutes is also an emergency.

Management: Start with A B C of resuscitation procedure

Diazepam: 0.2 to 0.3 mg/kg slow I V injection over 3 to 5 minutes (Caution: apnea may occur if given rapidly).

Also load **Phenytoin** sodium 15- 18 mg/kg (1 mg/kg/mt) with cardiac monitoring. Alternatively Fosphenytoin can be used. This can be given at a faster rate like 3mg/kg/mt. It acts faster and even can be given intramuscularly. In case seizures continue additional 5mg/kg can be given.

In Neonatal age use **Phenobarbital** 18 mg/kg.

Lorazepam 0.1-0.2 mg/kg, it is a long acting benzodiazepine and there is no need to give Phenytoin or Phenobarbital. When seizures continue after loading Phenytoin or Phenobarbital, the status becomes a refractory one. There are few alternatives available. Intubation with paralysis, thiopental infusion etc. however in recent years midazolam has been used widely.

Midazolam is a Benzodiazepine commonly used as preanesthetic with a wide safety margin, and Quick arousal after use. It rapidly diffuses across brain capillaries in CNS. Midazolam has easy mixing with saline or glucose. It is also an effective & potent suppressor of seizures. Initial bolus of 0.1 to 0.15 mg /kg followed by 1 Microgram/kg/mt. continuous infusion, increase as required by 1 mcg/kg/minute every 15 to 20 minutes until the seizures are controlled then maintain same rate for 24 hours afterwards taper by 0.25 mcg/kg/minute every 2 hours.

Summary of Management of Status epilepticus:
1. ABC
2. Diazepam 0.2 mg/Kg IV slow bolus, with respiratory monitoring followed by:
3. Phenytoin sodium under ECG monitoring 18 mg/kg (below 4 years), 15mg/kg (above 4 years). In neonates use Phenobarbital 18 mg/Kg instead.
4. If seizures not controlled in 15 – 20 minutes, consider using IV Phenobarbital or
5. Midazolam infusion under PICU care (see above for doses).

Note: A. If patient is coming first time and not known to be epileptic, Test blood sugar bedside and correct Hypoglycemia if needed. The dose is 5 ml/kg of 10% dextrose. Also keep in mind Ca++ and Mg++ if status does not respond and may be by that time the electrolyte profile is already with you.

B. If the patient is a known epileptic and on drugs:
    The status could be due to sudden withdrawal of the drug, concurrent infections, or drug interactions. Therapeutic drug levels should always be performed. This is important because the patient can be given the missed drug parenterally and a status can be aborted fast.

13.8 Cerebral Palsy

Definition: A disorder of movement and posture due to a **non-progressive** lesion (insult) in the brain during the phase of its rapid development (embryo to 3 years postnatal age). This could present at any time starting from neonatal to early childhood depending upon the severity and timing of the lesion. To avoid the stigma, these children should preferably be termed as *physically challenged persons*. The clinical course is static or slowly improving with time, hence it is also known as Static Encephalopathy.

It is quite important to differentiate cerebral palsy from **progressive disorders** like neurodegenerative or metabolic diseases, where in the course will be progressive (i.e. becoming worse with time). One should always bear in mind that the cerebral palsy is **not a familial condition** and all such cases deserve detailed investigations to find underlying treatable cause.

Prevalence Varies from 1-4/1000 population.
> Cerebral palsy is mainly a motor handicap but one third patients do have associated mental retardation, one third have seizures and nearly half have learning difficulties, language problems and hearing defects.

Clinical types: Depending upon the site of lesion in the brain the types are:
> **1. Spastic** (damage to the motor pathway) accounts for 70-80 % all cases,
> Depending upon the extant of involvement it is further sub classified as:
> * Quadriplegic type: Upper limbs are involved more severely than lower
> * Hemiplegic type: Involvement of Right or Left half of the body
> * Tirplegic type: involvement of three limbs
> * Diplegic type: lower limbs are involved more severely than upper
> * Monoplegic type: Involvement of a single limb only
>
> **2. Choreo-athetoid or dyskinetic** (damage to the extra pyramidal system) 10 % of all cases
> **3. Ataxic/hypotonic** (damage to the cerebellum), 10 % of all cases
> **4. Mixed** (Wide spread damage) as in hypoxic ischemic encephalopathy

Invariably children with bipyramidal involvement also have **pseudo bulbar palsy.**
Feeding difficulties, delayed motor milestones and abnormal gait may be the presenting features. Examination reveals **upper motor neuron signs** (hypertonia, exaggerated deep tendon reflexes, up going planters and clonus).

Causes: The cerebral palsy is caused by a Non-Progressive lesion (insult) during the rapidly growing phase of the brain. *In a significant number of patients, identifiable cause is not clearly understood.* In cases where the cause is known, the insult occurs during
> **Antenatal period (in 70-80% cases)**
> **Intrapartum period (in 10% of cases) and**
> **Postnatal (in 20-30% of cases).**

Main causes are:
* Prematurity, multiple births
* Hypoxic ischemic encephalopathy (Perinatal asphyxia)
* Infections (meningitis/encephalitis, congenital infections)

- Trauma
- Vascular insults to brain
- Congenital Brain malformations and various syndromes
- Maternal systemic diseases
- Drugs and toxins
- Fetal distress for any cause
- Difficult delivery leading to hypoxia
- Hypothyroidism
- Any severe systemic illness leading to brain insult

Diagnosis:
A detailed history may identify underlying the cause, history must highlight significant **events during pregnancy, birth or after the birth until early childhood**.
Antenatal history may reveal occurrence of significant maternal fever, rash, drug intake, systemic diseases, radiation exposure esp. in first trimester.

A detailed account of events surrounding the delivery should be noted especially if there was any fetal distress, need for emergency caesarian section, significantly low **APGAR** scores especially at or after 5 minutes after the birth and need for neonatal resuscitation should be enquired or gathered from the pink card or other birth records.

A good NICU discharge summary will highlight relevant post natal problems like neonatal infections, hypoglycemia, prematurity, hyperbilirubinemia, seizures and need for artificial ventilation.

Investigations: are usually not required as the diagnosis is usually based on the history and examination. In selected cases investigations like Neuro-imaging (MRI) for malformations and extent of brain damage, EEG (if seizures), thyroid screen for hypothyroidism, TORCH profile (up-to 6 months age) and Chromosomal analysis in a dysmorphic child may be needed.

Problems associated with CP:
- Feeding problems due to pseudo bulbar palsy,
- Aspirations leading to repeated pneumonia
- Problems related to mobility due to weakness
- Epilepsy
- Mental sub normality, learning difficulties and attention deficit hyperactivity syndrome
- Hearing and visual impairment
- Language and learning problems

Management:
General Management is provided through a **multidisciplinary team** approach. Pediatrician has a central role in organizing all the ancillary services as well as to treat any ongoing problems and complications. Other members of the team could be from any of the following specialties depending on the presence of associated disabilities: Ophthalmologist, ENT surgeon, Orthopedician, Physiotherapist, Speech therapist, Psychologists, Social worker and special educationist etc.

Role of Medications: the drugs, which reduce the spasticity like **baclofen**, are used in case of mild to moderate spasticity. **Botulinum toxin (Botox)** can be used in selected cases. Anticonvulsant drugs are required for control of epilepsy.

Prevention: Good antenatal and perinatal care is of utmost important.

13.9   Mental retardation (Mental sub normality)

Definition: Delay in attainment of the higher mental functions (Insufficient development of mental capacities). To avoid the stigma, these children are also termed as **mentally challenged persons**

Prevalence: almost one per thousand in general population.

Classification: based on IQ assessment mental retardation can arbitrarily divided into:

  Mild IQ 50-70, Educable group i.e. can be educated to achieve a sheltered job and living

  Moderate IQ score 25-50, can be trained to perform their daily routines.

  Profound IQ <25, Can not be trained therefore are completely dependent or need institutional care.

The children are tested on several developmental scales available. It is difficult to grade them below 2 years of age. Poor achievement of Psychosocial and language developmental milestones is more indicative of mental sub-normality.

Etiology: May be in isolation or associated with other neurological or systemic dysfunction. Occasionally the condition is familial. Mental retardation can result from varied causes due to:

Cerebral insult/damage due to prenatal, natal or postnatal causes (See cerebral palsy).

Genetic syndromes

Neuro-cutaneous disorders and

Chromosomal anomalies.

Examination: one must look for microcephaly, dysmorphism, neurocutaneous markers, and other neurological findings. Testing for hearing, vision, and language must be done.

Investigations: are directed on the suspected cause. These may include brain imaging, metabolic screening, detailed chromosomal examination, and genetic studies.

Other specific investigations are planned according to the associated neurological or systemic involvement.

Management: depends on the IQ assessment, other associated systemic abnormalities and seizures.

13.10 Meningitis

Meningitis is an inflammation of the leptomeninges and underlying subarachnoid cerebrospinal fluid (CSF). It can be useful to divide symptom onset into acute, sub acute and chronic categories. Depending on age and general condition, these gravely ill patients acutely present with signs and symptoms of meningeal inflammation and systemic infection. Patients may decompensate quickly and require emergency ICU care.

History: It is important to remember that younger the child, less specific are the symptoms.

Symptoms in older children:
- o Headache
- o Neck stiffness (generally not present in children <1 y)
- o Fever and chills
- o Photophobia
- o Vomiting
- o Prodromal upper respiratory infection (URI) symptoms (viral or bacterial)
- o Seizures (in 30-40% children)
- o Focal neurological symptoms (including focal seizures)
- o Altered sensorium (confusion may be sole presenting symptom)
- o Signs of shock
- o Purpuric rash of meningococcemia

Symptoms in infants
- o Fever
- o Lethargy and/or change in level of alertness
- o Seizures
- o Poor feeding and/or vomiting
- o Respiratory distress, apnea, cyanosis

Physical Examination findings are widely variable depending on age and infecting organism. Systemic examination occasionally reveals a pulmonary or otitis media co-infection.

- Signs of meningeal irritation:
  - o Nuchal rigidity or discomfort on neck flexion
  - o **Kernig's sign:** Passive knee extension in supine patient elicits neck pain and hamstring resistance.
  - o **Brudzinski sign:** Passive neck or single hip flexion is accompanied by involuntary flexion of both hips.
- Papilledema is present in only one third of meningitis patients with increased Intra cranial pressure; it takes at least several hours to develop.
- Focal neurological signs:
  - o Isolated cranial nerve abnormalities (principally III, IV, VI, VII) in 10-20% of patients
  - o Is associated with a dramatic increase in complications from lumbar puncture (Coning) and indicates a worse outcome
- Systemic findings
  - o Extra cranial infection (e.g., sinusitis, otitis media, mastoiditis, pneumonia, urinary tract infection) may be noted.
  - o Arthritis is seen with *N meningitidis,* less commonly with other bacteria.

- o Non-blanching **petechiae** and cutaneous hemorrhages are seen classically with *N meningitides;* however, these may occur with other bacterial and viral infections.
  - o Endotoxic shock with vascular collapse is characteristic of severe *N. meningitidis* infection.
- Altered mental status, from irritability to somnolence, delirium, and coma
- Infants
  - o Bulging fontanel (if euvolemic)
  - o Paradoxical irritability (i.e., quiet when stationary, cries when held)
  - o High-pitched cry
  - o Hypotonia
  - o Always examine skin over entire spine for dimples, sinuses, nevi, or tufts of hair, which may indicate a congenital anomaly (Occult Spina Bifida) communicating with the subarachnoid space.

Causes: Meningitis is caused by the following pathogens specific in each age group:

Infants less than 2 months of age:

- Group B streptococcus,
- E. Coli and other Gram-negative organisms
- Listeria monocytogenes
- S. Pneumoniae
- N. Meningitides
- Haemophilus influenzae type b.

Children over 2 months of age:

- Streptococcus pneumoniae,
- Neisseria meningitidis
- Haemophilus influenzae type b (Uncommon after age 6).

Risk factors

- o Children below 5 years, especially with diabetes mellitus, renal or adrenal insufficiency, hypoparathyroidism, or cystic fibrosis
- o Immunosuppressed patients are at increased risk of opportunistic infections and acute bacterial meningitis.
- o Over crowding (e.g., military recruits and college dorm residents), Large conglomeration of people e.g. during Hajj are prone for meningococcal meningitis.
- o Splenectomy and sickle cell disease patients are at increased risk of pneumococcal meningitis.
- o Recent exposure to others with meningitis, with or without prophylaxis
- o Children with facial cellulites, periorbital cellulitis, and septic arthritis.
- o Dural defect e.g., traumatic (Head injury with damage to nasal cribriform plate, surgical or congenital (Spina bifida occulta or Meningomyelocele) in recurrent meningitis.
- o Thalassemia major
- o Bacterial endocarditis
- o Ventriculo peritoneal shunt
- o Malignancy (increased risk of *Listeria* species infection)

Differential Diagnosis:
- Brain abscess
- Febrile Seizures
- Encephalitis
- Intracranial space occupying lesions

Lab Studies:
- Complete blood count (CBC) with differential
- Blood cultures
- Coagulation studies
- Serum glucose
- Erythrocyte sedimentation rate (ESR)
- Electrolytes
- Serum and urine osmolalities
- Bacterial antigen studies can be done on CSF, Urine or Serum in partially treated cases

Imaging Studies:
- Head CT scan with contrast or MRI with gadolinium:
  - Imaging is indicated in patients with evidence of head trauma, altered mental status, or focal findings.
  - Presence of Papilledema and inability to fully assess fundi or neurologic status are indications for **CT scan prior to LP.**

Procedures:
- The most important laboratory study is examination of CSF. The lumbar puncture (LP) study should include:
  - Opening and closing pressure in the cooperative patient.
  - Cell count
  - Gram stain
  - Culture and sensitivity
  - Glucose
  - Protein
  - Bacterial antigen test to diagnose partially treated meningitis as a result of previous course of antibiotic given for fever or URTI

Interpretation of abnormal lumbar puncture results:

	White cell count		Biochemistry	
	Neutrophils (x 10^6 /L)	**Lymphocytes (x 10^6/L)**	**Protein (g/L)**	**Glucose (CSF: blood ratio)**
Normal (>1 month of age)	0	5	< 0.4	0.6 (or 2.5 mmol/L)
Normal term neonate	0	11	<1.0	0.6 (or 2.1 mmol/L)

Bacterial meningitis	100-10,000 (may be normal)	Usually < 100	> 1.0 (may be normal)	< 0.4 (may be normal)
Viral meningitis	Usually <100	10-1000 (may be normal)	0.4-1 (may be normal)	Usually normal

Traumatic tap
- Some guidelines suggest that in traumatic taps you can allow 1 white blood cell for every 500 to 700 red blood cells and 0.01g/L protein for every 1000 red cells. However, rules based on a 'predicted' white cell count in the CSF are not reliable.

Antibiotics prior to lumbar puncture
- Prior antibiotics usually make CSF falsely sterile, therefore bacterial antigen test is more important in such cases
- Antibiotics are unlikely to significantly affect the CSF cell count or biochemistry if samples taken <24 hours after antibiotics.

Management
- **Antibiotics:** Ideal antibiotic therapy is based on a clearly identified organism on CSF Gram stain. Age and underlying conditions dictate empiric treatment.
  - **In neonates to age 1 month**, the most common microorganisms are group B or D streptococci, Enterobacteriaceae (e.g., *E coli*), and *L monocytogenes*.
    - Primary treatment is a combination of Ampicillin (age 0-7 d: 50 mg/kg IV q8h; age 8-30 d: 50-100 mg/kg IV q6h) plus Cefotaxime 50 mg/kg IV q6h.
    - Alternative treatment is Ampicillin (age 0-7 d: 50 mg/kg IV q8h; age 8-30 d: 50-100 mg/kg IV q6h) plus Gentamycin (age 0-7 d: 2.5 mg/kg IV or IM q12h; age 8-30 d: 2.5 mg/kg IV or IM q8h).
    - Most authorities recommend adding Acyclovir 10 mg/kg IV q8h for suspected Herpes simplex encephalitis.
  - **In infants (1-3 mo)**, the most common microorganisms are those listed under neonates above and under older infant/child below.
    - Primary treatment is Cefotaxime (50 mg/kg IV q6h, up to 12 g/d) or Ceftriaxone (initial dose: 100 mg/kg, 50 mg/kg q12h up to 4 g/day) plus Ampicillin (50-100 mg/kg IV q6h).
    - Alternative treatment is Chloramphenicol (25 mg/kg PO or IV q12h) plus Gentamycin (2.5 mg/kg IV or IM q8h).
    - If prevalence of Cephalosporin-resistant *S pneumoniae* (DRSP) is >2%, add Vancomycin (15 mg/kg IV q8h).
    - Strongly consider Dexamethasone (0.4 mg/kg IV q12h for 2 d or 0.15 mg/kg IV q6h for 4 d) starting 15-20 minutes before first dose of antibiotics.
  - **In older infants or young children (3 mo - 7 y)**, the most common microorganisms are *S pneumoniae, N meningitides,* and *H influenzae*.
    - Primary treatment is either Cefotaxime (50 mg/kg IV q6h up to 12 g/d) or Ceftriaxone (initial dose: 100 mg/kg, then 50 mg/kg q12h up to 4

g/d). If prevalence of resistant Strept. Pneumoniae (DRSP) is >2%, add Vancomycin (15 mg/kg IV q8h). In countries with low prevalence of DRSP, consider Penicillin G (250,000 U/kg/d IM/IV in 3-4 divided doses). Due to DRSP, Penicillin G is no longer recommended in the US.

- Alternative treatment (or if severely Penicillin allergic) is Chloramphenicol (25 mg/kg PO/IV q12h) plus Vancomycin (15 mg/kg IV q8h).
- Strongly consider **Dexamethasone** (0.4 mg/kg IV q12h for 2 d or 0.15 mg/kg IV q6h for 4 d) starting 15-20 minutes before the first dose of antibiotics.

o **In an older child or an otherwise healthy adult**, the most common microorganisms are *S pneumoniae, N meningitides,* and *L monocytogenes.*

- In areas where prevalence of DRSP is >2%, primary treatment is either Cefotaxime (Pediatric dose: 50 mg/kg IV q6h up to 12 g/d; adult dose: 2 g IV q4h) or Ceftriaxone (pediatric dose: initial dose: 75 mg/kg, then 50 mg/kg q12h up to 4 g/day; adult dose: 2 g IV q12h) plus Vancomycin (pediatric dose: 15 mg/kg IV q8h; adult dose: 750-1000 mg IV q12h or 10-15 mg/kg IV q12h). Some add Rifampin (pediatric dose: 20 mg/kg/d IV; adult dose: 600 mg PO qd). If *Listeria* species is suspected, add Ampicillin (50 mg/kg IV q6h).
- Alternative treatment (or if severely penicillin allergic) is Chloramphenicol (12.5 mg/kg IV q6h: not bactericidal) or Clindamycin (pediatric dose: 40 mg/kg/day IV in 3-4 doses; adult dose: 900 mg IV q8h: active in vitro but no clinical data) or Meropenem (pediatric dose: 20-40 mg/kg IV q8h; adult dose: 1 g IV q8h: active in vitro but few clinical data; avoid Imipenem as it is proconvulsant).
- In areas with low prevalence of DRSP, use Cefotaxime (pediatric dose: 50 mg/kg IV q6h up to 12 g/d; adult: 2 g IV q4h) or Ceftriaxone (pediatric dose: 75 mg/kg initial dose then 50 mg/kg q12h up to 4 g/d; adult: 2 g IV q12h) plus Ampicillin (50 mg/kg IV q6h).
- Alternativetreatment(orifseverelypenicillinallergic)isChloramphenicol (12.5 mg/kg IV q6h) plus Trimethoprim/Sulfamethoxazole (TMP/SMX; TMP 5 mg/kg IV q6h) or Meropenem (pediatric dose: 20-40 mg/kg IV q8h; adult dose: 1 g IV q8h).

Role of Steroids still remains controversial issue but current recommendation is still in favor of steroids use.

- Current evidence suggests that steroids protect against neurological sequelae from bacterial meningitis (particularly deafness) and may reduce mortality.
- The benefit is probably greatest if steroids are given at least 15 minutes before the first dose of antibiotics.

Accordingly, children (>4 weeks old) who are being treated for possible meningitis (who have not yet received parenteral antibiotics, or who have received their first dose less than 1 hour ago) should be given Dexamethasone.

- Give Dexamethasone 0.15mg/kg iv 6 hourly for 4 days
- Wait 15 minutes before giving antibiotics after the first dose.
- Antibiotics must not be delayed more than 30 minutes after a decision is made to treat.

Steroids should be ceased if a decision is made to cease antibiotic treatment for meningitis before 4 days (e.g. if cultures are negative at 48 hours, and CSF microscopy is not supportive).

From a practical point of view, it may be appropriate to give Dexamethasone at the time of lumbar puncture in children who are felt to be very likely to have meningitis.

Admission to ICU

Admission to ICU should be discussed with the ICU team in the following circumstances:

- Coma
- Cardiovascular compromise
- Intractable seizures
- Hyponatremia

Prevention:

- Routine childhood immunizations have been shown to effectively decrease the incidence of certain types of meningitis and encephalitis.
- Antibiotic prophylaxis is recommended for all household contacts in those households with at least 1 unvaccinated child younger than 48 months in patients with *H influenzae* meningitis.
- Treat all contacts in the household if any child is younger than 12 months.
    - Prophylaxis should be started as soon as possible.
    - Rifampin is the drug of choice.
    - Careful observation of any contacts and immediate evaluation is warranted if a fever develops.
- Prophylaxis is recommended for all persons in contact with oral secretions of patients with *N meningitidis* meningitis. This includes a health care worker who performed mouth-to-mouth resuscitation, intubation, or suctioning. Rifampin is the drug of choice.

Complications:

- Despite early aggressive management, the complications from bacterial meningitis remain significant.
    - In the neonatal period, the mortality rate is 15-25%.
    - After the neonatal period, the mortality rate drops to about 5% with appropriate care.
    - The morbidity rate is up to 40% depending on the causative organism and delay in therapy.
    - Hib meningitis has up to 15% rate of permanent neurological sequelae.
- Most children with enteroviral meningitis have an uncomplicated course.

Prognosis:

- The prognosis for appropriately treated meningitis has improved, but there is still a 5% mortality rate and significant morbidity.
- The prognosis varies with the age of the child, clinical condition, and infecting organism.
- The prognosis from viral meningitis usually is very good.

Follow-up:

All children should have hearing assessment done 6-8 weeks after treatment
Children should be followed for mental retardation or learning disabilities.

13.11 Approach to a comatose child

Introduction

Coma is a challenging medical emergency. There is an urgent need to diagnose and treat potentially reversible disease.

Definitions

Consciousness may be defined as a state of awareness of self and surroundings.

Stupor is defined as unresponsiveness from which the subject can be aroused only by vigorous and repeated stimuli.

Coma is defined as a sleeplike state with total absence of awareness of self and the environment from which person can not be aroused even after vigorous external stimulation.

Drowsiness lies between alertness and stupor.

States related to coma:

Akinetic mutism is similar to the vegetative state, except, these patients have little spontaneous or induced movements.

Catatonic patients are mute with little or no motor activity. Unlike stupor or coma, these patients maintain posture in a sitting or standing position. This state is caused by schizophrenia, drugs, or frontal lobe disease.

Pseudo coma (psychogenic unresponsiveness) occurs in patients who do not respond to vigorous stimulation because of psychiatric disease. Conversion reaction and malingering are common causes of pseudo coma.

Pathophysiology

Coma results from one of two Pathophysiologic mechanisms:
1. Diffuse insult to both cerebral hemispheres.
2. Focal lesion involving the ascending reticular activating system (ARAS) located in the upper pons, midbrain, and diencephalon. A lesion in one cerebral hemisphere will not produce coma; bi hemispheric dysfunction is required.

Causes

To assist in evaluation of coma, causes can be divided into two broad categories:
Structural or surgical (table 1)
Metabolic or medical (table 2).
Structural coma is usually associated with diffuse damage to both hemispheres from increased intracranial pressure or diffuse vascular damage. There may be a lesion in or displacement of the ARAS in the upper brainstem. In non-traumatic coma, there is a diffuse insult to both cerebral hemispheres from either an endogenous or exogenous toxin. This includes infectious causes (sepsis), drug overdose, and metabolic abnormalities, such as hyponatremia and hyper natremia.

Table-1 Causes of surgical or structural coma
Trauma
Subdural injury
Epidural injury
Diffuse axonal injury
Brain contusions
Penetrating head injury
Intracranial hemorrhage
Subarachnoid hemorrhage
Intracerebral hemorrhage
Posterior fossa (pontine, cerebellar)
Supratentorial (basal ganglia, lobar)
Ischemic stroke
Large middle cerebral artery infarction with brain herniation
Brainstem stroke involving bilateral rostral pons or midbrain
"Top of the basilar" syndrome with bilateral infarction of thalami and rostral midbrain
Diffuse microvascular abnormality
Thrombotic thrombocytopenic purpura
Cerebral malaria
Tumor
large tumor with herniation
Multiple metastatic lesions
Other disorders
Osmotic demyelination syndrome (central pontine myelinolysis)

Table 2, Causes of metabolic or medical coma
Drug overdose
Benzodiazepines, barbiturates, opioids, tricyclic agents
Infectious disease
Sepsis
Bacterial meningitis
Encephalitis (e.g., herpes simplex, arboviral infection)
Endocrine disorders
Hypoglycemic reaction
Diabetic ketoacidosis
Hyperosmolar coma
Myxedema
Hyperthyroidism
Metabolic abnormalities
Hyponatremia
Hypernatremia
Uremia
Hepatic encephalopathy
Hypertensive encephalopathy
Hypomagnesemic pseudocoma
Toxic reactions
Carbon monoxide poisoning
Alcohol poisoning
Acetaminophen overdose
Ethylene glycol poisoning
Medication side effects
Reye's syndrome
Neuroleptic malignant syndrome
Central anticholinergic syndrome
Serotonin syndrome
Isoniazid intoxication
Deficiency states
Thiamine deficiency (Wernicke's encephalopathy)
Niacin deficiency (pellagra)
Hypothermia
Psychogenic coma

Mnemonic for Causes of Coma: "SPITE ME NOT"		
S space-occupying lesions P psychiatric I infectious/inflammation. T trauma E endocrine	M metabolic E electrical/epileptic	N neoplastic O oxygen/other T toxic

Clinical evaluation

Coma is an acute, life-threatening situation. Evaluation must be rapid, comprehensive, and undertaken while urgent steps are taken to minimize further neurological damage. Emergency management should include: resuscitation with support of cardiovascular and respiratory system; correction of immediate metabolic upset, notably control of blood glucose, control of seizures and body temperature; any specific treatments—for example, naloxone for opiate overdose.

Assessment now should comprise:

- History through friend, family or emergency medical personnel
- General physical examination
- Neurological assessment to define the nature of coma

Pediatric Coma Scale:

Eyes open	Best verbal response	Best motor response
Spontaneously (4) To speech (3) To pain (2) None (1)	Orientated (5) Words (4) Vocal sounds (3) Cries (2) None (1)	Obeys command (5) Localizes pain (4) Flexion to pain (3) Extension to pain (2) None (1)

Normal aggregate score

0-6 months	9
> 6 - 12 months	11
> 1 - 2 years	12
>2 - 5 years	13
> 5 years	14

Clinical assessment of coma

General examination
Skin (for example, rash, anemia, cyanosis, jaundice)
Temperature (fever-infection /hypothermia-drugs/circulatory failure)
Blood pressure (for example, septicemia/Addison's disease)
Breath (for example, acetone breath)
Cardiovascular (for example, arrhythmia)
Abdomen (for example, organomegaly)

Neurological (general)
Head, neck and eardrum (trauma)
Meningism (SAH/meningitis)
Funduscopy
Level of consciousness
    As determined by using *Glasgow coma scale for older children or Pediatric coma scale for small children*

Brain stem function
 Pupillary responses
Spontaneous eye movements
Oculocephalic responses
Caloric responses
Corneal responses

Motor function
Motor response
Deep tendon reflexes
Muscle tone
Planters

Respiratory pattern
Cheyne Stokes: hemisphere
Apneustic: Rapid with pauses/lower: pontine
Central neurogenic hyperventilation: rapid/midbrain

Diagnostic Evaluation:
The immediate goal is to detect a treatable cause for the coma. Following tests are advised for all patients with coma.
- CBC
- LFT
- Renal profile
- Ammonia
- ABG

Specific Investigations:
    Antiepileptic drug levels should be determined in known patients.
    In febrile patient, septic screen be performed to rule out infection

CT brain is an important first test to be done in all comatose patients. A contrast-enhanced CT scan should be considered if mass lesion or bleeding is suspected.

Decision to perform **LP** depends on clinical situation and after ruling out Space Occupying Lesion on CT brain

MRI is ideal but is more difficult to perform in the emergency situation.

The **EEG** has a distinct role in the evaluation of comatose patients by identifying the patient with sub clinical seizures who may benefit from anticonvulsive therapy

Evoked potentials namely, BAEP and SSEP can provide evidence of brainstem involvement.

Treatment

- Treatment of specific cause
- Specific Management
  - Stop seizures
  - Treat metabolic disturbances
  - Lower intracranial pressure
  - Treat infection
- General Management
  - ABC
  - Take blood test as putting in lines
  - Nursing attention to pressure areas and eyes
  - Monitoring - vital signs/neurology

Prognosis

Regardless of the coma, recovery of higher cortical function and motor skills depends on the etiology and the duration of coma. The shorter the comas, from 1 hour to less than 1 to 2 weeks, better the outcome. When coma is of non traumatic origin, the chance of recovery from persistent vegetative state is poor if consciousness has not returned by 3 months from the initial insult.

13.12 Large and Small Head

Introduction:

The measurement of head circumference, a direct reflection of head growth, is an important step in the evaluation of childhood growth and development. Abnormal head growth is defined as a head circumference (also called fronto-occipital circumference) greater than three standard deviations above or below the mean for a given age, gender, and gestation.

- **Microcephaly** is defined as head circumference > 3 standard deviations below the mean.

- **Macrocephaly** is a head circumference > 3 standard deviations above the mean.

- **Megalencephaly** is an abnormally large brain.

- **Microencephaly** is an abnormally small brain.

Head size measurement

Head circumference should be measured at health maintenance visits between birth and three years of age. It should be measured at the widest points. The measuring tape should encircle the head and include an area 1 to 2 cm above the glabella anteriorly and the most prominent portion of the occiput posteriorly. The accuracy and consistency of measurement are improved if the same individual performs sequential measurements

Average postnatal head growth: Refer to anthropometric measurements in appendices

Microcephaly

Defined as head circumference three standard deviations below mean for age, body size, race and sex

Etiopathogenesis

The etiology of Microcephaly is complex and includes conditions that:

1-Restrict brain growth (such as the craniosynostosis)
2-Brain damage due to any cause (e.g., hypoxic-ischemic insults and TORCH infections)
3-Intrinsically impaired brain growth. This could be the result of a metabolic insult or a defect in the process of brain formation itself (as in the "primary" or genetic Microcephaly and chromosomal syndromes).

Diagnostic workup for Microcephaly

1. Karyotype of child for suspected congenital abnormality

2. Head imaging (Cranial Ultrasound/ CT brain)

3. Metabolic screen: Tandem MS, Maternal Phenylalanine level (where indicated)

Causes of Microcephaly:

Primary Small Brain Size	Restriction of Brain Growth
Non-genetic insults (pre, peri or post-natal) ⊠ Infectious ⊠ Vascular disruption, hypoxic-ischemic insult, Irradiation, Toxins and Teratogen ⊠ Malnutrition ⊠ Metabolic ⊠ Trauma (including shaken baby) *Genetic conditions* ⊠ Primary Genetic: Autosomal Recessive or dominant ⊠ Chromosomal disorders (e.g., trisomy 21 and 18 ⊠ Metabolic and degenerative conditions with onset before completion of brain growth (e.g., PKU, Smith Lemli Opitz syndrome, infantile neuronal ceroid lipofuscinoses) 5p- [cri du chat] syndrome) ⊠ Chromosomal breakage and premature ageing disorders (e.g., Bloom syndrome, Cockayne syndrome, Nijmegen breakage syndrome) ⊠ Monogenic or sporadic "syndromic" disorders (e.g., Cornelia de Lange syndrome, Meckel syndrome, Rubinstein-Taybi syndrome; and microcephalia Vera	*Disorders of bone and cartilage* *Non-genetic* ➢ Endocrinopathies *Genetic* ➢ Craniosynostosis, skeletal dysplasias *External restriction of skull growth in utero*

Outcome and prognosis

Microcephaly is often equated with developmental delay and mental retardation. However, not all children with Microcephaly are mentally retarded. The development of motor skills and speech may be delayed. Convulsions may also occur in some cases. Motor ability may be impaired and range from clumsiness in some children to spastic quadriplegia in others.

Treatment

There is no specific treatment for Microcephaly. If an underlying cause is found i.e. metabolic disease, should be treated Treatment is otherwise symptomatic and supportive. Accurate genetic counseling is most important and requires establishment of exact etiology.

Macrocephaly

Macrocephaly is diagnosed when the head circumference is more than three standard deviations above the mean for the child's age, sex, race, and gestation. It is distinguished from hydrocephalus in that there is no increase in pressure within the head.
Mental deficiency, seizures, and movement disorders are common in macrocephalic children.

Causes and symptoms

Most common causes for an enlarged head are Megalencephaly, or an enlarged brain, and hydrocephalus or excessive cerebrospinal fluid (CSF) in the brain. When Macrocephaly is a result of Megalencephaly, it is often impossible to determine the cause. However, Megalencephaly is often associated with metabolic diseases such as ***Canavan's disease or Alexander's disease*** or with syndromes such as **G***igantism, Achondroplasia* (dwarfism or small stature), *Osteogenesis Imperfecta*, **N***eurofibromatosis*, and some **C***hromosomal anomalies*. In all of these disorders, there is an enlargement of brain tissues.

In **Hydrocephalus**, excess CSF collects in the ventricular system due to impaired circulation, absorption or occasionally due to excessive production. The causes include Chiari malformation, abnormal cysts within the brain, and as a complication of meningitis.
In some cases, a child may have Familial large head. These children do not have an underlying condition and usually do not have any additional complications.

Children with macrocephaly may be asymptomatic or have delay in development or mental retardation.

The pediatrician usually diagnoses macrocephaly during physical examination. Some children will require additional diagnostic imaging procedures, such as computed tomography scan (CT scan), X ray, and MR, to determine the cause.

Treatment

There is no specific treatment. Management of developmental delay and mental retardation and treatment of the primary underlying condition is important.

Prognosis

For children with benign familial Macrocephaly, the prognosis is excellent. These children usually do not have any complications and have normal intelligence. The prognosis depends upon the cause that may cause delayed development, seizure disorders, and limited intelligence.

Common Surgical Problems

14.1 Common Pediatric Surgical Problems

A. Acute Appendicitis

Definition and Incidence:
Acute appendicitis is the commonest disease in childhood requiring abdominal surgery. It is unusual in infancy. The incidence peaks in teenage and young adult years. The frequency increases in autumn and spring months.

Etiopathogenesis:
Acute appendicitis is almost always caused by obstruction of lumen of the appendix, but the mechanism of obstruction varies and it may be due to:

    Hard concretions and appendiceal *fecalith*

    Hyperplasia of the submucosal lymphoid tissue, due to intercurrent infections.

    Fibrous stenosis resulting from an earlier inflammation or a carcinoid tumor

Nonobstructive appendicitis is rare and some reported cases are probably due to fecaliths that have dislodged.

Clinical manifestations:
Obstruction of the appendix initially produces central-abdominal cramps and reflex vomiting. A young child often indicates pain around umbilicus. Later as peritonitis sets in it lead to severe tenderness over the appendix, fever, tachycardia, and leukocytosis. The pain of peritonitis is made worse by movement and cough. Retrocolic appendix may irritate neighboring colon mimicking as acute gastroenteritis, similarly, pelvic appendicitis can cause urinary frequency and urgency by irritating the bladder mimicking as UTI. Rarely acute retrocecal or retroileal appendicitis may present with hip joint symptoms due to spasm of the right psoas muscle thus mimicking as septic arthritis of hip joint.

Physical Examination:
Inspection: The child with appendicitis frequently lies very quietly. The child may protect the right lower quadrant with a hand and may be reluctant to climb on the examination table. Abdominal examination may indicate complication such as intestinal perforation or obstruction.

Palpation of the abdomen should be gentle and aided by distraction. The right lower quadrant (McBurney point) should be palpated last; **McBurney point** is the junction of the lateral and middle thirds of the line joining the right anterior-superior iliac spine and the umbilicus. The most important finding is persistent direct tenderness, rigidity of the overlying rectus muscle and rebound tenderness. Rectal examination is done if the diagnosis is in doubt, especially in female adolescent excluding gynecological causes .

Laboratory findings:
CBC and urinalysis is must in all cases. The imaging studies that may be helpful include plain radiograph, ultrasonography and/or CT of the abdomen.

Management:
Children with non-perforated appendicitis require intravenous fluids and antibiotics. Appendicectomy should be done within a few hours of establishing the diagnosis. If the appendix has perforated with generalized peritonitis, significant fluid resuscitation and broad spectrum antibiotics with anaerobic coverage is required. Nasogastric suction should be used if the patient has significant vomiting or abdominal distension.

B. Hernia

Definition:
Hernia is a protrusion of the contents of a body compartment through the wall that normally encloses it.

Common types:
Most common hernia of the groin in infancy and childhood is the *indirect inguinal hernia (IIH)*. Femoral and direct inguinal hernias are rare in children (<1%). Other hernias in childhood are Esophageal, Diaphragmatic and Umbilical hernia.

Mechanism of Indirect inguinal hernia:
During the later stages of fetal development the processus vaginalis, an out-pouching of peritoneum originating at the internal ring, extends medially down each inguinal canal, leaving an obliterated passage through which intestines can protrude to the inguinal canal or scrotum. It is 3 times more common in premature babies then term infants

Common underlying causes:
Prematurity, (developmental uro-genital anomalies, increased Intra-abdominal pressure, Hypotonia and connective tissue weakness.

Clinical Manifestations:
Usually a swelling is noted at the external ring, but it may extend for a variable distance downward into the scrotum or the labia majora. The lump may be apparent only with raised intra-abdominal pressure, such as when the infant cries, or strains at stool and disappearing when baby relaxes with a bottle, or when an older child lies down. The diagnosis of inguinal hernia in infancy and childhood may be made from history alone even if significant physical findings are absent when the child is seen by the doctor, so long as the typical swelling is described by a competent observer. The older child with a hernia is likely to have had hydrocele in early infancy. The observation of an inguinal or inguino-scrotal mass which reduces either spontaneously or with manipulation is diagnostic. The diagnosis of hernia may be supported by palpation of a thickened spermatic cord on the side in question.

Management:
As there is no spontaneous resolution of indirect inguinal hernia, the treatment of choice is surgical repair at first available opportunity at a convenient time when the baby can tolerate the risk of surgery. Any inguinal hernia that cannot be reduced needs emergency surgical repair to avoid acute loss of blood supply and gangrene formation.

C. Hydrocele

Hydrocele in infants is the accumulation of fluid in the tunica vaginalis. It is found in 1-2 % newborns. It is mostly non-communicating with peritoneal cavity due to segmental closure of the processus vaginalis producing small hydrocele of the spermatic cord; sometimes it communicate with the peritoneal cavity leading to a reducible swelling that resembles inguinal hernia; swelling vary in size at different times and when distended, can be readily transilluminable. Most non-communicating Hydrocele disappears by one year age and requires no treatment. Hydroceles that persist (usually communicating type) after 1 year of age need be repaired by herniorrhaphy.

D. Phimosis, Paraphimosis and Circumcision

Phimosis is physiologic in early infancy, most prepuce become retractile by the 3 years of age. After this time a non-retractile prepuce or one with a tight tip is defined as Phimosis. This may be physiological or may result from fibrosis of prepuceal tip from forcible retraction of the prepuce in the past. Any prepuce that produces ballooning on voiding should be released surgically.

Paraphimosis is tightening of a phimotic prepuce behind the glans penis causing local pain and swelling. Reduction is by firm pressure against the glans with counter-traction on the prepuce. If unsuccessful, immediate surgical incision of the constricting band or circumcision is indicated.

Major medical indications for circumcision are persistent Phimosis or balanitis. Most circumcisions are performed on religious grounds. It is well documented that circumcision does give protection against UTI in under five children. UTI are reported 10 to 15 times more common in un-circumcised males then their counterparts.
Risks of circumcision are bleeding, wound infection, meatal stenosis, Phimosis and removal of insufficient skin. Prior to circumcision, a careful inspection of the penis should be made for anomalies such as epispadias, hypospadiasis, isolated chordee and anomalies of the penile skin; if any of these are present circumcision should be avoided, because the prepuce skin is needed for a reconstructive surgery.

E. Cryptorchidism (Undescended Testis)

Failure to find one or both testis in the scrotum may indicate absent, undescended or retractile testis. Cryptorchidism means hidden or undescended testes

Incidence:
One or both testes are undescended in about 30 percent of low birth weight infants, 4 percent of term infants. Most testis subsequently descend down by 6 months thus reducing incidence to about 0.8 percent at 6 months of age. Any testis not descended by 6 months age is unlikely to come down. Unilateral mal-descent is more common (90%) than bilateral.

Differential diagnosis:
Undescended testes must be differentiated from temporary or retractile testis due to hyperactive cremasteric muscles reflex which is a benign condition. Bilaterally impalpable testis could be due to ambiguous genitalia in a virilized female.

Pathology:
The ectopic testis may be located intra-abdominally or in the superficial inguinal region, perineum, thigh, femoral area, or at the base of penis.

Clinical examination:
To evaluate undescended testes adequately, examine in a warm relaxed environment with lubricated fingers. Exam may need to be repeated if failed once. Examination in squatting position may help in locating a highly placed testis.

Management:
Retractile testis require no treatment, gradually it will descend to scrotum.
The undescended testis is likely to be smaller than its mate, is more susceptible to malignant degeneration (Seminoma), and is a poor sperm producer leading to infertility. To detect bilateral testicular agenesis and thus avoid unnecessary surgery, children with bilateral undescended testes should have measurement of serum testosterone and urinary gonadotrophins after HCG challenge. When the testis is too high to be brought into scrotum and it appears salvageable, the choice is a 2 stage orchidopexy performed by 1 year of age. Orchidopexy does not appear to change the frequency of tumor, but makes the testis accessible to examination. A cosmetic result of orchidopexy is generally good but if fertility is apt to be improved is undetermined. Hormonal treatment with LHRH analog (Buserelin) is used in Europe but the results are not very impressive.

F. Intussusception

Intussusception occurs when one part of the intestine invaginates (telescoped) into the lumen of the adjoining bowel. It is the most common cause of intestinal obstruction in children below two years of age. male children are 4 times more affected than females. Annual incidence is 4 per 1000 live births.

Pathophysiology:
Telescoping of an intestinal loop with its mesentery causes venous compression and obstruction to the venous return of the intussusceptum leading to swelling, edema, and necrosis of the bowel wall. If neglected this usually ends up in arterial obstruction, ischemia necrosis, bowel perforation, peritonitis and death.

Causes:
The process begins with a lead point in the bowel, but the recognizable "lead points" are found in less than 10% of cases, and include:
- Meckel's diverticulum
- Neurofibroma or hemangioma
- Intestinal polyp
- Intestinal duplication
- Lymphoma
- Suture line of previous surgery
- Ectopic pancreas
- Thick impacted stools attached to the intestinal wall as in cystic fibrosis patients
- Intestinal wall hemorrhage as in hemophilia or Henoch Schonlein purpura.

In 90% of patients, hypertrophied Payer's patches accompanying URTI, otitis media, or gastroenteritis serve as the lead point. Adenoviral infections are mostly implicated. Rota viral infections and more importantly Rota viral vaccination were associated with increased incidence.

Clinical types:

Ileo-colic (at the ileocaecal junction) is the most common type
ileo-ileo-colic
Ceco-colic
Exclusively ileal.

Clinical picture:

1- Abdominal. Pain: Sudden severe, colicky pain causing the child to flex his knees and hips over the abdomen, it presents in intermittent bouts with pallor and circumoral cyanosis.

2- *Vomiting*: occurs early in the course; if neglected it becomes bilious or even fecal,

3- Bloody stools: Due to ulceration of the ischemic mucosa, occurs only in 60 % of patients, leading to the classical "red current jelly-like stools."

Always remember that the patient may be clinically free of symptoms in between the episodes of pain early in the disease. Palpation of the abdomen frequently reveals the presence of a tender sausage-shaped mass in the right hypochondrium or in the epigastrium, with absence of bowel in the right lower quadrant. Per rectal examination is mandatory and it may reveal the red current jelly-like stools. Rarely, the intussusceptum may prolapse through the rectum. If late, septicemia and shock may ensue. This condition can be fatal.

Diagnosis:

1- A careful history and examination gives enough clues for the diagnosis.
2- Plain X-ray of the abdomen may reveal sparse large bowel gas with a soft tissue mass in the area of the intussusception. X-ray may show signs of intestinal obstruction. X-ray is mandatory to rule out intestinal perforation before attempting reduction.
3- Ultrasound of the abdomen is the cornerstone for the diagnosis and for monitoring of reduction. Diagnostic findings include "a target, donut, or pseudo-kidney" appearance formed by the multilayered central echoes (intussusceptum) surrounded by the peripheral hypo echoes (intussuscepient).
4- Barium or water-soluble or air contrast enema show the filling defect (cupping), with a thin rim of contrast trapped around the invaginating intestine. This procedure may be curative reducing the intussusception back to normal.

Treatment:

1- Notify the surgical team, however,
2- **Medical management** before referral is of utmost importance and includes:
   a) Correction of dehydration, electrolyte disturbance and metabolic acidosis.
   b) Pain management,
   c) Cross-matching blood for children with profuse bleeding or those prepared for open surgery. Patients with severe bleeding may need to be transfused,
   d) Broad-spectrum antibiotic with good anaerobe coverage if perforation or sepsis suspected.
   e) If perforation, keep the patient NPO and insert a nasogastric tube for drainage.

3- After stabilization, refer the child for reduction (Hydrostatic or surgical):
   a) **Ultrasound monitored air or hydrostatic reduction.** Air reduction is preferred **in early cases.** Successful reduction is marked by free reflux of air into multiple loops of small intestine, and symptomatic improvement.
   b) **Open surgical approach** through a right lower quadrant incision is indicated either after failure of the air reduction or in late cases with high incidence of actual or suspected intestinal perforation.
   c) **Laparoscopic reduction** is a new trend for the treatment of intussusception. Is has satisfactory outcome in experienced hands.

Important Points to remember:
1- A child who appears normal at the time of examination, however, with a typical history and description of intussusception should be put under close observation, even if the initial clinical examination reveals no abnormal findings.
2- The signs and symptoms of acute gastroenteritis can mask the evolution of intussusception. Following should alarm you for the possible presence of intussusception:
   a) Change in the nature and course of illness, pain and vomiting
   b) Onset of rectal bleeding.
3- Exclude intestinal perforation before rushing to air or hydrostatic reduction.

G. Pyloric stenosis

As the name suggests this is a gastric outlet obstruction due to hypertrophy of the pyloric muscle mass from an unknown etiology.

Etiology, pathology and pathogenesis:

Infantile hypertrophic pyloric stenosis (HPS) varies in incidence in different ethnic groups. In USA it is reported as 3 per 1000 live born infants. It is 4 times more common in boys and classically occurs in a first child in a family at around 3 and 6 weeks of age.

A familial link was suggested; an increased incidence is observed in infants with blood group B or O, or after the administration of erythromycin or prostaglandin E2 in early infancy. Abnormal muscle innervation, elevated serum levels of prostaglandins, reduced levels of pyloric nitric oxide synthetase, and hypergastrinemia have been implicated in its pathogenesis. All these factors lead to hypertrophy of both the longitudinal and circular muscle layer, leading in turn to the elongation and thickening of the pylorus into an olive shaped mass causing gastric outlet obstruction.

Clinical Picture:
- The most important clue for diagnosis is non-bilious, usually projectile, progressively worsening **vomiting**, which occurs immediately after feeding, and classically starts by the third week of life (however, this can occur as early as the first week and as late as the fifth month of life).
- Patients are failing to thrive, wasted, dehydrated, constipated but are usually very eager to feed.
- They may have prolonged jaundice due to the inability to maintain glucuronyl transferase levels.

- Clinical examination:
    a) **Test Feed:** Feeling of the olive shaped mass, above and to the right of the umbilicus in the mid epigastrium beneath the liver edge during the feeding. The mass becomes more firm and is best felt just prior to onset of vomiting during a feed
    b) Visible peristalsis can be seen across the upper abdomen from left to right.

Laboratory Findings:

These mainly include *hypochloremic hypokalemic metabolic alkalosis*, occasionally pre-renal impairment secondary to the severe dehydration, and indirect hyperbilirubinemia may be seen (see before).

Diagnosis:

1. Clinical examination is sufficient to diagnose HPS in 60-80% of cases, *needing no further investigations.*
2. Abdominal ultrasound classically shows a pyloric length of 14 mm and a pyloric wall thickness of 4 mm.
3. Upper GI contrast (barium) study shows gastric dilatation, delayed gastric emptying, parallel streaks of barium in the narrowed elongated pyloric channel (string sign or rat tail sign), a bulge of the pyloric muscle into the antrum (shoulder sign), and an upturned pyloric curve.

Differential Diagnosis:

1. Faulty feeding, Inexperienced or anxious mothers
2. Pyloric atresia, antral web or membrane,
3. Gastric duplications, Gastric volvulus,
4. GERD with or without hiatal hernia,
5. Duodenal stenosis proximal to the ampulla of Vater (Down syndrome),
6. Salt-loosing congenital adrenal hyperplasia

Treatment:

1. Medical Treatment:

Fluid therapy- Correction of electrolyte imbalance and alkalosis is most vital prior to surgery. Commonly used fluid is 5% Dextrose in 0.45% saline + Potassium chloride 2-4 mEq/kg/day infused at a rate of 150-175 ml/kg/day. Correction of alkalosis is essential to prevent postoperative apnea. Keep the patient NPO with possible nasogastric suction. The patient should be ready for operation within 24 hours.

2. Surgical Treatment:

The "**Fredet-Ramstedt Pyloromyotomy**" is the gold standard. It is done either through an open or a laparoscopic approach. It entails splitting the pyloric muscle until the submucosa is seen bulging upwards. Persistent vomiting suggests incomplete pyloromyotomy, gastritis, GERD, or another cause of obstruction.

14.2 Common Pediatric ENT Conditions

The otolaryngology consultation and examination
This examination differs from other examinations as the regions of interest are rather inaccessible. The otoscope is the most useful instrument used for examination.

Clinical examination starts while taking the **history** from parent, by assessing the airway, general alertness, inspection of the head, neck, nose, ears and face. If the child is uneasy, proceed slowly as once confidence is lost it takes long to recover.

Examination Position: Small children are examined sitting on the mothers lap with one arm of mother is cuddling across the chest and arms of the child while the other hand steadies the fore-head of the child.

The examination includes; inspection and palpation of the head and neck for masses, lymph nodes, and salivary glands. Ear examination includes examination of external ear, otoscopic examination, and auditory acuity. Nasal examination includes anterior rhinoscopy with otoscope, lastly the oral cavity and oropharynx is examined by tongue depressor. For examination of the nasopharynx, hypopharynx and larynx child needs a specialist evaluation by flexible pediatric direct laryngoscopy with fiber optic nasopharyngolaryngoscope.

Airway obstruction in children

The signs and symptoms of airway obstruction in children include stridor, respiratory distress, feeding difficulties and aspiration. The quality and timing of **stridor** can give a clue as to the site of obstruction; if the obstruction is in the hypopharynx or larynx child will have an inspiratory stridor, if the site is in the trachea a biphasic stridor is noticed. Obstruction at level of bronchi and bronchioles presents with expiratory stridor.
Causes of airway obstruction are classified according to the age group:

> **Neonates-** Laryngomalacia is the most common cause of stridor in neonates and infants, other congenital causes include choanal atresia, nasopharyngeal dermioids, glioma, encephalocele, laryngocele, vocal cord palsy, glottic web, subglottic stenosis, laryngeal cleft, tracheomalacia, hemangioma, and glossoptosis in Pierre-robin and Downs syndrome.

> **Infants-** Foreign body inhalation is the most common cause of accidental death in children. Other causes include croup, bacterial tracheitis, and acute epiglottitis.

> **Young children-** Foreign body, infections like pertonsilar-parapharyngeal abscess, Ludwig's angina, Laryngeal trauma, tumors of airway and angioneurotic edema can all produce airway obstruction

The **signs of respiratory distress** include nasal flaring, supra clavicular, intercostals in drawing, sternal retraction use of accessory muscles of respiration with tachypnea and cyanosis.

Otitis Media

Otitis media is defined as inflammation in the middle ear. Based on the duration of disease, it can be acute, sub acute, and chronic:

1.   Acute Otitis media:

60-70% children usually have one episode before 3 yrs age;
Microbiology: *S. Pneumonia, H.influenzae, M. catarrhalis, and S. aureus* are the common organisms besides viruses.
Predisposing factors are – Eustachian tube dysfunction and obstruction, bottle feeding, passive smoking, and overcrowding. Obstruction of Eustachian tube leads to air absorption in middle ear causing negative middle ear pressure, resulting in middle ear mucosal oedema and exudates, and later infection of exudates.
Infants and toddlers present with ear-pulling and irritability due to otalgia, fever and hearing loss, *acute otitis media may be the hidden cause in a febrile children* and diagnosis can be missed unless otoscopy is routinely performed. If the Tympanic membrane is perforated there will be mucopurulent discharge (otorrhea). Otoscopy of tympanic membrane reveals retraction of the tympanic membrane in early stages with loss of bony landmarks followed by hyperemia (Redness), bulging of the tympanic membrane with reduced mobility and some times perforation.
Treatment is symptomatic with antipyretics, analgesics, decongestants, and antihistamines. Systemic antibiotics – Amoxicillin, Erythromycin and Cephalosporins may hasten resolution. Antibiotic drops instilled locally have no role. In children with recurrent acute otitis media, complicated otitis media, Myringotomy and tympanostomy tubes are indicated.
Complications include; TM perforation, chronic suppurative OM, Cholesteatoma, mastoiditis, labyrinthitis, sigmod sinus thrombophlebitis. The serious intracranial complications include meningitis, brain abscess and facial nerve paralysis.

2.   Otitis media with effusion (OME):

Also called as **Glue ear.** It is defined as fluid in the middle ear without signs or symptoms of ear infection. Frequently follows acute otitis media and adenotonsilar disease in children. Risk factors, predisposing causes and pathogenesis are similar to Acute suppurative otitis media. The child usually presents with delayed speech hearing loss and, poor school performance. On otoscopy TM appears dull, grey, often with air bubbles behind the TM. Diagnosis can be confirmed by tympanometery where a flat curve is obtained due to poor TM mobility.
90% cases resolve spontaneously by three months, medical therapy by antibiotics, antihistamines, nasal decongestants often help in resolution, for refractory cases myringotomy, ventilation tubes with or without adenoidectomy is the surgical treatment

The Adenoids and Adenoiditis

In children repeated URTI and allergies can lead to chronic adenoiditis and adenoid hypertrophy. The size peaks at 3-5 years of age and resolves by 12-15 yrs with maturity of the immune system. Clinical features include adenoid facies (dull facial expression, open mouth, and hyper nasal voice). There is a history of snoring and obstructive sleep apnea in severe cases. Chronic nasal obstruction, nasal discharge, postnasal drip and cough are invariably present in children with adenoiditis and adenoid hypertrophy. Diagnosis is usually clinical but can be confirmed by enlarged adenoid shadow seen on plain Lateral X-Ray of neck and face taken in position of retracted neck. Complications of adenoid hypertrophy are sleep apnea with or without cor pulmonale. Adenoidectomy is indicated if child has chronic upper airway obstruction with sleep disturbance, sleep apnea, medically refractory chronic nasopharngtis, recurrent or refractory acute otitis media, and Otitis media with effusion and chronic suppurative otitis media.

Tonsillitis

1.   Acute tonsillitis

The etiology of acute tonsillitis is infection by *Group A beta hemolytic streptococcus. S. pneumonia, S.aureus, H Influenza M.catarrhalis and EB Virus* . Child presents in acute attack with severe sore throat, dysphagia, fever and malaise. Throat examination reveals inflamed tonsils often with follicles (Pustules), and cervical lymphadenopathy of the submandbular and jugulodigastric glands. A throat swab and CBC are indicated in a child with acute tonsillitis. Treatment advised is bedrest, analalgesia, antipyretics and antibiotics; penicillin, amoxicillin, erythromycin.

2.   Chronic tonsillitis

 is diagnosed if more than 3 attacks of tonsillitis occur for past 3 years or more than 6 attacks for past one year. For these children tonsillectomy is indicated, other absolute indications for tonsillectomy include sleep apnea with corpulmonale and excisional biopsy for suspected malignancy like lymphomas.

15

Common Gynecologic Problems

15.1 Gynecological History and Physical examination

A detailed gynecological history or examination is routinely not required unless there is specific concern or complaint is made. On a routine basis, one may enquire about H/O urinary symptoms or vaginal discharge or rash in children or about the menarche and menstrual disorders in adolescent girls.

Gynecologic examination in children should be done very gently and after explanation and verbal consent from the child and parents. Children need lot of reassurance in order to avoid a long lasting psychological trauma.

A. Examination of Neonate:

Breast size may normally be enlarged and there may also be a nipple discharge (Witches milk) in newborn due to the effects of maternal estrogens. The parents must be reassured about the self limiting nature of this condition and need strictly be warned not to press or squeeze the breast swelling as this may encourage the development of breast abscess.

The abdomen must be palpated gently to rule out any organomegaly.

External genitalia are assessed for any ambiguity (Clitoromegaly, fused labia or presence of gonad in the labial folds). Inspection of the Labia and introitus usually reveals a thin white mucoid discharge and a normal protuberant hymen.

In the first few days of life there may be a small amount of vaginal bleeding due to declining levels of circulating maternal estrogens, again the parents need be counseled and reassured about the self-limiting and benign nature of this condition.

B. Pre-pubertal child:

The initial gynecological assessment of a child must be in a friendly, relax and safe environment in presence of an attendant usually the mother.

An adequate explanation to the child as well as the mother is important before and during the examination.

Inspection of vulvo-vaginal area is best done in frog –leg position. Look for any *abnormal discharge, trauma, foreign body and condition of hymen*. If needed, aspirate can be collected for examination under microscope and for culture. In some cases when detailed examination is needed, it could be performed under sedation or anesthesia by a competent gynecologist.

C. Adolescent:

History must be taken in details from the patient as well as the parent. Confidentiality must be highly regarded in this age group. Patient must be offered a separate interview to speak to physician in confidence if required. Concerns for *vaginal discharges (STI), pregnancy, or menstrual disturbances* should be explored. A competent and experienced physician should only perform examination at this age after verbal consent and in presence of an attendant preferably the mother. Dorsal lithotomy position is preferred position for examination.

15.2 Sexual abuse in children

Child sexual abuse is on rise globally and yet it is universally under reported.
Definition: (Shecter & Roberge 1976): Involvement of children in sexual activities that they can not understand, for which they are not developmentally prepared, to which they can not give informed consent and/or that violate the normal social norms.
Sexual abuse may also be associated with physical or emotional abuse and child neglect.

Incidence:

This condition is on rise and grossly under-reported.
In USA 150,000 cases are reported each year
80% of reported cases were females
Most vulnerable age is between 7 to 13 years

Clinical evaluation:

History:

Acute presentations are rare; mostly the problems are long standing and repetitive.
Separate account must be obtained from the child as well as the family
Ask only non leading questions
Questions to the child should be developmentally appropriate
Clinician must gain the child's trust by creating a non-threatening atmosphere. A non-judgmental approach that focuses on child is important.
Ask about the symptoms like local trauma, bleeding, pain, discharge, and pain on defecation.
Ask about the relationship with the perpetrator, methods used, single or repeated episodes, any threats made
Ask about any psychosexual impacts, performance at school, in small children there is some tell tail signs like excessively clinging, anxiety, nightmares, and loss of bowel/urinary control

Physical examination:

Examination is performed according to the age (see before)
In small pre-pubertal children simple inspection is enough
Note any injuries, discharge, bleeding or foreign body, blood staining
Bite marks
Note any hymen loss / attenuation
Note if any Healed tears / scars, tear of the hymen and forchette
Note any signs of sexually transmitted disease
Few physical signs are quite suggestive of abuse: Presence of semen or sperm, genital injuries without any accidental explanation, Syphilis or culture proven gonorrhea infection
Labial adhesions, mild hymen trauma or Candida are not indicative of abuse

Laboratory tests:

Take the secretion for microscopy for sperm and organism
Culture for Gonorrhea, Chlamydia and other genital culture
Test for syphilis (RPR),
Hepatitis serology and HIV if indicated
Other forensic tests

Management:

> Ensure child safety and inform social authorities for child protection
> Always involve the senior doctor
> Counsel the parents
> Involvement of child psychologist
> Painkillers and sitz bath may help relieve inflammation
> Treatment of identified STD
> Prevention of pregnancy in adolescents by Hormonal treatment

Complications:

> Sexually transmitted diseases
> Emotional trauma leading to various social problems like mistrust, suicide attempt, school failure, depression etc
> Drug abuse
> Pregnancy
> Aggressive hypersexual behavior

Long-term sequels of sexual abuse are:

> Sexual precociousness, reckless sexual behavior, and sexual dysfunction
> Difficulties in trust, isolation and a dislike of intimacy
> Depression, phobias, and re-victimization
> Self harm, substance abuse, delinquent behavior

15.3 Vaginal discharge in children (Vulvovaginitis)

Vulvovaginitis: Is the most common gynecological problem in children and pre-pubertal girls

Reasons for high incidence:
>   Lack of protection due to lack of labial fat, pubic hair and thin labia minora
>   Vaginal alkaline pH
>   Thin vaginal mucosa due to lack of estrogen effect
>   Close proximity to rectum and inadequate cleaning

Clinical Manifestations:
>   Vaginal discharge
>   Erythema
>   Pruritus
>   Dysuria

Causes of vaginal discharge in children:
>   Physiologic/Non-specific: a normal variant and self-limiting, discharge is clear, non-irritating and not foul smelling.
>   Bacterial: Gardnerella, Anaerobes, Enterococci and Group B Strept.
>   Protozoa: Trichmonas
>   Fungal: Candida
>   Viral
>   Helminthes: Pinworms and scabies
>   Foreign body, irritants like bubble bath, talk, detergents, tight fitting synthetic clothes etc
>   Sex abuse

Management:
>   Good history and examination
>   Swabs for microscopy and cultures
>   Local hygiene and avoidance of all precipitating factors
>   Proper cleaning after toilet, cleaning the perineum from front to back
>   Check for foreign body (Sand, tissues etc)
>   Sitz bath and use of mild soap, keeping area dry
>   Treat the pathogen
>   Topical estrogen cream can prevent reoccurrence by improving local epithilization.

Labial adhesions

This condition is commonly seen in preschool girls.
The labia minora recurrently get adhered centrally by a line joining from clitoris to forchette.
This happens due to recurrent local inflammation as a result of low estrogenic state in pre-pubertal girls.
The condition is usually asymptomatic but may be associated with pooling of urine in the vagina leading to recurrent vulvovaginal and Urinary tract infections in 20-40% of girls.
Topical Estrogen cream applied for 1 week, followed by bland ointment of petrolatum or zinc oxide for 1month, is effective in 90% of cases.
Mechanicals separation of the adhesions is done if easy followed by examination for any vaginal septum.

Foreign body

Foreign body in the vagina are the common causes of blood stained/fowl smelling vaginal discharge in children; the object may be a cotton wool, a small toy, sand from the beach or a fragment of toilet paper.

Hymenal trauma, or repetitive self-insertion of foreign objects should raise suspicion of exposure to sexual abuse.

Foreign bodies in the vagina need to be removed carefully, vaginal discharge be treated as outlined above and advice given for prevention in future.

16

Preparation for Examination

16.1   Extended Matching Questions (EMQ)

What are Extended Matching Questions?
- They are also known as type (R) questions.
- They are reasonable alternative to MCQ or free response questions.
- Are based on the idea of matching two items from different lists as in simple matching questions, but in EMQ the list of options contains more items than the other (stem) list, which is written as clinical scenario or vignette.
- Questions are matched to a list of options where any number of answers from a long list may be correct or incorrect.
- Examinees may also rank from a list of options those that are more correct.
- The same list of options can pertain to any number of independent test items.

Advantages of EMQ
- Objective and easy to mark
- Reliability of scoring is high
- It is used to test both knowledge and application of knowledge.
- Relative to MCQ format there is less cuing & less chance of examinees guessing

Drawbacks of EMQ
- Difficult to construct.
- Do not test understanding & reasoning very well compared to short essay and oral examination, which test reasoning best.
- Higher order skills can't be assessed without some writing from the students.
- Neither EMQ nor MCQ are adequate for assessing generative skills. Short essay & MEQ are used for this purpose.

Amplified EMQs
- To make EMQ useful tool for assessing students reasoning abilities & to reduce "sneak-a-peek" cheating, amplified EMQ format is used in some medical schools.
- Students are asked to justify each answer of EMQ in a 1-2 sentences
- Justifications are written on separate paper & are used to assign partial credit.

Steps in Writing EMC
- Identify the theme & outcome you wish to assess
- Prepare the list of options first and then think about the appropriate scenarios for each.
- Write the lead-in statement.
- Write the stems or scenarios; usually 5 or 6 stems for each theme.
- Review the items carefully.

Identify the Theme
Theme is a topic addressed by a set of items. It may be
- Clinical sign
- Chief complaint or complication
- Emergency or bedside procedure
- Treatment or class of drug
- Diagnostic test

- Patho-physiological concept
- Lab data or microbiology organism
- Genetic or mode of inheritance
- Biochemical defect or compound

The Option List

- It provides the response choices that apply to the theme-related items.
- Sets can be made more or less difficult by altering the option list in terms of number & the degree of discrimination.
- Options may be single words, short phrases or more creative forms such as pictorial material.

Prepare the list of options

- Options should be homogeneous, concise & approximately of equal length.
- Usually double the number of items (usually, number of items +3).
- It should be arranged alphabetically or in a logical order.
- Avoid subtle differences and uncommon diagnoses & consider examinee level.

Write the lead-in

- A single lead-in statement is used for all items in a set.
- It provides directions for the set and indicates the relationship between the stems and the options.
- Care must be taken to give explicit directions and to avoid ambiguity.

Write the stems

- A useful form of item stem is the clinical vignette, which describes a patient or a clinical situation.
- EMQ can be written in a non-vignette format, but when so written it should not focus on recall of isolated facts or on simple associations.
- To minimize cuing, stems within a set should be of similar structure.

Review the items

- Ensure one single best answer for each question.
- Usually not more than 5 or 6 stems per theme.
- Check that all stems are relevant to the theme and are in accordance with the lead-in.

Example

Theme: Breathlessness in children
Options:

    A. Lateral neck X-ray
    B. Prepare to establish an airway
    C. Sweat chloride test
    D. Serum Ig E level
    E. Throat swab for gram's stain
    F. Emergency tracheostomy
    G. Bronchoscopy
    H. Humidified oxygen

    I. Aerosolized racemic adrenaline

    J. Oral theophylline

Lead-in: For each patient, select the initial intervention or the investigation.

Item stems:

1. A 10-yr-old boy presents with breathlessness & infra orbital swelling. O/E he has barrel chest, pale boggy nasal mucosa & expiratory wheeze.

2. A 9-month-old baby had a mild URTI. 4 days later he developed a brassy cough & intermittent stridor. O/E he has nasal flaring & retraction of intercostals muscles. There were no crackles or rhonchi.

3. A 6 yr old child with severe asthma is started on IV Aminophyllin drip. He is feeling sleepy & become less responsive. Auscultation revealed less wheezing than on admission.

4. A 5 yr old girl presents with high-grade fever, sore throat and inspiratory stridor. You note drooling of saliva from her mouth.

5. A 3-yr old boy presents with recurrent right lobe pneumonia and wheezing. Examination shows reduced air entry in the right infra mammary region.

Key: 1. D,   2. H,   3. B,   4. B,   5. G

16.2 Introduction to OSCE
(Objective Structured Clinical Examination)

Definition:
OSCE is an examination format or framework to assess student's clinical competence and performance. OSCE is more objective and reliable than long and short case, viva voce etc.

Basic format and general rules for the OSCE:
- There are multiple stations, usually 12-20, each testing different skills and competence
- All station have the same time limit, 5-10 minutes
- All students rotate through all the stations and thus are tested on the same material
- All students are judged by the same preset standards, usually using check lists or rating scales
- All students are assessed by the same examiner fixed to the individual station

Tests scenario commonly used in the OSCE:
- Test of clinical skills by:
  - History taking
  - Performance of physical examinations
  - Demonstration of a procedures (on models)
- Test of Knowledge and understanding by using:
  - Data Interpretation
  - Picture reading
  - Radiological images reading
  - Problem solving
- Test of counseling skills and attitude

Tests methods, which may be used
- Short cases (Real patients or surrogates)
- Oral examination
- Interpretation of laboratory result and images
- Computerized problem solving

Format of Pediatric OSCE Circuit

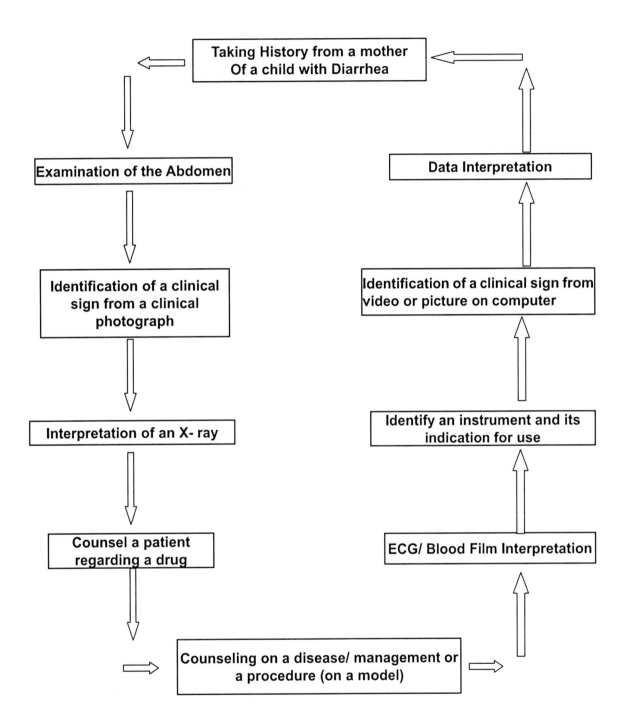

16.3 Communication Skills

Effective communication involves skills of questioning, active listening, and facilitating help.

Questioning:

1.   Always use open ended questions especially at the beginning of the interview.
2.   Obtain specific information using focused and closed questions.
3.   Use probing questions to clarify and check accuracy
4.   Avoid using leading questions
5.   Avoid asking several questions at once
6.   Give the patient time to answer
7.   Rephrase the questions in a simple language if they are not clear

Listening:

1.   Allow patients to talk without interruption
2.   Effective listening means concentrating on what the patient says and trying
to   understand their feelings as they speak.
3.   Be alert to verbal and non-verbal cues.
4.   Use appropriate body language to demonstrate your attention
5.   Allow pauses or silences

The interview between patient and doctor is to gain as accurate a picture as possible of the patient's problem. This information must then be processed in such a way that will enable the doctor to develop a plan of management and communicate it back to the patient.

Developing a Management Plan for a Patient
Establish a relationship with the patient

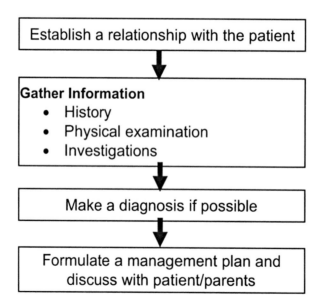

460

Guidelines for conducting an interview

At the beginning of the interview:
- Greet patient and shake hands if appropriate
- Ask to sit down
- Introduce yourself
- Explain purpose of interview
- Say how much time is available
- Explain need to take notes

Main parts of interview:
- Maintain a positive atmosphere; warm manners and good eye contact
- Listen carefully/Be alert and responsive to verbal and non-verbal cues
- Facilitate the patient both verbally *("tell me more")* and non- verbally *(Using posture and head nods)*
- Use specific (closed) questions when appropriate
- Clarify what the patient has told you
- Encourage the patient to be relevant

Ending the interview:
Summarize what the patient has told you and ask if your summary is accurate. Ask if they would like to add anything and thank the patient.

Giving information (Counseling)

The way, in which information is given, influences patient's satisfaction and compliance.
- Outline what information you plan to give
- Summarize your understanding of the patient's problem
- Before giving information find out their understanding of the condition
- Outline the structure of the rest of the interview *(diagnosis/treatment/ complication…)*
- Use appropriate language *(avoid medical jargons, avoid vagueness instead use short, simple words and sentences)*
- If relevant, use drawings to supplement the information
- Give the most important piece of information first
- Explore the patient's views on the information given
- Negotiate management
- Check the patient's understanding

Breaking the bad news

Giving bad news is most challenging of tasks in medical practice. The way it is given affects how people cope and adjust with their problem. Before giving bad news, consider the likely consequences of giving it and be prepared to response appropriately.
- Be familiar with the child's name, gender and parents' name.
- It helps to find out what the patient already knows and may want to be told. Making assumptions about either of these can lead to serious problems in management.

- Giving bad news requires time free from distractions or interruptions, empathy, active listening and humility to say that you may not have the answers to certain questions.
- Have lab results and relevant scans available
- Inform the parent candidly, clearly and completely
  - -Get to the point quickly
  - -Be comfortable with silence
  - -Name the diagnosis if possible
  - -Avoid medical jargon
  - -Individualize information to the specific situation
  - -Demonstrate empathy and caring
  - -Provide information about peer support groups
- Elicit the patient's own resources for coping / Instill realistic hope
- Be prepared to discuss prognosis and "next steps"
- Ensure that colleagues know what the patient has been told
- Provide support for the patient's relative and your professional colleagues
- Negotiate future plans
- Arrange follow-up meetings if needed

Telling parents they have an abnormal baby
- Parents should be told of the problem as soon as possible. Tell them together. A single mother should be asked if she would like someone with her.
- The most senior person should break the news
- It may be helpful to make a drawing of the abnormality. The explanation should be brief and simple avoiding too much detail at this stage.
- Parents are often afraid of what they will see. Encourage them to first hold the baby.
- The baby should be wrapped in a blanket with only its face showing. The parents should also be persuaded to name the baby, and the doctor and colleagues should use the name.
- Positive features should be emphasized, although a balanced and realistic view should be presented.

Communicating with children

Do's:
- Put yourself at the same physical level as the child when you examine or talk to them.
- Establish rapport before touching the child; gain their confidence e.*g.: by playing*
- Learn the child's terminology for their concerns and parts of the anatomy.
- Explain what you are going to do before doing them. Prepare the child for a strange noise or smell, a painful procedure, or change from a familiar routine.
- Keep talking, a calm voice is reassuring, even if it does not stop the child crying.
- Engage the help of a parent or guardian, especially when examining a child.

Don'ts:

- Rely too much on bribery or small gifts. Child will constantly expect a reward after treatment or medication.
- Make promises you can't keep, e.g. 'this will not hurt'
- Use complex language or medical terms. If appropriate, check the child understands by asking them to repeat what you have said, or to demonstrate using a doll or teddy.
- Allow the child to worry about a medical procedure. Try to carry it out immediately to prevent prolonged anxiety.
- Leave the child alone in an unfamiliar setting or with unfamiliar people.
- Encourage the child to be "good." Instead, allow them to cry or scream if appropriate.

16.4 Sharing the bad news with parents

Introduction:

Sharing bad news with the family of a child is painful part of pediatrics practice. Health care providers in all areas of the specialty face it but for some it is a daily chore e.g.: Oncologists and Neonatologists. Giving "Bad News" is amongst the most challenging of tasks in medical practice. Recent advances in treatment especially in cancer care have made it relatively easier to offer hope compared to a few years ago when prospects for cure of malignancies were bleak. The way bad news is given affects how people cope and adjust. The doctor may feel responsible and fears of being blamed. He may not know how best to do it. There may be an element of possible inhibition because of personal experience of loss and reluctance to spoil the existing doctor-patients' relationships. Parents vividly remember the manner in which the diagnosis of their child's illness was communicated to them for years after the event as the news may have resulted in a critical change in the future of child and family.

A proper strategy should be planned before breaking the bad news including the set-up of the interview and specific techniques of communications. Parent's intellectual and social background, ethical and legal imperatives should always be kept in mind. Undergraduates and postgraduates programs should have relevant courses included in the curricula and junior doctors should be encouraged to observe experienced colleagues in these encounters.

Definition of bad news

- Any information that adversely and seriously affects an individual's view and threatening his or her future mental or physical well-being.
- Bad news is always in the eye of the beholder.
- A relative concept could be an impending death (terminal illness), diagnosis of serious incurable illness or congenital abnormality and progressive disease or handicap.
- When an illness is serious or a child dies, parents deserve to be told in a way that helps them cope with their grief.

Why Is Delivering Bad News So Challenging?

- The way bad news is presented to a family may influence the parent's ability to cope.
- The experience tests the strength of the doctor-patients' relationships.
  The two participants: physician and parents are experiencing conflicts independent of each other.
- The Physician's Responsibility
  - Inform the parents candidly, clearly and completely
  - At the same time avoid hurting them unduly

  However, this can be particularly stressful when:
  - The clinician is inexperienced
  - The patient is young
  - There are only limited prospects for successful treatment

Remember that parents want to know **the truth**, though may resist it and be unprepared to accept it.
Besides there are cultural, ethical and legal imperatives in sharing Bad News.

Burden of Responsibility
- •How to be honest with the patient without destroying hope
- •Dealing with the patients' emotions
- •The news may sometimes create unwarranted optimum to patient or parent.

The Bearer of Bad News Often Experiences Stress
- Anxiety
  - Not having had any formal training in breaking bad news
  - No opportunity during training to observe bad news being delivered
- Being uncomfortable, physicians tend to avoid discussing distressing information but sometimes there is no choice but to convey the bad news.
- A plan for determining patient values and a strategy for addressing their distress when   the news is given
  - Can significantly increase the physician's confidence
  - Can significantly reduce stress and burn-out in the physician
  - May encourage parents to participate in difficult treatment decisions

Strategy for sharing bad news
- •Set-up an interview
- •Determine who will participate
- •Prepare to communicate the news
  - Check patients' understanding of the information
  - Identify patients' main concerns
  - Elicit patients' copying strategies
- •Use specific techniques for sharing the news
- •Anticipate parental reactions
- •Negotiate future plans
- •Arrange follow-up meetings
- •Health care team "debriefing"

1) Setting-up An Interview
- •Arrange for the meeting as soon as you are aware that a problem exists (without delay)
- •Choose a private place
- •Provide protected, uninterrupted time
- •Arrange the room so everyone can be seated
- •Make sure the person giving the news is at eye level with the people receiving it

2) Determining Who Participates
- •Have the physician most familiar with the child's medical condition break the news
- •Tell both parents at the same time if possible
- •Discourage initial participation of the child if you suspect strong parental reactions
- •Try to have a colleague available if he/she has a close relationship with the family
- •Have another health care professional present to provide support for the family
- •If language is a barrier, use an experienced translator, rather than a family member
- •Avoid unnecessary participants

3) Preparing to break the news

- Write down three or four most important points to be covered during the interview
- Prepare a plan for establishing the interview
- Be familiar with the child's name, gender and parent's name
- Have lab results and relevant scans available
- Be prepared to discuss prognosis and "next steps"
- Anticipate your own reactions to the encounter

4) Techniques for sharing the news

- Get to the point quickly
- Be comfortable with silence
- Active listening
- Name the diagnosis if possible
- Avoid medical jargon, use simple language
- Maintain optimism and realistic hope
- Find out what they want to know and elicit patients' own resources for copying
- Individualize information to the specific situation
- Demonstrate empathy and caring
- Provide families with information about peer support groups

5) Anticipate parental reactions

- Anticipate expressions of anger, sadness, guilt, blame, relief or a combination of these feelings
- Never judge a parents reaction
- Acknowledge the parents emotions and allow the parents to express them
- Try to comfort
- Be polite and firm
- If he stands up, beat his level of eyes

6) Negotiating future plans

- Work with parents as partners
- Assess parental concerns and perceived barriers
- Elicit parental input in developing the treatment plan
- Ask questions, don't make assumptions

7) Arranging follow-up meetings

- Parents will not absorb all the information at the first meeting
- Encourage them to write down questions
- Arrange a follow-up meeting to address and clarify key points
- A plan should be made for follow-up to provide a further opportunity to address concern
- Can refer to a Social Worker or Psychologist or Counselor for further management.

8) Health care team debriefing

- Debriefing members of the caring team after an event is helpful
- Inform about the meeting and summarize including the problems or reactions encountered
- The team may experience feelings of sadness, anger, guilt or relief

•They need to pay attention to their own emotions
•Support and comfort for the team should come from valued colleagues or friends

Should Children Be Told?
- Most children know when something serious is going on
  - Over time experience similar distress as older more informed children
  - Figure it out themselves
  - Non disclosure tends to make them feel isolated

- Children are often told little about their illness
  - To protect them from fear and feeling of being overwhelmed
  - Cultural issues, family hierarchy, relationships among family members influence decisions on how much to tell
  - Younger children have limitations in reasoning
- It is beneficial to have open lines of communication between parents, the child and physician. Sensitivity to cultural norms, age and developmental stage of child

Poor delivery of bad news
•Being too blunt
•Discussing at an inappropriate time and place
•Conveying the sense that there was no hope or giving unrealistic hope

Guidelines (Summary of the main points)
- Parents should be told of the problems as soon as possible
- First check how much they are aware of and what they want to know
- The most senior person responsible in the care of patient, should break the news
- It may be helpful to make a drawing of the abnormality
- Positive features should be emphasized, although a balanced and realistic view should be presented
- Take it seriously. You may say in firm tone
- "I'm sorry to have to give you this news. I realize that you were not expecting to hear this." However, you may also want to speak to someone else and get their opinion
- As a last resort, if you fear for your safety, open the door, or leave the room
- If the patient threatens suicide: In most cases, patients can be talked out of harming themselves or resorting to suicide. However, this demands patience, care and re-assurance
- Not discharged or left alone, get help of psychiatrist

Conclusion
Communicating "Bad News" is a fundamental physician's skill. Doctors should be aware that their own sense of a good encounter may differ from that of their patients especially when cultural backgrounds differ.

These conversations when handled well taking into consideration of cultural and religious backgrounds can help patient being informed, hopeful and physicians affirmed their commitment to their care of patients.

Appendices

I. Normal values in Pediatrics

Normal Respiratory Rate (per mt.):

Infant   30 - 40
Toddler   24 - 40
School Age   18 - 30
Adolescent   12 - 16

Normal Heart Rate (per mt.):

Age	Awake	Mean	Sleeping
< 3 months	85 - 205	140	80 - 160
3 mo to 2 yr.	100 - 190	130	75 - 160
3 yr. to 10 yr.	60 - 140	80	60 - 90
> 10 yr.	60 - 100	75	50 - 90

At any age HR > 220, consider SVT.

Normal Blood Pressure *(from Hazinski MF 1992)*

	Systolic	Diastolic
Day 1 (< 1000g)	39 - 59	16 - 36
Day 1 (> 3000g)	50 - 70	25 - 45
Neonate	60 - 90	20 - 60
Infant	87 - 105	53 - 66
Toddler	95 - 105	53 - 66
> 7 years	97 - 122	57 - 71
> 15 years	112 - 128	66 - 80

Blood Pressure in Hypertension: See chapter on hypertension
Hypotension: if systolic BP is

         0 - 1 month   < 60
         1 mo - 1 yr.   < 70
         Older   < 70 + (2 x age in years)

$$Body\ Surface\ Area\ (m_2) = \sqrt{\frac{Ht\ (cm)\ x\ Wt\ (Kg)}{3600}}$$

Hematology
a) Routine Hematological Values

Age	Hb (g/dL)	PCV (%)	Retics	MCV (fL) Lowest	MCH (pg/cell). Lowest	TWBC (x1000)	Neu (Mean)	Lymp (Mean)
Cord Blood	13.7–20.1	45-65	5.0	110		9-30	61	31
2 wk	13.0–20.0	42-66			29	5-21	40	63
3 mo	9.5–14.5	31-41			27	6-18	30	48
6 mo – 6 yr	10.5–14.0	33-42	1.0	70-74	25-31	6-15	45	48
7-12 yr	11.0–16.0	34-40		76-80	26-32	4.5-13.5	55	38
Adult Male	14.0–18.0	42-52	1.6	80	27-32	5-10	55	35
Adult Female	12.0–16.0	37-47			26-34			

Eosinophils: 2-3%, Monocytes: 6-9 %

Platelets are mildly decreased in 1st few months, by 6 months have reached 250 - 300 x 10$_9$.
ESR should be < 16 in childhood provided PCV at least 35%.
b) Differential WBC

< 7 days	**Neutrophils > Lymphocytes**
1 wk - 4 yr.	**Lymphocytes > Neutrophils**
5 yr - 7 yr.	**Neutrophils = Lymphocytes**
> 7 yr.	**Neutrophils > Lymphocytes**

Normal values in clinical chemistry:

Acid-Base	PH 7.3-7.45 PCO$_2$ 4.5-6 kPa (32-45 mmHg) PO$_2$ 11-14 kPa (78-105 mmHg) Bicarbonate 18-25 mmol/L Base Excess -4 to +3 mmol/L
Alanine Amino-Transferase (ALT) Albumin	Newborn 1 month up to 70 IU/L Infants and children 15-55 IU/L Preterm 25-45 g/L Newborn (term) 25-50 g/L 1-3 months 30-42 g/L 3-12 months 27-50 g/L 1-15 years 32-50 g/L
Alkaline Phosphatase	Newborn 150-600 u/L 6 months-9 years 250-800 u/L
Ammonia	Newborn <80 µmol/L Infants and children <50 µmol/L
Amylase	70-300 IU/L
Aspartate Amino-Transferase (AST)	<45 IU/L
Base Excess	See Acid-Base
Bicarbonate	See Acid-Base
Bilirubin	Full term day 1 <65 µmol/L Day 2 <115 µmol/L 3-5 days <155 µmol/L > month <10 µmol/L
Calcium (Ionized)	Adult Value is 1.19-1.29 mmol/L Preterm 1.5-2.5 mmol/L Infants 2.25-2.75 mmol/L >1 year 2.25-2.6 mmol/L Correction for protein binding-measure Ca^{2+} + (40-Albumin/40 g/L) mmol/L
Calcium (Urine)	Children <0.1 mmol/kg per 24 hours
Chloride	95-105 mmol/L
Creatine Kinase	Newborn <600 IU/L 1 month <400 IU/L 1 year <300 IU/L Children <190 IU/L (male), <130 IU/L (female)

Creatinine	0-2 years 20-50 μmol/L
	2-3 years 25-60 μmol/L
	6-12 years 30-80 μmol/L
	>12 years 65-120 μmol/L (male), 50-110 μmol/L (female)
Creatinine Clearance	0-3 months 17-50 ml/min/m²
	3-12 months 26-75 ml/min/m²
	12-18 months 36-95 ml/min/m²
	2 years – adult 50-85 ml/min/m²
Creatinine (Calculation of GFR from serum level)	GFR = (49.5 x ht (cm)/plasma Creatinine (μmol/L)
C-Reactive Protein	<20 mg/L
Gamma Glutamyl Transferase (GGT)	Neonate <200 IU/L
	1 month –1 year <150 IU/L
	>1 year <30 IU/L
Glucose	Newborn – 3 days 2-5 mmol/L
	> 1 week 2.5-5 mmol/L
Glycosylated Hemoglobin	4.5-7.5%
Lactate	0.7-1.8 mmol/L
Liver Function	See Bilirubin, AST, GGT and Protein
Magnesium	Newborn 0.7-1.2 mmol/L
	Child 0.7-1.0 mmol/L
Serum Osmolality	275-295 mmol/kg
Phosphate	Preterm first month 1.4-3.4 mmol/L
	Full term newborn 1.2-2.9 mmol/
	1 year 1.2-2.2 mmol/L
	2-10 years 1.0-1.8 mmol/L
	>10 years 0.7-1.6 mmol/L
Potassium	0-2 weeks 3.7-6 mmol/L
	2 weeks-3 months 3.7-5.7 mmol/L
	>3 months 3.5-5 mmol/L
Protein (Total)	1 month 50-70 g/L
	1 year 60-80 g/L
	1-9 years 60-81 g/L
Sodium	135-145 mmol/L
Urea	1-1 year 2.5-7.5 mmol/L
	1-2 1-7 years 3.3-6.5 mmol/L
	1-3 7-17 years 2.6-6.7 mmol/L (male), 2.5-6.0 mmol/L (female)

II. Glasgow Coma Scale (GCS)

TEST	GRADE
Best Motor Response	1 = none 2 = extensor response to pain 3 = abnormal flexion to pain 4 = withdraws from pain 5 = localizes pain 6 = responds to commands
Eye Opening	1 = none 2 = to pain 3 = to speech 4 = spontaneous
Best Verbal Response	1 = none 2 = incomprehensible sounds 3 = inappropriate words 4 = appropriate words but confused 5 = fully oriented
Maximum Score 15 **Minimum Score 03**	

Pediatric Coma Scale:

Eyes open	Best verbal response	Best motor response
Spontaneously (4) To speech (3) To pain (2) None (1)	Orientated (5) Words (4) Vocal sounds (3) Cries (2) None (1)	Obeys command (5) Localizes pain (4) Flexion to pain (3) Extension to pain (2) None (1)

Normal aggregate score

0-6 months	9
> 6 - 12 months	11
> 1 - 2 years	12
>2 - 5 years	13
> 5 years	14

III. Centile Chart for Hypertension in Boys

95 Percentile = Hypertension, >99 Percentile = Severe Hypertension, Adapted with modification from 2006 (AAP)

Age (years)	BP %ile	Systolic BP, mm Hg							Diastolic BP, mm Hg						
		Percentile of Height							Percentile of Height						
		5th	10th	25th	50th	75th	90th	95th	5th	10th	25th	50th	75th	90th	95th
1	90th	94	95	97	99	100	102	103	49	50	51	52	53	53	54
	95th	98	99	101	103	104	106	106	54	54	55	56	57	58	58
	99th	105	106	108	110	112	113	114	61	62	63	64	65	66	66
2	90th	97	99	100	102	104	105	106	54	55	56	57	58	58	59
	95th	101	102	104	106	108	109	110	59	59	60	61	62	63	63
	99th	109	110	111	113	115	117	117	66	67	68	69	70	71	71
3	90th	100	101	103	105	107	108	109	59	59	60	61	62	63	63
	95th	104	105	107	109	110	112	113	63	63	64	65	66	67	67
	99th	111	112	114	116	118	119	120	71	71	72	73	74	75	75
4	90th	102	103	105	107	109	110	111	62	63	64	65	66	66	67
	95th	106	107	109	111	112	114	115	66	67	68	69	70	71	71
	99th	113	114	116	118	120	121	122	74	75	76	77	78	78	79
5	90th	104	105	106	108	110	111	112	65	66	67	68	69	69	70
	95th	108	109	110	112	114	115	116	69	70	71	72	73	74	74
	99th	115	116	118	120	121	123	123	77	78	79	80	81	81	82
6	90th	105	106	108	110	111	113	113	68	68	69	70	71	72	72
	95th	109	110	112	114	115	117	117	72	72	73	74	75	76	76
	99th	116	117	119	121	123	124	125	80	80	81	82	83	84	84
7	90th	106	107	109	111	113	114	115	70	70	71	72	73	74	74
	95th	110	111	113	115	117	118	119	74	74	75	76	77	78	78
	99th	117	118	120	122	124	125	126	82	82	83	84	85	86	86
8	90th	107	109	110	112	114	115	116	71	72	72	73	74	75	76
	95th	111	112	114	116	118	119	120	75	76	77	78	79	79	80
	99th	119	120	122	123	125	127	127	83	84	85	86	87	87	88
9	90th	109	110	112	114	115	117	118	72	73	74	75	76	76	77
	95th	113	114	116	118	119	121	121	76	77	78	79	80	81	81
	99th	120	121	123	125	127	128	129	84	85	86	87	88	88	89
10	90th	111	112	114	115	117	119	119	73	73	74	75	76	77	78
	95th	115	116	117	119	121	122	123	77	78	79	80	81	81	82
	99th	122	123	125	127	128	130	130	85	86	86	88	88	89	90
11	90th	113	114	115	117	119	120	121	74	74	75	76	77	78	78
	95th	117	118	119	121	123	124	125	78	78	79	80	81	82	82
	99th	124	125	127	129	130	132	132	86	86	87	88	89	90	90
12	90th	115	116	118	120	121	123	123	74	75	75	76	77	78	79
	95th	119	120	122	123	125	127	127	78	79	80	81	82	82	83
	99th	126	127	129	131	133	134	135	86	87	88	89	90	90	91

Centile Charts for Hypertension in Girls

95 percentile =Hypertension, >99 percentile =Severe Hypertension, Adapted with modification from 2006 AAP

Age, (years)	BP Percentile	SBP, mm Hg Percentile of Height							DBP, mm Hg Percentile of Height						
		5th	10th	25th	50th	75th	90th	95th	5th	10th	25th	50th	75th	90th	95th
1	90th	97	97	98	100	101	102	103	52	53	53	54	55	55	56
	95th	100	101	102	104	105	106	107	56	57	57	58	59	59	60
	99th	108	108	109	111	112	113	114	64	64	65	65	66	67	67
2	90th	98	99	100	101	103	104	105	57	58	58	59	60	61	61
	95th	102	103	104	105	107	108	109	61	62	62	63	64	65	65
	99th	109	110	111	112	114	115	116	69	69	70	70	71	72	72
3	90th	100	100	102	103	104	106	106	61	62	62	63	64	64	65
	95th	104	104	105	107	108	109	110	65	66	66	67	68	68	69
	99th	111	111	113	114	115	116	117	73	73	74	74	75	76	76
4	90th	101	102	103	104	106	107	108	64	64	65	66	67	67	68
	95th	105	106	107	108	110	111	112	68	68	69	70	71	71	72
	99th	112	113	114	115	117	118	119	76	76	76	77	78	79	79
5	90th	103	103	105	106	107	109	109	66	67	67	68	69	69	70
	95th	107	107	108	110	111	112	113	70	71	71	72	73	73	74
	99th	114	114	116	117	118	120	120	78	78	79	79	80	81	81
6	90th	104	105	106	108	109	110	111	68	68	69	70	70	71	72
	95th	108	109	110	111	113	114	115	72	72	73	74	74	75	76
	99th	115	116	117	119	120	121	122	80	80	80	81	82	83	83
7	90th	106	107	108	109	111	112	113	69	70	70	71	72	72	73
	95th	110	111	112	113	115	116	116	73	74	74	75	76	76	77
	99th	117	118	119	120	122	123	124	81	81	82	82	83	84	84
8	90th	108	109	110	111	113	114	114	71	71	71	72	73	74	74
	95th	112	112	114	115	116	118	118	75	75	75	76	77	78	78
	99th	119	120	121	122	123	125	125	82	82	83	83	84	85	86
9	90th	110	110	112	113	114	116	116	72	72	72	73	74	75	75
	95th	114	114	115	117	118	119	120	76	76	76	77	78	79	79
	99th	121	121	123	124	125	127	127	83	83	84	84	85	86	87
10	90th	112	112	114	115	116	118	118	73	73	73	74	75	76	76
	95th	116	116	117	119	120	121	122	77	77	77	78	79	80	80
	99th	123	123	125	126	127	129	129	84	84	85	86	86	87	88
11	90th	114	114	116	117	118	119	120	74	74	74	75	76	77	77
	95th	118	118	119	121	122	123	124	78	78	78	79	80	81	81
	99th	125	125	126	128	129	130	131	85	85	86	87	87	88	89
12	90th	116	116	117	119	120	121	122	75	75	75	76	77	78	78
	95th	119	120	121	123	124	125	126	79	79	79	80	81	82	82
	99th	127	127	128	130	131	132	133	86	86	87	88	88	89	90

IV. Anthropometrics measurements in children

Regular anthropometric measurements in children are essential part of clinical examination. Any child who is growing normally is less likely to have any serious illness Therefore; any deviation from the norm should be looked seriously to determine the underlying cause. The usual parameters measured in children are:

4.   Weight
5.   Height (length, in infants)
6.   Head circumference

1. Weight:

The average weight at birth is 3-3.5 Kg. <2.5 kg birth weight of a term baby is termed as IUGR (Intra uterine growth retardation)

After birth, there is an initial period of weight loss in the first 3-4 days of life due to redistribution of body fluids with loss of fluid in the extra-cellular fluid compartment. Most full term infants regain their birth weight by 10 days of age.

During the first year of life the body weight increases as follows:
In the first 4 months weight increases by 20 to 30 Grams per day
Then ½ kg every month from 4 to 8 months
and ¼ kg every month from 8 to 12 months

Double Birth Weight by 5 month age.
Triple Birth Weight by 1 year of age.

After the first year, the average weight of a child can be calculated by:

(Age in years x 2) + 8 = Weight in kg

As a rough guide the normal weight at various ages is:

Age	Birth	1 Y	5 Y	10 Y
Wt in kg	3.5	10.0	20.0	30.0

2. Length (Height):

The average length at birth is 50 cm.
During the first year of life, the length increases as follows:
3 cm per month in the first 3 months.
2 cm per month between the 3rd and 6th month.
1.5 cm every month from the 6th – 12th months of age.

Length at birth	*50 cm*
1 year	*75 cm*
2 yr.	*87 cm*

After the second year, the average length is calculated by:

(Age in years x 5) + 80 = Length in cm.

3. Head Circumference:

The head circumference is measured routinely in a child below 2 years of age or if the size of child's head growth warrants it. Place the tape around the head at points just above the eyebrows and the ear to the most prominent point of occiput.

Normal Head circumference at birth is 35 cm, increasing by 2 cm per month in first three months, then 1 cm per month from 3 to 6 months and ½ cm per month from 6 to 12 months

<u>Age</u>	<u>Head growth</u>	
Birth	35 cm	
1 - 3 mo.	2 cm per mo.	(41 cm at 3 months)
4 - 6 mo.	1 cm per mo.	(44 cm at 6 months)
6 - 12 mo.	0.5 cm per mo.	(47 cm at 1Y)
1 - 2 yr.	2 cm per yr.	(49 cm at 2Y)
2 - 7 yr.	0.5 cm per yr.	(51.5 cm at 7Y)
7 - 12 yr.	0.3 cm per yr.	(53 cm at 12 Y)
Adult	54-56 cm	

Index

T

Tandem MS 189
Tardive dyskinesia 407
Test feed 444
Tetanus 36, 38
Tetralogy of Fallot 281
Thalassemia 300
Thyroid 378
Thyroid cancer 383
Tics 407
Tonsillitis 447
TORCH infections 434
Total parenteral nutrition (TPN) 133
Transient neonatal diabetes 364
Translocation 147
Trisomy 146, 147, 148, 149, 151
Tricyclic antidepressant poisoning 75
Tuberculosis 36, 213
Tumor lysis syndrome 310
Turner syndrome 148
Typhlitis 314

U

Ulcers 205
Unconjugated Hyperbilirubinemia 129, 130
Undescended Testis 440
Upper respiratory tract infection 250
Urea cycle diseases 176
Urinary tract infection 358
URTI 250
Urticaria 204

V

Vaginal discharge 452
Ventricular septal defect 279
Vesicles 204
Viral hepatitis 222
Viral pneumonia 272
Vision assessment 18
Vitamin D 31-33
Vitamin D dependent Rickets 33, 34
Vitamin D resistant rickets 34
Von Willebrand disease 321
Vulvovaginitis 452

W

Warning signs in development 16
Weaning 20, 21
Weight 7, 475
Wheals 204
Wheezing 267
Whipple's triad 185

X

X-Linked agammaglobulinemia 194
X Linked Recessive Inheritance 145

Printed in the United Kingdom
by Lightning Source UK Ltd.
130684UK00001B/13-36/P

9 781434 317421